The West Riding Asylum and the Origins of British Neurology 1866-1876

Andrew J. Larner

The West Riding Asylum and the Origins of British Neurology 1866-1876

When Neurology Became a Science

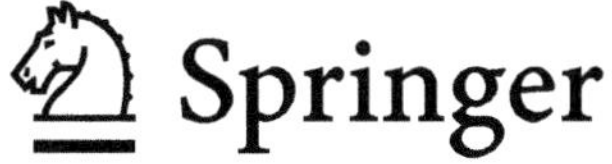

Andrew J. Larner
Department of Translational Neuroscience and Stroke
University College London
London, UK

ISBN 978-3-032-12590-3   ISBN 978-3-032-12591-0   (eBook)
https://doi.org/10.1007/978-3-032-12591-0

Persevere and prosper

Dedicated to the people of Wakefield

Foreword

The West Riding Pauper Lunatic Asylum was opened on November 23, 1818, a mile outside the town of Wakefield at Stanley-cum-Wrenthorpe, two hamlets on the banks of the Calder, and accommodated 150 mentally disturbed people. It was one of the first county mental asylums to be funded by the public purse, but otherwise there was little to distinguish it from the many other "grand stone goliaths" that had started to sprout up in the British countryside. Samuel Tuke, the Quaker reformer whose family founded The Retreat, 30 miles away in York, was charged by the Leeds Magistrates Court to advise on the new asylum's design and approach to care. His son, Daniel Hack Tuke, later wrote that Wakefield had become the "legitimate child" of the Retreat with its philosophy of moral management and enthusiasm for occupational therapy. Only with the appointment of the 25-year-old James Crichton-Browne (1840–1938) as its fifth medical superintendent in 1866 did it become exceptional.

James Crichton-Browne was born in Edinburgh, the son of W.A.F. Browne, the alienist and phrenologist and pioneer of art and music therapy for the treatment of the insane. James read medicine at Edinburgh University and after graduation followed in his father's footsteps and spent time studying asylum medicine in Paris. Alienists and "mad doctors" were regarded by the medical establishment as "second-rate" managers with negligible interest in research. When he arrived at the West Riding Lunatic Asylum it had become the largest institution of its kind in England with 1130 overcrowded inmates. Despite his administrative responsibilities he determined to try to correct the stigma which his father had experienced during his career. He managed to find funding for a pathological service, a small research laboratory and photographic studio and was appointed a lecturer on mental illness at the nearby

Leeds Medical School, where he endeavoured to interest students in the opportunities for research offered by asylum medicine. He also raised money for evening "conversaziones" intended to educate and open up the asylum to local general practitioners. Like his father he had an interest in phrenology and taught the students that Gall and Spurzheim had never really achieved recognition for their contributions to cerebral physiology. Charles Darwin had studied medicine at Edinburgh and been a contemporary of Crichton-Browne's father but it was through a mutual acquaintance, Henry Maudsley, that the two men began to collaborate. In addition to an active correspondence Crichton-Browne sent Darwin a large number of photographs of the physiognomy of the insane from the West Riding Lunatic Asylum as source material for Darwin's book on expression of the emotions in man and animals.

But by far the most important initiative of Crichton-Browne in his efforts to put the asylum on the map was to offer David Ferrier facilities to carry out experimental animal research in a small room at the asylum. Ferrier held an academic post in medical jurisprudence at King's College Hospital and later was an assistant physician at the National Hospital for the Paralysed and Epileptic in London. Hughlings Jackson, an early acquaintance in London and later a colleague at Queen Square, believed in cerebral localisation in relation to the march of cortical epilepsy and aphasia and Ferrier determined to find supportive scientific evidence for this notion based on Jackson's clinical studies. In the Spring of 1873 he started to carry out experiments in which he used faradic stimulation of the cerebral hemispheres of cats and dogs followed by lesioning experiments which provided strong support for cortical localisation. Over the next 2 years Ferrier continued this line of physiological study on various animals including monkeys. Sceptics like Goltz continued to challenge Ferrier's findings, particularly at the International Medical Congress held in London in 1881 where Ferrier demonstrated a monkey rendered hemiplegic by a focal brain lesion and which led Jean-Martin Charcot, who was in the audience, to comment "C'est un malade". Ferrier's findings would ultimately pave the way for the first surgical removal of brain tumours.

Between 1871 and 1876, 62 of the 80 articles published in the *West Riding Lunatic Asylum Medical Reports* were concerned with research conducted in the asylum. As well as Ferrier's publications, the six volumes included five contributions from Hughlings Jackson, four on epilepsy and one on optic neuritis. Clifford Allbutt, a leading physician in Leeds at the time, who had previously published his work on the clinical usefulness of the ophthalmoscope in studying the retinal vessels in general paralysis of the insane, contributed the results of his use of electrical stimulation administered to the head and neck that had been inspired by his time in Paris with Duchenne de

Boulogne. As well as editing the journal Crichton-Browne wrote articles on cranial injury and mental illness, the neuropathology of general paralysis, delirium, and the use of amyl nitrate in status epilepticus.

In the historical introduction to his Ferrier lecture of 1939, given to the Royal Society in London, Lord Adrian remarked that neurology, as a science, first emerged in Great Britain at the West Riding Lunatic Asylum. Alastair Compston, in similar vein in an editorial in *Brain* in 2007, wrote that "Modern British neurology had been born in the wards, laboratories and soirées of the West Riding Lunatic Asylum". William Bynum, a historian of medicine, has also argued that the flowering of neurology in London during the years 1870–1890 had its roots in West Yorkshire. Despite this, most British neurologists of my generation were brought up believing that it was the clinical-pathological approach of physicians like Rudolph Virchow, William Osler and Jean-Martin Charcot that had lit the neurological flame in Great Britain, and that its two cradles were the National Hospital for the Paralysed and Epileptic in Queen Square and the London Hospital in Whitechapel. Whatever the truth, the influence of the county of Yorkshire in the emergence of British neurology as a separate speciality needs to be acknowledged.

Thomas Laycock (1812–1876), the son of a Wesleyan Methodist preacher, was born in the small West Yorkshire market town of Wetherby close to the Great North Road. After completing his apprenticeship as a surgeon apothecary in 1833 he studied medicine at the University Dispensary at University College London before completing his training in Paris and Göttingen. He then took up a post as physician at the York Medical Dispensary where he took an interest in hysteria. His theoretical "romantic neuroscience" led him to the conclusion that the nervous system represented a continuous series of structures that obeyed the laws of reflex function, and that the brain, although the organ of consciousness, did not differ from other nervous ganglia in the body. Two of his protégés in York, Jonathan Hutchinson and Hughlings Jackson, both Yorkshire-born like Laycock, were influenced by his teaching and when they later left York and were appointed to the staff of the London Hospital both studied nervous disease. In 1855 Laycock was appointed to the chair of medicine at Edinburgh University where both Crichton-Browne and the younger David Ferrier were his students. Crichton-Browne later acknowledged Laycock as his most important mentor at medical school and Ferrier worked as his clinical assistant and through him would have been made familiar with the new scientific developments occurring in Germany's state-sponsored research hospitals where laboratory-based microscopical work and experimental cerebral physiology research were starting to have clinical ramifications. Many of the early leading lights in British neurology including several of the first members of the staff at the National Hospital, including Jabez Spence Ramskill, Charles Bland Radcliffe, John Russell Reynolds, and William Gowers, were members of a non-Conformist minority all with strong Yorkshire connections.

Apart from the subliminal effects of Laycock's teaching, Crichton-Browne's time in France from 1862 to 1863 would become a lasting influence on his research. During his time visiting the Paris hospitals he could not have failed to be impressed by the changes in approach to the management of the insane that had occurred since his father's visit to Esquirol's department at the Salpêtrière asylum 30 years earlier. Detailed serial clinical assessments and subsequent clinico-pathological correlations were changing the nosography and understanding of brain disorders. Clifford Allbutt, Crichton-Browne's collaborator in Wakefield, had also spent time in Paris with Trousseau and Duchenne de Boulogne. In 1869 Brown-Séquard, the first physician appointed to the staff of the National Hospital for the Paralysed and Epileptic in Queen Square, and his friend Jean-Martin Charcot travelled from Paris to attend the British Medical Association meeting held in Leeds but it is not known if they also participated in the optional tour of the West Riding Lunatic Asylum or the dinner held in the central hall.

After Crichton-Browne's resignation from Wakefield and move to London in 1876 to become Lord Chancellor's Visitor in Lunacy, the physiological research at the West Riding Lunatic Asylum ceased abruptly and nothing of lasting substance came out of subsequent work in the pathological laboratory. Crichton-Browne now saw himself as a neurologist, despite never becoming a fellow of the Royal College of Physicians, but unlike Ferrier and Jackson he kept a foothold in the medical psychology camp through friends like Henry Maudsley, another Yorkshireman, who had worked for 9 months at the Wakefield asylum before Crichton-Browne's arrival. He also had strong connections in the literary world becoming friendly with both Thomas Carlyle and Thomas Hardy.

By the start of the twentieth century there were four separate West Riding asylums with the same generic name. The Wakefield asylum remained the largest, becoming known as Stanley Royd Hospital after it joined the National Health Service in 1948. The second to be built, in 1872, was known as the Wadsley Asylum (Middlewood) and was built on farmland three miles north of Sheffield. In 1888 in the village of Menston near Leeds a self-supporting facility with its own library and orchestra, butchers and baker's shops, upholstery and shoemaker workshops, dairy and a laundry, large farm and railway line, was constructed and became known as High Royds. Storthes Hall opened near Huddersfield in 1904 and expanded to accommodate over 3000 patients in the middle of the twentieth century. All four institutions have now closed and been converted to residential property.

As a 9-year-old child, the council van that would come and take me to the "loony bin" in Menston if I got into trouble was, unlike the bogeyman, a real threat because I had watched a mad woman at the top of our street being taken away screaming and resisting. I pictured High Royds as a gloomy dungeon shrouded in a shadow of horror. At medical school after my psychiatry elective, I came to appreciate asylums as places of refuge and protection. Claybury Hospital was a therapeutic community with egalitarian rules which applied equally to patients and staff. Its founders, the physician superintendent Denis Martin and psychiatrist John Pippard, had, since the asylum days, broadened and diversified occupational rehabilitation, opened mixed gender wards and forged greater links with the outside world through outings into town and holidays. They also encouraged family visits especially for the isolated chronic long stay patients. Physical treatments were used but sparingly. In the early 1980s I walked the long corridor of Friern (the old Colney Hatch Asylum), later to be called "the North Circular of the Soul" by Will Self in his novel *Umbrella*. In the rambling wards with their high ceilings and lofty windows, Bill Gibb and I examined 170 patients with schizophrenia in an attempt to better classify their kinesics and hyperkinetic movements. This sort of research was not something which was considered as part of neurology at the National Hospital where I worked at that time as a young consultant.

Although I carry no romantic ideas about asylums, I have seen the untold damage that was done by the precipitate closing of psychiatric hospitals like Stanley Royd and Claybury. The "chemical approach" to mental illness, combined with "halfway houses" or imprisonment, has not been an enlightened advance. If money can be found to revisit the notion of the therapeutic community that grew out of the more enlightened asylums and an eclectic approach to treatment with research facilities made available, then I believe as Crichton-Browne did that inroads could be made into the treatment of psychosis.

The fruitful scientific exchanges between asylum doctors and physicians with an interest in brain pathology and cerebral physiology at the West Riding Lunatic Asylum have served as the impetus for Andrew Larner's scholarly work. As befits a neurologist he has understandably focused on its importance in the origins of his speciality. The importance of scientific research as part of the apprenticeship of a British neurologist lives on, although it is no longer a pre-requisite for a consultant neurology post.

Larner's deep excavations have turned up evidence to show that although Hughlings Jackson was interested and supportive of the work going on at the West Riding Lunatic Asylum, there is no evidence that he ever went there. Furthermore, he has confirmed that the famous soirées (conversaziones) occurred once a year, rather than monthly. He also provides compelling evidence in favour of his view that the *West Riding Lunatic Asylum Medical Reports* were not only an antecedent of *Brain*, the world's first clinical neuroscientific journal, but its direct precursor. It is to be hoped that Andrew Larner's book will set the record straight in relation to the importance of the West Riding Pauper Lunatic Asylum in relation to the stirrings of British neurology and also provide a reminder that these later dreaded Victorian institutions provided in their time a needed control and protection for mentally disturbed patients from their own destructive impulses and from the ostracism, aggression and abuse often visited upon them in the outside world. For those readers who after reading this book may also become interested in the lives of some of the inmates at the time when Crichton-Browne became superintendent I would recommend David Scrimgeour's self-published 2015 book *Proper People* which uses transcribed extracts from patients' surviving case records, other original asylum reports and newspaper articles.

The National Hospital, Queen Square   Andrew J. Lees
London, UK
August 2025

Preface

To the accusation levelled by Professor Michael Shepherd that "a medical education conduces to an emphasis on factual information rather than on theoretical speculation",[1] I enter the plea of guilty, and the following work will serve to convict me. In mitigation, if Hilary Morris's view that "a collaboration between those who are fascinated by the history of medicine, regardless of their academic credentials"[2] is deemed acceptable, then the following work might be found not entirely devoid of interest, and possibly of value.

Early in my education I learned from reading E.H. Carr that "The historian and the facts of history are necessary to one another. The historian without his [sic] facts is rootless and futile; the facts without their historian are dead and meaningless".[3] Without its factual basis, all historical theoretical speculation is surely at best moot and at worst void. The imaginative, story-telling (fabulist) approach to history may have a place and may be enjoyed by some, but I think it invites a tendency to fill in the gaps in the historical record with the speculations and preferences of the author, sometimes masquerading as fact. Later in my education, as a clinician, I learned that factual errors may lead to faulty diagnostic reasoning, with potentially adverse consequences for patients.

So, at risk of being envisaged as a successor of Dickens's Mr. Gradgrind, it may seem that an emphasis on facts is unduly prominent in this text (and, as a corollary, the indication of what I believe to be factual errors in previously published materials). But the reader may rest assured that, like Anthony Nuttall, "I know that there is a special demon who lies in wait for people who

---

[1] To be found in Shepherd's Foreword to Cashman (1992:vii).
[2] Morris (2021:4).
[3] Carr (1981:30).

make a thing of accuracy as I do in this book. This means that certain errors—all mine—will have survived. The demon will have his victim".[4] So it goes.

Perhaps unwisely, in view of the commitment to factual accuracy, a little theorising has been included in the final chapter, which I may be ill-equipped to attempt; indeed, the whole book may be read as promoting a specific thesis related to the origins of British neurology. This may ensure that the overall result is a hybrid work which pleases neither medical historian (i.e. primarily educated in medicine) nor historian of medicine (i.e. primarily educated in history).

Perhaps it would be better to think in terms of probabilities rather than facts. The historical record may be opportunistic, and hence absence of evidence does not equal evidence of absence. We may fail to detect something that did happen, an error of omission or a false negative (a type II error); or, worse still to my way of thinking, we may think we detect something that did not happen, an error of commission or a false positive (a type I error).

On a practical note, in an endeavour to combine scholarship with readability, much material has been placed in the footnotes, to be available to those who desire such critical apparatus but easily ignored (subliminal?) for those who just want the story.

By the nature of its subject matter, this book includes terminology which was in common usage in the period under discussion, roughly from 1810s to 1870s, to describe medical conditions, mental health and learning disabilities, which is now outdated and may be considered offensive. Some of these terms are retained here, specifically in direct quotations from the contemporary sources, because to do otherwise risks a form of ahistoricism or anachronism, but elsewhere these terms are eschewed in favour of modern terminology.

Andrew J. Larner

---

[4] Nuttall (2003:xi).

Acknowledgements

I am indebted to the staff members at various institutions who have facilitated my access to resources, specifically: the Liverpool Medical Institution, Liverpool (especially Anna Jackson and Sean Martin); the West Yorkshire Archive Service at Wakefield; the Wellcome Collection, London; Wakefield Museum and Local Studies Library, Wakefield; Chester Record Office, Chester; Medical Society of London, Chandos Street, London; Cadbury Research Library, University of Birmingham; library of the Royal College of Physicians of Edinburgh; Royal Society of Medicine, London; and the Royal Society, London.

No research related to the West Riding Asylum can ignore the thesis by Michael Finn dating from 2012. Although I have disagreed respectfully with some of his conclusions and find occasional errors, the frequency of reference to his work in the footnotes is indicative of how indebted I am to his work as a catalyst for my own approach, albeit from a different perspective. All remaining errors are strictly my own work.

Continuing encouragement and support of many colleagues and friends is gratefully acknowledged (in alphabetical order, with apologies to any inadvertently omitted): Guleed Adan, Alasdair Coles, Crispin and Kari Fisher, Tim and Philippa Griffiths, Tom Hughes, Mari Huws-Edwards, Chris Jones, Thomas Larner, Elizabeth Larner, Andrew Lees, Michael and Sally Mansfield, Gashirai Mbizvo, Hilary Morris, Michael Swash, Lazaros Triarhou. At Springer, I thank Melissa Morton.

For forbearance above and beyond reasonable expectation, and with apologies for my occasional inability to work peacefully, my greatest debt and deepest love to Lauren Fratalia.

Abstract

Neurology as practised in the United Kingdom has long been recognised as a clinical discipline with a strong commitment to research. How did this bipartite structure, encompassing both clinical and research expertise, evolve?

It is generally accepted that neurology as a distinct medical discipline originated in the 1860s and 1870s. Much of the existing historiography of British neurology has focused on the role of the National Hospital, Queen Square, London, the first institution specifically dedicated to the care of those with neurological disease, founded in 1860. In contrast, it is the argument of this book that work undertaken at the West Riding Pauper Lunatic Asylum at Wakefield in West Yorkshire in the decade 1866–1876 was a decisive contributor to the origins and evolution of British neurology in ways which differed from those enacted at Queen Square, in particular in its orientation to research.

In his desire to pursue a scientific approach to insanity, James Crichton-Browne, the Medical Superintendent at West Riding Asylum, inaugurated changes which rendered it a "birth-place for neurology rather than as a stimulant for psychiatry". Firstly, institutional change: building a dedicated pathological laboratory wherein research studies, both clinical and experimental, could be pursued. Secondly, changes to faculty: employing unpaid clinical clerks or assistants who could devote time to research studies. Thirdly, founding a house journal: the *West Riding Lunatic Asylum Medical Reports* was a medium for the publication and hence dissemination of research undertaken at the Asylum and also included material from established physicians working elsewhere, some of whom were invited to avail themselves of the clinical and experimental resources of the Asylum. Fourthly, arranging annual medical gatherings: termed *conversazione*, these meetings were another medium for

"

the dissemination of research undertaken at the Asylum, as well as for the education and entertainment of local practitioners. In the corresponding time period, Queen Square remained an entirely clinical institution, lacking laboratory, clinical assistants, house journal or public medical meetings.

The source materials are synthesised into a new formulation of the shared past of neurology and psychiatry, establishing the work undertaken at the West Riding Asylum in this period as contributing decisively to the research ethos of the nascent discipline and thus forming an integral component in the origins of British neurology.

Contents

Part III   Journal

Abbreviations

AMO	Assistant Medical Officer
AMOAHI	Association of Medical Officers of Asylums and Hospitals for the Insane
BMJ	*British Medical Journal*
MPA	Medico-Psychological Association
n.d.	not dated
n.p.	not paginated
NSL	Neurological Society of London
ODNB	*Oxford Dictionary of National Biography*
WRA	West Riding Asylum, Wakefield
WRLAMR	*West Riding Lunatic Asylum Medical Reports*

List of Figures

List of Tables

1

Introduction: The Origins of British Neurology and the West Riding Asylum 1866–1876

Neurology and Neurologists

As every neurologist knows (or certainly should know!) the term "neurology" originated in the seventeenth century in the work of Thomas Willis (1621–1675), specifically as "Neurologie" in his book *Cerebri anatome cui accessit nervorum descriptio et usus* of 1664. In the English translation of 1681 by Samuel Pordage, this word was rendered as "the doctrine of the nerves".[1] The word "neurology" itself was, however, little used until the nineteenth century, when it came to denote that branch of medicine concerned with diseases of the nervous system.[2]

But whence the term "neurologist", to denote a medical specialist in the diagnosis and treatment of disorders of the nervous system?[3] As few neurologists may know (and certainly this one did not!), the earliest reference to the word "neurologist" listed in the *Oxford English Dictionary* dates from 1832, from the writings of John Thomson (1765–1846), physician and surgeon, and sometime President of the Royal College of Physicians of Edinburgh (1834–6).[4] It appeared in Thomson's biography of William Cullen (1710–1790).[5]

---

[1] Feindel (1962:295).

[2] Casper (2014:5–6) tracked this evolution of "neurology".

[3] The evolution of the word "neurologist" is explored in Larner (2025a).

[4] For biographical material on John Thomson, see Doyle (2009). Neither this work nor his Wikipedia entry mentioned his coining of the word "neurologists".

[5] Thomson (1832:443). For Thomson's biography of Cullen, see Shuttleton (2014).

These two origins beg a third: when and how did neurology emerge as a distinct specialty and neurologists as a distinct professional group?

The Origins of British Neurology

It has been stated that "the story of how the field of neurology emerged in Britain is one that defies easy retrospective reconstruction of the process".[6]

It is perhaps uncontroversial to say that this emergence occurred in the years after around 1860: "This was the period when neurology began to form as a medical specialty, arising from both general internal medicine and psychiatry".[7] The year 1860 saw the opening of the National Hospital for the Paralysed and Epileptic in Queen Square, London,[8] an institution which has loomed large in (what one might call) the standard creation story (or myth?) of British neurology, being the first hospital dedicated to the care of patients with neurological disorders. The years following 1860 have been characterised as the "splendid seventies"[9] and part of a "memorable decade in the history of neurology".[10] This included the inauguration of *Brain: a journal of neurology* in 1878, sometimes characterised as "the world's first neuroscientific journal",[11] the "first truly neurological journal published in English",[12] and "the first academic journal devoted to 'neurology' in Britain".[13] The first British society dedicated to the subject of neurology, the Neurological Society of London, was founded in 1886, becoming the Neurological Society of the United Kingdom in 1903.[14]

This brief history might be deemed an adequate outline of the origins of British neurology.[15] However, whilst few might disagree with the suggested time frame, the locus/loci from which neurology emerged may be more open to question. A case has been made that the origins of British neurology in fact

---

[6] Casper (2014:14).

[7] Shorvon (2023:30).

[8] Shorvon and Compston (2019).

[9] Luria (1973:22, 23). Crichton-Browne (1937:123) claimed in retrospect that "science … crowed so lustily in the seventies".

[10] Spillane (1974a, b) dated the years 1874–1884 as "a memorable decade in the history of neurology".

[11] Jellinek (2005:429–430).

[12] Finn (2012:188).

[13] Casper (2014:12).

[14] Schurr (1985), Casper (2014:37–57), Shorvon and Compston (2019:291–292), Reynolds and Broussolle (2022:292), Larner (2026a).

[15] Some neurologists may still regard "Queen Square" as the Neurology "mother ship" (Larner 2019a). I thank Professor Jonathan Schott for introducing me to this idea.

lie within a psychiatric, rather than a general medical, setting.[16] It is in this context that the West Riding Pauper Lunatic Asylum located in Wakefield, West Yorkshire, demands consideration.

West Riding Asylum

Institutions designated specifically as places for the care of the insane date to the medieval period but the major programme of asylum building in the United Kingdom dates from the nineteenth century, initially under the auspices of the discretionary County Asylums Act of 1808. The Asylum at Wakefield opened in 1818 to serve the population of the West Riding of Yorkshire. Over the following five decades, under the superintendence of successive medical directors, the West Riding Asylum expanded significantly, not only in terms of patient numbers but also in the extent and diversity of its facilities. From 1866 onwards, during the superintendency of James Crichton-Browne, construction of a dedicated pathological laboratory was indicative of his desire to foster a new scientific approach to insanity.

A number of informative and scholarly books, chapters, and theses related to the West Riding Asylum at Wakefield (WRA), its history, personnel, and patients, have been published, many of which have contributed to the ideas to be discussed in this book.[17] Many of these works have been facilitated by the excellence of the extant archives of WRA available through the West Yorkshire Archive Service located at the West Yorkshire Heritage Centre in Wakefield.[18]

Although occasional publications have summarised, sometimes very briefly, some of the activities which occurred and some of the research contributions which emerged from WRA in the 1860s and 1870s,[19] it remains (in this author's view) curiously neglected in the existing historiography of neurology and of neurologists in the United Kingdom.[20] The central proposition of this book is that the collective endeavours of those clinicians working at and/or

---

[16] Bynum (1985) (reprinted Bynum (1990)).

[17] In alphabetical order, these include (but are certainly not limited to): Ashworth (1975), Bolton (1928), Davis (2013a), Finn (2012), Gatehouse (1981), Pearce (2003a), Russell (1988), Scrimgeour (2015), Sloffer (2023), Todd and Ashworth (1991, n.d.), Viets (1938), Wallis (2017a), WFN Research Group on the History of the Neurosciences (1997), Wilkins (1997).

[18] See West Yorkshire Heritage | West Yorkshire Archive Service (wyjs.org.uk) (accessed 08/10/2024).

[19] For example: WFN Research Group on the History of the Neurosciences (1997), Wilkins (1997), Snaith (1998), Pearce (2003a), Pearce and Lees (2013), Rollin and Reynolds (2018), Mindham (2020). The most detailed account is the unpublished thesis by Finn (2012).

[20] There is only a single, passing mention in Casper (2014:29). See also Spillane (1981:387–389), Shorvon and Compston (2019:140).

associated with WRA during the decade from 1866 to 1876 were fundamental to the origin of neurology as a clinical and research discipline and profession in the United Kingdom; or, in the words of E.D. Adrian (1889–1977), to "a classical period in the history of medicine, the period when neurology became a science".[21]

Professionalisation and Specialisation

Definitions of the concept of professions invariably encompass the idea that they are based on a body of specialised knowledge. For example, Abraham Flexner (1866–1959), renowned for his reform of American medical education as author of the Flexner Report of 1910, listed criteria characterising professions in 1915, hence probably those most proximate to the periodisation of the current work. These specified that professions involve "essentially intellectual operations with large individual responsibility; they derive their raw material from science and learning; this material they work up to a practical and definite end; they possess an educationally communicable technique; they tend to self-organization; [and] they are becoming increasingly altruistic in motivation".[22] One of the key arguments of this book is that many of these criteria may be adjudged to be fulfilled by the activities taking place at WRA between 1866 and 1876.

In turn, these criteria relate to the development of specialisation, specifically how this body of specialised knowledge is acquired and shared. In his analysis of medical specialisation in the nineteenth century, George Weisz noted that the "crux of this transformation was the creation of an unprecedented [*sic*] large and integrated community of doctors around an organized system of institutions and, most importantly, devoted to advancing medical knowledge through rigorous empirical clinical research".[23] Hence, in this formulation, specialisation required both an institution (or institutions) which allowed a specialist medical interest to emerge, and also a faculty dedicated, at least in part, to research activity in that specialism.

Furthermore, Weisz suggested that "Whether a field became widely recognized as a disciplinary specialty or not depended on the amount and quality

---

[21] Adrian (1939:433); also cited by Todd and Ashworth (1991:416).

[22] Of course, many other sets of criteria for a profession have been posited. Aside from his sphere of interest and the date of his criteria, the rationale for choosing Abraham Flexner, despite his absence of medical training, included his family connections: brother to a clinician (Simon Flexner) and uncle to a neuroscientist (Louis Barkhouse Flexner).

[23] Weisz (2006:11).

of knowledge that its practitioners were thought to produce".[24] Such judgments must needs rely not only on the production of knowledge through research but also the effective articulation and dissemination of that knowledge. Hence specialisation also required both social media and opportunities to broadcast research findings, such as a dedicated technical journal, or journals, and associational meetings. Again, many of these conditions may be adjudged as met at WRA.

Building a knowledge base strengthens a profession's claim to special expertise, to such an extent that individuals outside the profession are deemed not competent to judge its workings. Hence the core criterion of a profession: autonomy.[25]

Outline of the Work

This work seeks, then, to address the "usual historical enquiries: Why here? Why then? Why in this form?",[26] but more specifically, in light of the foregoing considerations, the focus is on four key areas:

- Part I: Institution: the evolution of WRA from its inception in 1818 to the early 1870s is examined, in particular the key infrastructural changes effected in the early years of the superintendency of Dr James Crichton-Browne, especially the construction and equipping of a dedicated pathological laboratory and a photographic studio. These changes are examined as a prelude to the description of the factors which coalesced at Wakefield Asylum in the early 1870s, in terms of faculty, journal, and meetings, which contributed decisively to the origins of British neurology.
- Part II: Faculty: the development of "the lunacy profession and its staff" at WRA from 1866 onwards is examined, particularly the employment of clinical clerks or clinical assistants and a dedicated pathologist to pursue research studies under the supervision of Crichton-Browne. An extended prosopography of the doctors involved in this work is included.

---

[24] Ibid., 15.

[25] Freidson (1970). I am grateful to Dr Tom Hughes who pointed out to me (05/12/2024) that in addition to institution(s), faculty, journal(s), and meetings, a profession needs some form of agreed curriculum for the appropriate education and training of its would-be members. This may perhaps be encompassed in Flexner's requirement for professions to "possess an educationally communicable technique".

[26] Pickstone and Marland (1989:198).

- Part III: Journal: the WRA house journal, the *West Riding Lunatic Asylum Medical Reports* (*WRLAMR*), edited by Crichton-Browne and published between 1871 and 1876, is examined, including the subject matter of the articles published in the journal and its critical reception by the extended medical community, both national and international. An extended prosopography of the doctors from outside the "lunacy profession" who were invited to work at WRA and/or who contributed material to *WRLAMR* is also provided.
- Part IV: Meetings: the annual medical *conversaziones*, held at WRA between 1871 and 1875, are examined, particularly the interactive demonstrations of clinical or experimental methods, and the exhibition of items from the WRA collections of pathology, photography, instruments, microscopy, and medicines. An extended prosopography of the keynote speakers and those contributing to the demonstrations is included.

Material is presented for the most part chronologically, although this should not be taken to indicate a commitment to a "linear vision of progressivism".[27]

In a concluding chapter, an attempt is made to synthesize these various strands to address the issue of the origins of British neurology between 1866 and 1876, in light of competing models based on emergence from general internal medicine and from psychiatry, and specifically Adrian's comment that this was "the period when neurology became a science".[28]

Why is such a proposed history of WRA required? Finn has, for example, already cogently documented the role played by WRA in making the physiological doctrine of cerebral localisation a "canon of medical practice".[29] A number of possible purposes might be adduced.

The clinical specialty of neurology as practiced in the United Kingdom has long comprised a bipartite or two-fold discipline in which the probabilistic nature of clinical practice (often masquerading as certainty) is balanced with the greater exactitude of clinical and/or experimental (laboratory) science. Acknowledged as a very academic subject, the expectation of a higher research degree (MD or PhD) as a necessity for advancement in UK neurology has only recently been diluted by changes in training programmes (sometimes fatuously deemed to be "streamlining"). Hence attempts to explain the origins of British neurology need to address both its clinical and its scientific basis.

---

[27] Ellis (2015:337).

[28] Adrian (1939:433).

[29] Finn (2012:passim) (quote at 12).

That, as per Adrian, WRA played a role in these developments is reason enough to anticipate an historical account; the moreso in light of the impression that WRA has been relatively overlooked, indeed neglected, in comparison to the developments at the National Hospital, Queen Square.

Part I

Institution

In the bleak countryside at a grim gothic [*sic*] mental asylum …[1]

To my eyes a Pauper Lunatic Asylum, such as may now be seen in our English counties, with its pleasant grounds, its airy and cleanly wards, its many comforts, and wise and kindly superintendence, provided for those whose lot it is to bear the double burthen of poverty and mental derangement—I say this sight is to me the most blessed manifestation of true civilization that the world can present.[2]

---

[1] Haig (2017:202). The full quotation reads: "In the bleak countryside at a grim gothic [*sic*] mental asylum called the High Royds Hospital, a woman had been locked up for telling people the truth of her condition." (I thank Dr Michael Mansfield for drawing my attention to this reference, 27/04/2019.) Hence it refers to a different part of the West Riding Asylum system, the third such asylum to be opened, at Menston in 1888, rather than to the one to be discussed here (see text for further details).

[2] Paget (1866:34–35). Scull (2019:43) erroneously ascribed the quotation to Sir James Paget (1814–1899) rather than to his brother, Sir George Edward Paget (1809–1892).

2

The West Riding Pauper Lunatic Asylum 1818–1866

Introduction/Prologue: Origins

One very striking change within my recollection is the difference in the treatment accorded to lunatics. Asylums purposely for pauper lunatics were unknown in the beginning of this [19th] century, and the poor creatures were kept along with other paupers and vagrants in work-houses; the barbarous inhumanity with which they were treated by those in authority over them, would hardly be believed in these days when every gentle and skilful method is resorted to for their cure. The West Riding Asylum was the first one, I believe, specially for paupers, and I very well recollect its foundation stone being laid in about 1817, by Mr. Godfrey Higgins, of Skellow, one of the magistrates who had been particularly active in forwarding the scheme, and who, sad to say, became deranged himself before the building which his philanthropic efforts had so greatly helped was completed. It was a very small building at first, and it has been found necessary to enlarge it again and again, till it has reached its present gigantic size.[1]

So recalled the octogenarian Henry Clarkson, of Alverthorpe Hall, Wakefield, in his book of *Memories of Merry Wakefield* first published in 1887. He must have been a very small boy when the foundation stone of the Asylum was laid, but evidently such was the occasion that something of it remained in his memory for many decades.

---

[1] Clarkson (1887:200–201).

A. J. Larner, *The West Riding Asylum and the Origins of British Neurology 1866-1876*,
https://doi.org/10.1007/978-3-032-12591-0_2

However, contrary to Clarkson's recollections, the Asylum's foundation stone was actually laid in February 1816.[2] According to the Asylum's historians, John Todd and A. Lawrence Ashworth:

The first stone of the new Asylum was laid on Thursday, 1st February, 1816 (some six months after the Battle of Waterloo) by Mr. John Foljambe, the Clerk to the Visiting Magistrates and "Superintendent of Building erection".[3]

This is confirmed, very briefly, in a contemporary notice appearing in a local newspaper:

Yesterday, Mr. Foljambe, Deputy Clerk of the Peace, laid the first stone of the Pauper Lunatic Asylum, for the West Riding. Every feeling heart must be grateful to the magistrates for their humanity and exertion in procuring so desirable an Institution for the cure or alleviation of the severest affliction incident to human nature.[4]

Clarkson might possibly have confused the laying of the foundation stone with the opening of the Asylum. This event occurred over 2½ years later, on 23rd November 1818. In the previous week's local paper, a notice appeared "By order of J. Foljambe, Clerk to the Visiting Justices dated Wakefield, 16th October 1818":

Asylum for Lunatic Paupers.
West-Riding of Yorkshire
To the Overseers of the Poor of Townships
within the said Riding

---

[2] Walker (1939:562).

[3] Todd & Ashworth, not dated (henceforward "n.d."):9. Finn (2012:222) cited this book as "1985" but this dating does not agree with that of a book review by Breathnach (1996). Perhaps Finn's "1985" was a typographical error for "1995"? The book was not referenced in Todd and Ashworth (1991), which I think would be surprising if it had been published in 1985, or indeed any time before 1991. Smith (1999) hazarded both "c.1990" (11) and "1993" (127, 186, 221, 300). A website devoted to High Royds Hospital at Menston (http://www.highroydshospital.com, accessed 22/10/2024), where John Todd (1914–1987) was Consultant Psychiatrist from 1955 to 1979, dated the book as 1993 (the material on this website was possibly derived from John Todd (whonamedit.com), accessed 22/10/2024). John Todd's many publications are also listed on both websites, of which the best remembered by neurologists is perhaps his characterisation of perceptual distortions, both visual (metamorphopsia) and somaesthetic, as the "Alice in Wonderland syndrome", named after Lewis Carroll's character (Todd 1955). Todd thus contributed to both medical history and neurology (Larner and Mbizvo 2025). Finn (2012:5) described Todd and Ashworth as "former employees at Wakefield" but as far as I am aware this is true only of Lawrence Ashworth.

[4] *The Wakefield and Halifax Journal; and Yorkshire and Lancashire Advertiser* Volume XIII, No. 768, 2nd February 1816, p.3 [my transcription].

Notice is hereby given,
That the Asylum of Wakefield, built for the reception of Lunatic Paupers will be ready to admit patients on Monday the 23rd day of November next between the Hours of Nine and four O'clock in the Day, and on every succeeding Monday and Thursday, at the same Hours ....[5]

A later historian of Wakefield, J.W. Walker, stated that the opening was performed by Godfrey Higgins.[6]

Also contrary to Clarkson's recollections, the West Riding Asylum at Wakefield (henceforward WRA) was the sixth, not the first, county asylum in England to be opened specifically for pauper lunatics. This construction followed the permissive, discretionary, enabling County Asylums Act of 1808 (48 Geo. 3. c. 96), often known as Wynn's Act in recognition of the efforts of Charles Watkin Williams-Wynn (1775–1850) who promoted the Act.[7] The building at Wakefield, which received its first patients on Monday 23rd November 1818, was the first public asylum in the West Riding of Yorkshire, and hence was known as the West Riding Lunatic Asylum or sometimes the West-Yorkshire Lunatic Asylum.[8]

County Asylums were funded from the public purse (i.e. by the local rate-payers) as part of the Poor Law administration, and so generally accepted only those patients who were unable to pay, hence were dependent for their maintenance wholly or in part from public funds (i.e. "paupers"), unlike private asylums.[9] The institution at Wakefield was therefore sometimes known as West Riding Pauper Lunatic Asylum. As Hilary Marland has documented, the maintenance of paupers at Wakefield Asylum was a large financial burden

---

[5] *The Wakefield and Halifax Journal; and Yorkshire and Lancashire Advertiser* Volume XV, No. 914, 20th November 1818, p.1 [my transcription]. I could find no account of the opening of the Asylum in the following week's edition (27th November) of *The Wakefield and Halifax Journal.*

[6] Walker (1939:562). However, Walker then went on to state that "Dr. Corsellis was placed in charge as the first medical director"; as this statement is incorrect (*vide infra*), it may call into question his other material. This passage did not appear in the first edition of Walker's history of Wakefield (1934).

[7] Wakefield Asylum was preceded by Nottingham (February 1812), Bedford (August 1812), Norfolk (Norwich; May 1814), Lancaster (July 1816), and Stafford (October 1818). Digby (1983:230) erred in stating that Wakefield Asylum opened in 1819. Bewley (2008:7) peculiarly omitted Bedford from his chronological list of county asylums. A later Act, the County Asylums Act of 1845 (8&9 Vict. c.126), made the building of county asylums for pauper lunatics compulsory. The Irish system of district asylums predated the English system of county asylums.

[8] For general histories of the West Riding Asylum at Wakefield, to which this account is greatly indebted, see Bolton (1928), Ashworth (1975), and Todd and Ashworth (1991, n.d.) (see note 4 above for possible dating of the latter).

[9] The *ODNB* entry for Godfrey Higgins, Gordon, revised Lloyd, (https://doi.org/10.1093/ref:odnb/13232) stated that he "provided for the erection of a house for pauper lunatics near Wakefield", a wording which might perhaps suggest that private finance as well as public money was involved in meeting the costs of Asylum construction.

for ratepayers,[10] which may partly explain why, according to Robert Ellis, up to one third of patients were not paupers since their relatives paid a weekly charge for them.[11]

The need for a dedicated institution for the insane poor of West Yorkshire had become increasingly apparent during the early years of the nineteenth century as a consequence of the apparent increase in the numbers of those afflicted with "insanity".[12] The 1808 Bill:

> also required their numbers to be returned by the parish officers. These lists, though very defective, showed so many more to be suffering under this most deplorable disease than was at all calculated upon, that, in different parts of the country, the feelings of some truly philanthropic gentlemen being excited, they sought out their situations, and discovered that nearly half of them were chained in the most wretched holes, in workhouses and in prisons, and even in the institutions professedly established for their cure.[13]

One of these "philanthropic gentlemen" was, in all likelihood, the magistrate Godfrey Higgins (1773–1833).[14] Higgins had been instrumental in exposing the failings at the York Lunatic Asylum in 1813–1814, following the mistreatment of a pauper he had committed there.[15] He also gave evidence to a Parliamentary Inquiry (the Select Committee on Madhouses) of 1815–1816 into the provisions, both private and public, for the insane and which recommended the monitoring of asylums by an independent inspectorate.[16]

---

[10] Marland (1987:64).

[11] Ellis (2001:61–63).

[12] Andrew Scull has dissected the possible causes for the increasing numbers of those labelled insane and hence consigned to asylums in the nineteenth century and suggested that the principal cause was a changing definition of those so labelled (Scull 1979:221–253).

[13] Bolton (1928:599). Movement of pauper lunatics between workhouse and asylum in the nineteenth century was examined by Ritch (2023). For prisons, see material on William Dyson Wood in Chap. 5 and on Henry Clarke in Chap. 7.

[14] For biographical material on Higgins, see Gordon, revised Lloyd, https://doi.org/10.1093/ref:odnb/13232; Scull 1979:73; Digby 1983:224, 225, 226–227, 233, 235, 239; 1985:240–242; Smith 1999:28–29; Brown 2006:441, 444–447; Finn 2012:64n214 . He even has a mention in Foucault (2006:146). Digby (1983:224) gave Higgins's date of birth as 1773, presumably following *ODNB*, but Wikipedia has 1772.

[15] For the York Lunatic Asylum scandal of 1813–1815, see Digby (1983), Brown (2006), and Adams (2025:35–64). Digby (1983:239) seemed to imply that Higgins's actions of March 1814, when he visited the York Asylum unexpectedly early one morning and discovered four hidden cells only eight feet square and inches deep in excremental filth where thirteen old women had spent the night, were the inspiration for the episode in Charles Reade's novel of 1863, *Hard Cash*, in which Alfred Hardie discovers a receptacle "filled with chains, iron belts, wrist-locks, muffles, and screw-locked hobbles" hidden there just prior to the arrival of the visiting justices (at Chap. 33).

[16] Scull (1979:77).

Higgins's work in connection with the York Lunatic Asylum had brought him into contact with the Tuke family and with the York Retreat, wherein a different policy of treatment of the insane to that at the York Asylum was pursued.[17]

Sometime after 1813, the West Riding visiting magistrates requested Samuel Tuke (1784–1857), grandson of William Tuke (1732–1822), the founder of the York Retreat, to prepare instructions for the architects of a proposed Wakefield Asylum. These instructions were subsequently published, along with the winning design, that of Watson and Pritchett, architects of York.[18] The successful design for the Asylum building conformed to a symmetrical H-plan or shape, as seen in an engraving by John Landseer.[19]

Writing in the *Monthly Magazine, or, British Register* for December 1815, Higgins explained that Wakefield's new pauper lunatic asylum had emerged from the York scandal and was shaped by advice from Samuel Tuke, whose recommendations for its design rested on "the easy and complete classification of the patients" who were intended to be "150 of the very worst" of the West Riding's 650-plus lunatics.[20] Many years later, Daniel Hack Tuke (1827–1895),[21] Samuel Tuke's son, reported on a letter:

> written by Mr. Higgins to my father in April, 1815, which is very brief, but announces a fact of greatest importance. It reads thus: "I write in great haste to inform you that it was the unanimous wish of the magistrates (at the quarter sessions) to accede to the proposal to build a place for our pauper lunatics, and we have proceeded as far as it was in our power according to law; indeed, I believe a little further. There was but one opinion."[22]

The site selected for construction was "within one mile of the central town of the West Riding, in a cheerful and healthy situation combining the convenience of contiguity to a market town with the salubrity and quietude

---

[17] For York Retreat, see Digby (1985).

[18] Tuke (1815). Samuel Tuke had also advised on Lancaster Asylum (Walton 1981:167). Smith (1999:33–34). Charles Watson (1771–1836) designed a number of buildings in Wakefield aside from the Asylum (https://wakefieldcivicsociety.org.uk). In later life he developed psychiatric disease and died in the York Asylum, parts of which he had designed (Adams 2025:92).

[19] WYAS C85/1361. Landseer's engraving is reproduced in Mindham (2020).

[20] Higgins G. *Monthly Magazine, or, British Register*. December 1815, pp. 405–406. Cited in Wynter (2015:16–17).

[21] Biographical material on Daniel Hack Tuke may be found in Hare (1987:53–58) and Beveridge (1998).

[22] Hack Tuke (1889a:368, 1889b:9). Godfrey Higgins was one of the dedicatees of the latter publication, along with Samuel Tuke.

of the rural districts".[23] This was in the township of Stanley-cum-Wrenthorpe,[24] a location which was "then some distance from the nearest habitation".[25]

If it was indeed the case, as stated by Andrew Scull, that "To some extent, the treatment the patients in these new asylums received depended on which older institution their asylum was modelled after",[26] the patients admitted to Wakefield Asylum were fortunate in that it was modelled on the York Retreat. The links were several. In addition to the roles of Godfrey Higgins and Samuel Tuke in its inception and design, the inaugural superintendent at WRA, William Ellis (*vide infra*), visited the York Retreat on four occasions, including shortly before taking up his post at Wakefield.[27] Hence, Daniel Hack Tuke was later to describe the Asylum at Wakefield as the "legitimate child" of the Retreat.[28] In this particular respect, Henry Clarkson's recollections proved to be largely correct, in that WRA substituted "barbarous inhumanity" with "every gentle and skilful method" in the treatment of the insane.[29]

---

[23] Hack Tuke (1889a:368, 1889b:10).

[24] White (1866:857).

[25] Todd and Ashworth (1991:389). The siting may also have taken into account the guidance of the 1808 County Asylums Act to locate asylums in an "airy and healthy situation".

[26] Scull (1979:61).

[27] Digby (1985:244). Caleb Crowther, visiting physician to WRA (*vide infra*), also visited the Retreat, in December 1817 (Digby 1985:316n33).

[28] Hack Tuke (1889a:367, 1889b:8). Wakefield Asylum as the "legitimate child" of York Retreat was also quoted in the report of Hack Tuke's address to the Section of Psychology at the British Medical Association meeting reported in *Illustrated Medical News* 1889;4:190 (24th August). Smith (1999:39) considered Hack Tuke's opinion "an overstatement". As the quote from Scull suggests, such asylum "genealogy" may possibly have been locally determined: for example, the Bedford Asylum appears to have been greatly helped in its early stages by Thomas Dunston, Master of St Luke's Hospital in London (Cashman 1992:9,10,16,23,54; Smith 1999:33).

[29] Incidentally, Clarkson's suggestion that Higgins "became deranged himself before the building which his philanthropic efforts had so greatly helped was completed" is highly questionable, and indeed incorrect if "completed" meant by the time of its opening in 1818. The *ODNB* entry for Higgins (https://doi.org/10.1093/ref:odnb/13232) stated that he attended a meeting of the British Association at Cambridge in June 1833, two months before his death, which hardly seems the action of someone deranged. Perhaps Clarkson viewed as a marker of derangement Higgins's work entitled *Anacalypsis: An Attempt to Draw Aside the Veil of the Saitic Isis or an Inquiry into the Origin of Languages, Nations and Religions*, published posthumously in 1836 but to which Higgins had reportedly applied himself for "nearly ten hours daily for almost twenty years". For possible links between Higgins and the character of Edward Casaubon in George Eliot's novel *Middlemarch*, see Larner (2025b). A similar suggestion was made independently and contemporaneously by Adams (2025:310n20).

Institution: Development of the West Riding Asylum, 1818–1866

As Henry Clarkson noted of the Asylum at Wakefield, it was subsequently "found necessary to enlarge it again and again".[30] Writing around the same time as Clarkson, Daniel Hack Tuke considered it "wearisome to enumerate the successive enlargements of the original building which were found to be necessary".[31] However, some brief account (NB not an institutional history) must be given of these developments in the built environment at WRA, and its administration, in order to appreciate the form of the institution at the outset of the time period to be considered hereafter in greater depth. This may be most conveniently done by considering the physical changes accruing during the incumbencies of the successive superintendents of the Asylum.[32]

William Charles Ellis (Superintendent 1818–1831)[33]

The foundation medical superintendent of WRA at the time of its opening on 23rd November 1818 was William Charles Ellis (1780–1839). His medical training in Hull had been as an apprentice to a surgeon-apothecary, possibly John Alderson (1758–1829),[34] and here he obtained the basic qualification of the Membership of the Royal College of Surgeons (MRCS, 1800). An interest in mental disorders was fostered by his work at the Sculcoates Refuge, which had been founded by Alderson,[35] where treatment methods were based on those used at the York Retreat.

Following the revelations of mistreatment of patients at the York Lunatic Asylum in 1815, Ellis published an open "letter" addressed to Thomas

---

[30] Clarkson (1887:201).

[31] Hack Tuke (1889a:368, 1889b:10).

[32] Herein I follow the plan used by Todd and Ashworth (n.d.) Information on the history of WRA may also be found in Bolton (1928), Ashworth (1975), and Todd and Ashworth (1991).

[33] Biographical material on William Ellis may be found in Bolton (1928:596–604), Ashworth (1975:61), Bickford and Bickford (1983:37–38), Todd and Ashworth (n.d.:7–47); Smith https://doi.org/10.1093/ref:odnb/53734, and Howe (2017).

[34] Bickford and Bickford (1983:3–4).

[35] Bickford and Bickford (1976:14–19), for details of the Sculcoates Refuge (open 1814–1840). Bickford and Bickford (1983:37) reported that the Refuge came about when "[John] Alderson sought his [Ellis's] help in founding a first hospital for mental patients, to serve Hull and district". Digby (1985:244) stated that "One of the founders of the Sculcoates Refuge was William Ellis". Sculcoates Refuge opened in May 1814. Other authors have reported that Ellis worked at a private asylum in Hull (Bolton 1928:588; Howe 2017:247).

Thompson MP, outlining his thoughts on how asylums should be managed.[36] Undoubtedly this aided his subsequent appointment at WRA. Godfrey Higgins, apparently a friend of Ellis, was largely influential in securing this post.[37] Ellis's wife, Mildred, was appointed Matron at the same time (11th December 1817). Around this time, Ellis obtained the MD degree from St Andrews (1818)[38]; he was apparently the only county asylum superintendent thus qualified at this time.

From the opening of WRA in 1818, Ellis sought to exclude "those coercive measures, formerly used in other asylums".[39] The system of so-called moral management of the insane, free of mechanical restraints or coercive measures, had been pioneered from the 1790s in England at the York Retreat by the Tuke family. Similar policies had been pursued contemporaneously by Philippe Pinel (1745–1826) at the Bicêtre and Salpêtrière hospitals in Paris and by Vincenzo Chiarugi (1759–1820) in Florence. In addition, Ellis sought to secure "the employment in some way or other, of every patient", for example experimenting "with agricultural work as a form of occupational therapy for his patients".[40] In 1820, Ellis was able to report that "The employment in some way or other, of every patient, has been constantly persevered in, during the year, and this has been attended with the best effects".[41] These employments included weaving which provided the cloth for patients' and attendants' clothing, farm work, and brewing.[42]

The Asylum building had been designed to accommodate 150 patients, 75 male and 75 female. This was in keeping with Ellis's "rule that from 100 to 120 patients are as many as ought to be in any one house. Where they are beyond that number ... the individual cases cease to excite the interest they ought".[43] Moreover, the "disposition of the various day rooms was such that it was possible to classify the patients as to their illness or behaviour pattern, and to provide for progression in their treatment".[44] In 1823, Ellis reported that:

---

[36] The letter ran to 48 pages and 11,000 words according to Todd and Ashworth (n.d.:17).

[37] Bolton (1928:588). There were apparently no other applicants (Todd and Ashworth n.d.:12).

[38] Bolton (1928:589) reported that "Dr. Ellis obtained the degree of Doctor of Medicine" but does not say where from or when

[39] Bolton (1928:588).

[40] Bolton (1928:596–597) and Oppenheim (1991:57).

[41] Bolton (1928:596).

[42] Ashworth (1975:31).

[43] Hack Tuke (1889a:367).

[44] Ashworth (1975:17).

Two of the Wards for the males are set apart for the Maniacal, the fatuous and Epileptic: the other three are occupied by those who vary in their approaches to perfect sanity.[45]

By this time the asylum population had reached 230, well above Ellis's stipulated maximum.

Despite the implementation of a meliorative regime, both morbidity and mortality in the Asylum were high. A contemporary account of dysentery at the Asylum in 1826, 1827, 1828, and 1829 from a "Physician of the Establishment" ascribed its prevalence, often fatal, to "the crowded state of the asylum" prompting alterations to the wash-house and drains.[46] In a work of 1837 it was reported that "There die in Wakefield Asylum 24 in 100 patients, or 1 in 4".[47] Hence, as per the standard practice at other asylums at this time, in addition to the medically qualified superintendent, visiting physicians and surgeons were also appointed on the opening of Wakefield Asylum, two of each.[48] Such honorary posts were status-conferring and much sought after. Throughout the nineteenth century Wakefield "contained a high proportion of middle-class inhabitants" which included "considerable numbers of … members of the medical profession, some of whom were employed by the asylum".[49] The first visiting surgeons to the Asylum were Mr. Samuel Marshall and a Mr. Sevindin, but the latter soon resigned to be replaced by Mr. Joseph Bennett.[50] The visiting physicians were Dr. James Richardson, who died in 1820 to be succeeded by Dr. Disney Alexander, and Dr. Caleb Crowther.

Ellis subscribed to the beliefs of phrenology, founding a Phrenological Society in Wakefield in 1820.[51] Hence, a notice which appeared many years later to the effect that "Dr. Spurzheim, one of the founders of the science of phrenology, made post-mortem examinations at the asylum to demonstrate the possibility of unfolding the convolutions of the brain"[52] is entirely credible.

---

[45] Smith (1999:193).

[46] Gilby (1830–1831).

[47] Browne (1837:75).

[48] Bolton (1928:589).

[49] Marland (1987:22). Marland also reported (261) that "By the mid-nineteenth century approximately one-third of all medical practitioners resident in Wakefield were full-time employees or part-time honorary attendants at the Asylum".

[50] Ashworth (1975:63) has "Mr. I. Bennett" but Marland (1987:passim) has "Joseph Bennett".

[51] Cooter (1976a:5,17) and Marland (1987:213). The influence of phrenology at WRA is examined in Chap. 10.

[52] *The Wakefield Express, and Barnsley, Normanton, Pontefract, Ossett, Horbury & Dewsbury Advertiser* Volume 22, No. 1126, 29th November 1873, p.2, col. 4 (Medical conversazione at the West Riding Asylum. Speech by Lord Houghton. Lecture by Dr. Carpenter).

Johann Gaspar Spurzheim (1776–1832) was, along with Franz Josef Gall (1758–1828), one of the founders of phrenology.

William Ellis left Wakefield in 1831 to move to Hanwell Asylum in Middlesex.

He was the first superintendent of a lunatic asylum to be knighted (1835),[53] but left Hanwell under difficult circumstances in 1838.[54]

Disney Alexander (1769–1844)

Disney Alexander (1769–1844) was appointed honorary physician to the Asylum in 1820.[55] Like Ellis, he was an enthusiastic phrenologist and lectured to the Wakefield Dispensary on the subject.[56] According to Marland, he "acted as Superintendent of the Wakefield Asylum between 1831 and 1836"[57] but he is not mentioned in this capacity, or indeed at all, by other sources.[58]

Caleb Crowther (1772–1849)[59]

Caleb Crowther was honorary physician to the Asylum, possibly from the time of its foundation.[60] Whilst he supported many philanthropic activities in Wakefield, as well as maintaining a large and prosperous medical practice in the town, he "failed to see eye to eye with several other of his medical brethren",[61] including William Ellis.

It was Ellis's view of the Asylum that "It is absolutely necessary that to manage such a house and such inhabitants the heads of it ought to possess the most sovereign authority over all the rest, and, consequently, to be accountable for everything".[62]

---

[53] Todd and Ashworth (1991:390).

[54] Howe (2017).

[55] Finn (2012:67) stated that Disney Alexander was "Crowther's replacement as visiting physician" but the dates of Alexander's appointment (1820) and Crowther's resignation (1828) negate this.

[56] Cooter (1976a:5, 18–19). Marland (1987:351–353).

[57] Marland (1987:352).

[58] For example, Bolton (1928) and Ashworth (1975).

[59] Biographical material on Crowther may be found in Bolton (1928:590–596), Ashworth (1975:61, 63), Todd and Ashworth (n.d.:63–77), and Marland (1987:353–356).

[60] Ashworth (1975:61) stated that Crowther was appointed on the opening of the Asylum, 1818, ditto Todd and Ashworth (n.d.:63), but Bolton (1928:590) said 1819.

[61] Marland (1987:321), based on Walker (1939:569–570).

[62] Hack Tuke (1889a:367).

This was a view vigorously contested by Dr. Crowther: as a general practitioner of around 25 years standing in Wakefield, he "felt strongly that the visiting physician should have sole control over the medical and other treatment of the patients, and that an asylum director should be a sort of male head attendant, on a par with the matron", views perhaps buttressed by the fact that he was eight years Ellis's senior, and had trained as a physician in Edinburgh (MD 1793), rather than as a surgeon-apothecary.[63] Consequently, Crowther and Ellis were often at loggerheads, and appeal to the visiting magistrates was in favour of Ellis, his powers being increased in 1821.[64]

Crowther eventually resigned his post at the Asylum in February 1828.[65] An appeal to Higgins met with short shrift.[66] Crowther continued to agitate for asylum reform, petitioning Parliament in the 1830s for an Act to further regulate the management of asylums, including a requirement for inspections.[67] As late as 1849, he was still attacking the magistrates in print, satirically depicting Godfrey Higgins as "Major Vanteur".[68]

---

[63] Bolton (1928:590–591). William Browne (1837:6) mentioned that "Crowther", *inter alia*, entertained the opinion that "insanity is always connected with organic change" which, if this refers to Caleb Crowther, as assumed by Finn (2012:35n120), might possibly have put him at odds with the opinions of a phrenologist like Ellis.

[64] For the Ellis-Crowther dispute, see Smith (1999:66–68). It was Godfrey Higgins (1821) who revised the Asylum rules.

[65] Both Bolton (1928:591) and Ashworth (1975:61) dated Crowther's resignation as 1828, and Bolton reproduced his letter of resignation dated 16th February 1828, but Marland (1987:353) stated that he "acted as visiting physician to the Wakefield Asylum from 1818 to 1826" and elsewhere (292) that he was visiting physician for eight years, possibly following her (incomplete) quotation (cited at 321) from Walker (1939:569–570). This latter material does not appear in Walker (1934) (the only mention of Crowther therein, at 1934:463, is not related to the Asylum).

[66] Bolton (1928:591–592).

[67] Crowther (1830).

[68] Might this be a possible source for Henry Clarkson's assertion (*vide supra*) that Higgins was "deranged"? Long dead, Higgins was in no position to respond.

Charles Caesar Corsellis[69] (Superintendent 1831–1853)[70]

In 1831 the first addition was made, by the erection of an east wing, which was opened in the spring of that year, almost contemporaneously with a change of Directorship, by the retirement of Dr. and Mrs. Ellis, and the appointment of Dr. and Mrs. Corsellis as resident superintendents of the institution.[71]

In addition to this eastern wing, a western wing was added to WRA in 1841,[72] followed by a director's house (1843), and then the "New Asylum", partially occupied in 1846 and completed in 1848. These piecemeal enlargements permitted the accommodation of more patients, their number reaching 800 by the time of Corsellis's departure,[73] but to the detriment of the attractive symmetrical appearance of the original Georgian building.

Despite these changes, an American visitor *circa* 1841 noted that the Asylum "is pleasantly situated, about a mile from the town of Wakefield, and, when approaching it, is nearly hidden from view by the shrubbery and trees with which it is environed".[74] A ground plan of the Asylum "from the ready and accurate pencil of Mr. Naylor", dated July 1850 and illustrating both the Old Asylum and the New Asylum, appeared in a publication by Thomas Wright, the Visiting Physician (*vide infra*).[75] This confirmed the presence of

---

[69] In *J Ment Sci* 1863–1864;9(October 1863):456 he was recorded as "Nicholas C. Corsellis, Esq., M.R.C.S. Eng., late Medical Superintendent of the West Riding Asylum, Wakefield: Benson, Oxford." Ditto *J Ment Sci* 1865–1866;11:301 and 458. An indirect descendant of Corsellis was the neuropathologist John Arthur Nicholas Corsellis (Todd and Ashworth n.d.:51) who was known as "Nick" (John Arthur Nicholas Corsellis | RCP Museum, accessed 20/11/2024) but obviously this cannot explain the use of "Nicholas" for his predecessor in the 1860s. Neurologists may be familiar with the work of J.A.N. Corsellis (1915–1994): he described the brain pathology in certain of the dementias, as a consequence of boxing, in focal epilepsies, and in some psychoses (Kasper et al. 2010).

[70] Biographical material on Corsellis may be found in Todd & Ashworth, n.d.:49–62.

[71] Wright (1850:11).

[72] Smith (1999:179): "At Wakefield, after being shown the new wing in 1841, patients clamoured for a transfer".

[73] Bolton (1928:604).

[74] Earle (1841:10).

[75] Wright (1850, n. p.), but effectively x (ground plan) and xi (key), although the Contents page erroneously listed the Ground plan as at "ix" (in fact a blank page). G.F. Naylor was reportedly the Asylum House Surgeon (*vide infra*). He is not mentioned by Bolton (1928), but Scrimgeour (2015:147) called "Mr. George Frederick Naylor" the "visiting surgeon", a different role altogether, hence not correct in this instance.

buildings detached from the main Asylum (Fig. 2.1). Samuel Gaskell (1807–1886), the superintendent of Lancaster Asylum,[76] had read a paper at the 1847 meeting of the Association of Medical Officers of Asylums and Hospitals for the Insane (AMOAHI) advocating separation and detachment of asylum buildings in place of the existing model of one large and continuous structure.[77]

Shortly after the completion of the New Asylum, in 1849, a cholera outbreak afflicted Wakefield and the Asylum was not spared its effects. Within one month, from September to October, 100 of the 600 inmates had died.[78] An initial report by the Visiting Physicians, William Thomas and Thomas Wright, in November 1849, stated that "Not a single ward escaped; and there seemed no difference in any, as to the deadly nature of the poison or the rapidity of its operation. Almost every one attacked with livid collapse died". On the worst day, 19 patients died. The Visiting Physicians recorded "the unwearying and kind assiduity of Mr. Naylor (the House-Surgeon) and Miss Roseden (one of the Deputy-Matrons), in their respective arduous duties; and, generally, to the faithful and unshrinking exertions of every Servant, Nurse, and Keeper in the institution".[79]

Wright wrote an extensive report on the cholera outbreak, published in the following year, in which he attempted to analyse many of its aspects based on his experience and researches.[80] His conclusion was that cholera had been brought to the Asylum by infection, specifically through the medium of a patient, Elizabeth Fenton, admitted from the workhouse at Gomersal where cases of cholera had already occurred, although Fenton had not been in the workhouse hospital where the cholera patients died. Contrary to prevalent beliefs, Wright did not find that "defective drainage and ventilation, had a share in *generating* cholera".[81]

---

[76] For biographical material on Samuel Gaskell, see Scull et al. (1996:161–186) and Larner (2016) (reprinted in adapted form in Larner 2023a:69–76). He was brother-in-law to the novelist Elizabeth Gaskell (1810–1865).

[77] Bewley (2008:16).

[78] Anon. (1849), Wright (1850:vi), and Marland (1987:45).

[79] Wright (1850:3, 7).

[80] Wright (1850).

[81] Wright (1850:77, 78) [italics in original].

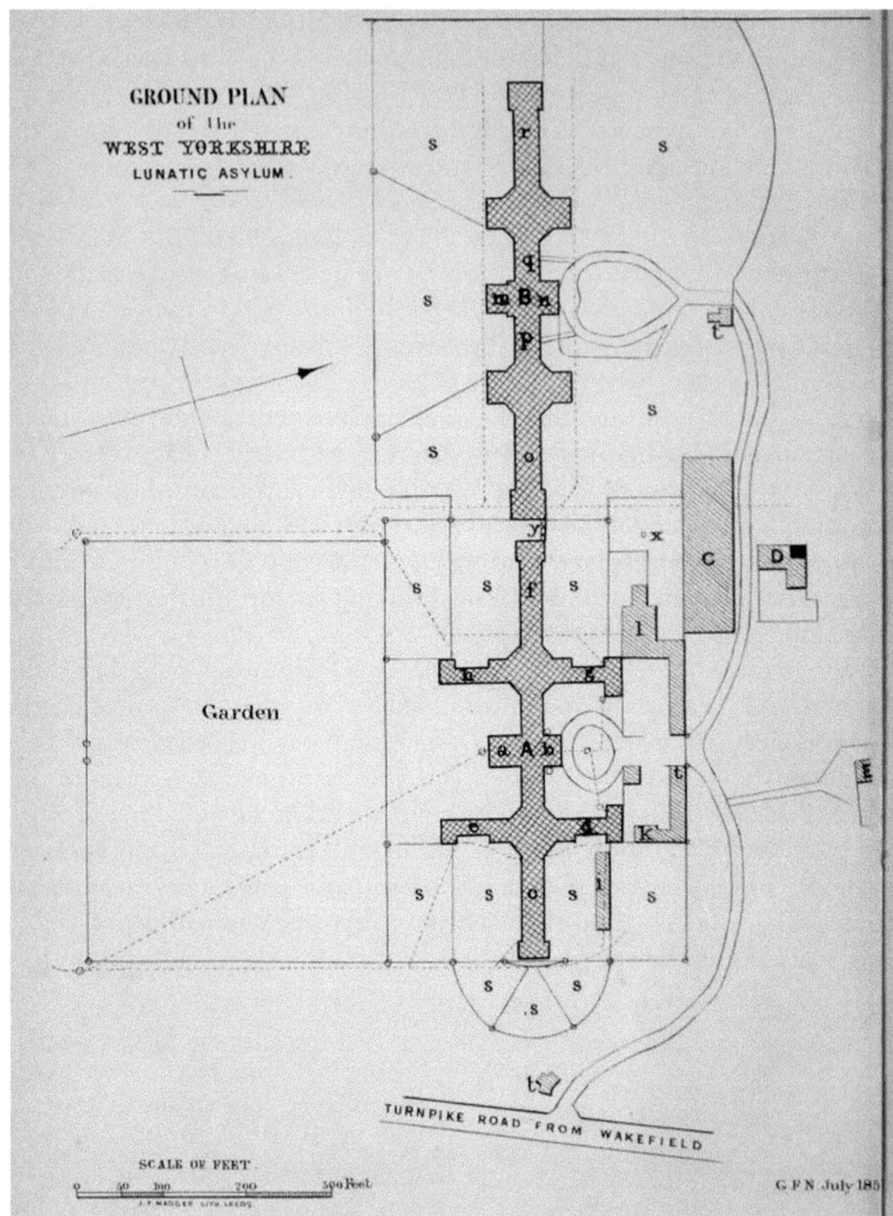

Fig. 2.1 Plan of West Riding Asylum, 1850, by GF Naylor

GROUND PLAN OF THE ASYLUM.

To facilitate reference to the wards and other arrangements alluded to in the ensuing reports, a ground plan is annexed, from the ready and accurate pencil of Mr. Naylor. In the following explanation, the apartments in each division of the buildings are described from the ground floor upward.

A The Old Asylum.

    a. The Director's residence.

    b. The office, entrance, and house-keeper's room: the chapel: and dormitories to ward 9.

Men's Wards.

    c. East wing; basement story: wards 1, 4, and 7; over the eastern end of which is the men's hospital.

    d. Wards 3, 6, and 9. In the airing-court of No. 3 are (i) the weaving shops.

    e. Wards 2, the shoemakers': 5, the tailors': and 8, which has occasionally been used as a separate ward, but is now a dormitory to Nos. 2, and 5.

Women's Wards.

    f. West wing; wards 18, 14, and 13; over the western end of which is a hospital.

    g. Kitchens, larder, &c: wards 16, and 12.

    h. No. 17, a dormitory to the wards above, viz: 15 and 11.

    k.l. Stables and out-offices.

    t.t. Porter's lodges.

B. The New Asylum.

    m. Apartments of the house-surgeon, and deputy matron.

    n. Entrance, surgery, &c.: chapel: dormitories.

Women's Wards, east wing.

    o. Wards 1, 2, 3, 4; and above them the hospital.

    p. Kitchens: wards 10 and 11.

Men's Wards, west wing.

    q. Offices: wards 9 and 8.

    r. Wards 5, 6, 7; and hospital.

s.s.s. Airing courts.

C. Brew-house, bake-house, engine-house, wash-house and laundry.

D. Gas-house; at the north-west angle of which is a large chimney, 128 feet high: into it pass flues from the adjoining offices; and also, since last autumn, air-flues from some of the chief drains.

E. Farm buildings: and dead-house.

x. The principal well, in which are forcing-pumps worked by a steam-engine, for supplying both asylums.

y. Passage uniting the two buildings.

The dotted lines indicate the course of the drains: and in connection with them is shewn the situation of the cess-pools for collecting the solid contents of the sewers. Five, that were in the entrance yard of the old building, are now disused and filled up.

The wards in the old building are ten feet six inches high; and in the new eleven feet: and the galleries ten feet, and ten and a half, wide. The bed-rooms for single patients, contain each about 800 cubic feet.

Fig. 2.1   (continued)

Like his predecessor as superintendent, Corsellis was criticised by Caleb Crowther, even though the latter was no longer a visiting physician, the allegations being that Corsellis "rode too frequently to hounds and was too often in the streets of Wakefield and Leeds".[82] Nevertheless, in 1838 Corsellis did produce a table, based on 20 years of admissions to the Asylum, identifying 55 distinct causes of insanity. More worryingly, Corsellis may have reverted to a more traditional coercive regime, considering "a moderate degree of mechanical restraint preferable to an increase of staff".[83]

The departure of Corsellis from WRA is reported to be "shrouded in mystery" and "seems to have been rather sudden".[84]

Thomas Giordani Wright (1808–1898)[85]

Thomas Giordani Wright settled in Wakefield in 1833 and was soon thereafter appointed Honorary Physician to the Asylum, a post he held for 65 years until his death in 1898. Trained as a physician (MD Leiden; LRCP 1841; MRCP 1859), he spent most of his working life in Wakefield, although he may perhaps be best known to posterity for the diary of his experiences written whilst he was an apprentice doctor in the 1820s in Newcastle-upon-Tyne.[86] He was the leading physician in Wakefield in the second half of the nineteenth century, charging a guinea fee for visits and retaining five household servants. He was one of the founders of the Wakefield Microscopic Society in 1854 and lectured at the Mechanics Institute.[87] His report on the 1849 cholera outbreak in the Asylum and his subsequent (1850) book have already been mentioned.

In later years, in 1872 and 1873, Wright was among those reported to be invited to the medical *conversazione* held at WRA and reportedly accepted

---

[82] Bolton (1928:605). Crowther's criticisms were one of the few instances in which Wakefield Asylum was mentioned by Kathleen Jones (1993:71), where it was also suggested that the resident director received a salary of £550 plus services valued at £400 a year.

[83] Smith (1999:106), Bolton (1928:605), and Walton (1981:167).

[84] Todd and Ashworth (1991:390).

[85] Biographical material on Wright may be found in his obituary: *BMJ* 1898;1:1493 (4th June); also Ashworth (1975:65–66) and Marland (1987:356–357). Contrary to the *BMJ* obituary, Bolton (1928:590) stated that Wright served the Asylum for 64 years. Ashworth (1975:65) gave his middle name as "Geordani", presumably a typographical error; ditto White's *Directory* (1858:580) which listed him as "J.G. Wright".

[86] Johnson (1999).

[87] Marland (1987:299, 284, 307, 338).

an invitation in 1875.[88] He was listed below the "Resident Medical Officers" of the Asylum as "Non-resident Consulting Physician" in the second volume of the *West Riding Lunatic Asylum Medical Reports* published in 1872 (II:308).[89]

John Septimus Alderson (Superintendent 1853–1858)[90]

John Septimus Alderson was Medical Superintendent at York Asylum (1842–1845)[91] and Nottingham Asylum before transferring to Wakefield. In 1844 he had been joint Chairman of the Association of Medical Officers of Asylums and Hospitals for the Insane (the organisation had no President before 1854), sharing the role with John Thurnam (1810–1873), the first medical superintendent of the York Retreat.

In his history of the WRA, Joseph Shaw Bolton reported that Alderson "died after a very short period of office"[92] and that this was "after a long period of ill-health". He was on sick leave from June 1857, and did not return, dying on 2nd January 1858. In his history of WRA, Ashworth credited Alderson with the discontinuance of restraint as a mode of treatment.[93]

Another innovation which appears to date from the years of the Alderson superintendency related to junior medical staffing at the Asylum. On the recommendation of the Lunacy Commissioners, a "Resident House Surgeon/

---

[88] For 1872: *Leeds Mercury* 17th October 1872, p.8 (Medical Conversazione at the West Riding Asylum). For 1873: *Yorkshire Post and Leeds Intelligencer* 27th November 1873, p.3 (West Riding Asylum. Medical Conversazione). For 1875: *Leeds Mercury* 20th November 1875, p.3 (Medical Conversazione at Wakefield Asylum). For details of the medical *conversazione* held annually at WRA between 1871 and 1875, see Part IV.

[89] For details of the *West Riding Lunatic Asylum Medical Reports* published annually between 1871 and 1876, see Part III.

[90] Biographical material on John Septimus Alderson is limited, for example, Bolton (1928:588, 605), Ashworth (1975:67), and Todd and Ashworth (n.d.:79–85); *Plarr's Lives of the Fellows online*, Alderson, John Septimus (- 1858) (rcseng.ac.uk). He barely features in Adams' history of the York Asylum (Adams 2025:71, 107, 112). I presume he was the son of John Alderson (1758–1829) of Hull, who was reported (Bickford and Bickford 1983:4) to have fathered eleven children, five of whom survived infancy, one of whom, John, married in June 1827 ("Septimus" presumably indicates that he was the seventh child).

[91] Based on this dating, Alderson may have encountered Thomas Laycock (for whom, see Chaps. 4 and 5) at York: the latter "regularly visited patients in the York psychiatric hospitals" where a "Mr. Alderson, the resident medical officer" assisted Laycock in timing a patient's movements. Laycock was "probably accompanied by medical students" in these visits according to Dewhurst (1982:8–9), but Alderson would not have encountered the young John Hughlings Jackson (see Chap. 7) as he was a student at the York Medical School a decade later (1852–1855).

[92] Thus Bolton (1928:588) considered five years (1853–1858) to be a "very short period", which presumably it must have seemed to him considering that he had already been Medical Director at Wakefield for 18 years at the time he was writing, and continued in post until his retirement in 1933, 23 years in all. Biographical material on Bolton may be found in Ashworth (1975:75).

[93] Bolton (1928:615–617), writing on the subject of "Wakefield and Restraint", said nothing of Alderson.

Apothecary" should be substituted following the resignation of a Visiting Physician or Surgeon.[94] The appointee, in November 1856, was John Chapman.[95]

It would appear the work of the Asylum was sustained during the period of Alderson's illness by the extra work done by the junior staff, supported by the visiting physician, Thomas Wright. John Chapman, named variously as Alderson's assistant or house surgeon,[96] was given an additional allowance for his efforts but was not subsequently elected superintendent after Alderson's death, apparently because he lacked the necessary medical qualifications stipulated by the regulations of the Asylum (namely, membership of one of the Royal Surgical Colleges).[97]

Henry Maudsley (1835–1918)[98]

It was during this difficult period of time that Henry Maudsley, a Yorkshireman, later to become one of the leaders of the profession and eventually the benefactor of the Maudsley Hospital in London, gained at Wakefield his first experience of asylum work. Bolton noted that he was appointed temporary house surgeon on 13th July 1857, and was in post until 29th April 1858 when Alderson's successor, Cleaton (*vide infra*), took office.[99]

Later sources differ in their interpretation of Maudsley's exact role during this time, ranging from his being "briefly the director",[100] to "locum superintendent" in the absence of Alderson though officially the "house surgeon",[101] to "assistant medical officer",[102] to merely the assistant to the resident medical

---

[94] Todd & Ashworth, n.d.:82. However, Mr. G.F. Naylor had been designated "the House-Surgeon" prior to this (*vide supra*).

[95] Chapman's appointment is noted in *Asylum J Ment Sci* 1857;3:284. However, Ashworth (1975:72) stated he was appointed in 1856. Scrimgeour (2015:213) did not specify an appointment date. In the *Medical Directory* for 1856 (109) "CHAPMAN, John, jun." is listed as "Assistant Medical Officer, Wilts County Asylum, Devizes—M.R.C.S. Eng. 1851; M.D. Aberd. 1855", ditto 1857 (164), but in 1858 (397) he is "House-Surg. West York Asyl. Wakefield, Yorksh.".

[96] Chapman was denoted as "house surgeon" in White's *Directory* of 1858 (580) and as Surgeon (601; as was Alderson). As noted previously, G.F. Naylor was "House Surgeon" during the cholera epidemic in 1849.

[97] Bolton (1928:605). However, Chapman's entry in the *Medical Directory* clearly contradicts this: "M.R.C.S. Eng. 1851".

[98] Biographical material on Maudsley may be found in Lewis (1951), Turner (1988), Scull et al. (1996:226–267), and Turner, https://doi.org/10.1093/ref:odnb/37747

[99] Bolton (1928:605).

[100] Pearce (2003a:1141).

[101] Walk (1990:15).

[102] Turner (1988:154).

officer, John Chapman.[103] Suffice it to say that Maudsley made sufficient impression that the Asylum's Committee gave him a testimonial expressing a high opinion of his ability, which may have been instrumental in his obtaining the superintendency at the Manchester Royal Lunatic Asylum at Cheadle in 1859 at the age of 24.

John Davies Cleaton (Superintendent 1858–1866)[104]

John Davies Cleaton (1825–1901), a Welshman and graduate of Guy's Hospital in London, worked at Lancaster County Asylum under Samuel Gaskell, an early proponent of non-restraint, before becoming Medical Superintendent of the Lancashire Asylum at Rainhill.[105] He moved to Wakefield in 1858. Bolton later opined that "during the next eight years the entire asylum was transformed under the influence of perhaps the most brilliant administrator our specialty has ever possessed". As for mechanical restraint, "Dr. Cleaton, in his first report (1858), advocates the disuse of restraint and of all things reminding patients of an asylum, and during his directorship it was never employed".[106]

This was certainly a period during which the fabric of the Asylum was greatly extended:

> a large new kitchen and dining hall were erected, together with store-rooms, cellars, offices, reception room and clock tower. A new weaving shed and new joiner's, upholsterer's and painter's shops were added. Quarters for medical officers, housekeeper and servants were erected, and a new entrance lodge was built. A large general lavatory for working-out patients with a covered way to it from the dining hall was provided. Lastly, a fine church with 700 sittings, identical with that built by the Great Northern Railway Company at Doncaster, was erected. In 1859 Ivy House was opened for quiet and parole

---

[103] Scrimgeour (2015:213). Ashworth (1975:67) stated that Maudsley was appointed to assist Alderson's (unnamed) deputy. Adams (2010:160), although technically correct chronologically, may be susceptible to misinterpretation when he stated that Maudsley was "Crichton Browne's [*sic*] predecessor at the Wakefield Asylum". My own (cynical?) suspicion, based on what is known of Maudsley's character, is that he was a young man in a hurry to rise quickly who, able as he undoubtedly was, could ingratiate himself to whomsoever he needed to ingratiate himself in order to gain advancement. Todd & Ashworth's (n.d.:83) characterisation of Maudsley as "whimsical and modest" does not ring true to my ears.

[104] Biographical material on Cleaton may be found in Bolton (1928:606–607), Ashworth (1975:69), and Todd and Ashworth (n.d.:87–113). Obituaries: *BMJ* 1901;2:653 (7th September); *J Ment Sci* 1901;47(October 1901):863.

[105] For Cleaton at Rainhill, see Regan (1986:43–44, 48–49, 50, 51).

[106] Bolton (1928:606 and 617).

patients, and in 1866 the large ward 20 for working-out patients was opened, and a detached hospital for contagious diseases was completed and ready for opening.[107]

These changes met with approbation in some quarters, for example the new Chapel.[108] Discussing the need to expand asylums to accommodate a population of more than 500 patients, Charles Lockhart Robertson (1825–1897) was of the view that:

> One has only to look at the transmutation of the West Riding Asylum on this principle, under the able superintendence of Mr. Cleaton, and its adaptation to the requirements of 1000 patients, to see how cheaply, yet well, these extensions and alterations can be carried out.[109]

Certainly, this was an era during which:

> Local magistrates almost universally adopted the practice of tacking on wing after wing, story upon story, building next to building, in a haphazard and fortuitous fashion, as they strove to keep pace with the demand for accommodation for more and more lunatics.[110]

As a result of these additions, by 1862 Cleaton was of the view that:

> the Institution has now, by the completion of the additions and alterations which have been in progress during the last four years, attained its final size and capacity.

a view which ultimately proved wrong. It did, however, coincide with the production of "a large and well-drawn bird's-eye view map of the now completed buildings"[111] executed by one of the patients, James Walker, an architect, which was adjudged to be a "very clear and faithful

---

[107] Bolton (1928:606).

[108] *J Ment Sci* 1863–1864;9(April 1863):116 ("He should visit the West Riding Asylum, and see how well the new detached chapel there has answered"). Prior to 1861 the chapel had been part of the main building (see ground plan of Wright 1850:x,xi).

[109] Robertson (1864–1865:484).

[110] Scull (1979:196). See also McCandless (1979).

[111] *J Ment Sci* 1862–1863;8(July 1862):278 (The West Riding of York Asylum).

isometrical drawing of the whole of the buildings"[112] and was subsequently lithographed.[113]

Perhaps the most significant of these additions at WRA was the Dining and Recreation Hall,[114] located to the west of the main building, first used for a Christmas function in 1859 and completed in 1861. As the Recreation Hall, it could reportedly accommodate several hundred people, possibly up to 1000, and was later described as "the capacious and beautiful Grecian hall, which is 108 feet long by 50 feet broad".[115] It also found uses other than simply as a refectory: Cleaton encouraged recreational activities, most particularly in terms of public musical concerts,[116] to which end the employment of attendants with musical abilities was encouraged from around this time (see Chap. 3: Attendants and Nurses). The hall later served for theatrical presentations, as well as for the medical *conversazione* (see Part IV).

As for the junior medical staff in this period, John Chapman, who had taken on additional duties during Alderson's illness, himself died in 1860 as a consequence of consumption.[117] Further appointments followed: William James Lancaster, formerly of St Bartholomew's Hospital, London, was appointed in Chapman's place and served until 1865.[118] "W.J. Lancaster"

---

[112] Scrimgeour (2015:311 and n22), citing "Annual Reports [*sic*] of the Superintendent. C85/1/12/7. 42nd Report for 1861. Page 21" (not seen by me). The annual *Reports* of the Commissioners and of the Medical Superintendent are henceforward denoted as "*Report*" and qualified by year of publication (as per the Bibliography), not by the preceding year to which they refer. This discrepancy is pointed out repeatedly in the text to avoid any misunderstanding.

[113] Discussed and reproduced in Ashworth (1975:57, 58), Finn (2012:57), and Scrimgeour (2015:310–313).

[114] So called by Ashworth (1975:53, 55). This may be seen in the lithograph plate based on Walker's drawing, dated as 1862 by Ashworth (1975:58) and Scrimgeour (2015:312) but as 1865 by Finn (2012:57, Figure 2.1; [WYAS C85/1363]). The images differ, the former two being more extensive and including the Chapel.

[115] *The Wakefield Express, and Barnsley, Normanton, Pontefract, Ossett, Horbury & Dewsbury Advertiser* Volume 22, No, 1126, 29th November 1873, p.2, cols. 4–7 (Medical conversazione at the West Riding Asylum. Speech by Lord Houghton. Lecture by Dr. Carpenter).

[116] The Asylum Church was also used for public concerts: *J Ment Sci* 1863–1864;9(October 1863):415–416 (Public concerts in the West Riding Asylum). The topic of music at WRA is covered at greater length in Golding (2021).

[117] *Report* (1861:13) (this is the 41st *Report*, for the year 1860) and Scrimgeour (2015:290). Chapman was still listed as a member of AMOAHI in *J Ment Sci* 1861;7(April 1861):unpaginated (after p.158).

[118] *Report* (1861:13) and Scrimgeour (2015:290, 359). The *Medical Directory* of 1865 (419) listed William James Lancaster as "Res. Asst. Med. Off. West Riding Co. Asyl." and the *Medical Directory* of 1866 (424) listed him with an address in Barnsley, Yorkshire, as "late Res. Asst. Med. Off. West Riding Co. Asyl.". A letter in the *Lancet* of 4th September 1875 mentioned in passing a "Dr. Lancaster" who "was for five years assistant medical officer at the West Riding Lunatic Asylum, and thus had special opportunity of being acquainted with the normal and abnormal appearances of the brain" (*Lancet* 1875;2:363).

from Barnsley was among those invited to the medical *conversazione* at WRA in 1872 and 1873, and accepted an invitation in 1875.[119] In addition, a Mr. P.W. Jones, formerly Assistant Medical Officer of the Kent County Asylum, was appointed as medical assistant in view of the large increase in the number of patients in the Asylum.[120]

Cleaton left Wakefield Asylum in 1866 to become a Commissioner in Lunacy,[121] in which capacity he was to return to Wakefield to make inspections on three occasions[122] during the superintendency of his successor.

---

[119] For 1872: *Leeds Mercury* 17th October 1872, p.8 (Medical Conversazione at the West Riding Asylum). For 1873: *Yorkshire Post and Leeds Intelligencer* 27th November 1873, p.3 (West Riding Asylum. Medical Conversazione). For 1875: *Leeds Mercury* 20th November 1875, p.3 (Medical Conversazione at Wakefield Asylum).

[120] Scrimgeour (2015:213–214). The *Medical Directory* of 1862 (471) listed Philip William Jones as "House-Surg. West Riding Asylum, Wakefield—L.R.C.P.Lond. 1861; M.R.C.S. Eng. 1859; late Asst. Med. Off. Kent Co. Asyl. Maidstone; and Path Prosector Queen's Hosp. Birmingham."; ditto 1863 (463) and 1864 (472), but in 1865 (410) there was no mention of Wakefield and his address was given as Waltham Abbey, Essex.

[121] *Lancet* 1866;2:27 (7th July; Medical Appointments); *BMJ* 1866;1:30 (7th July; Medical News); *J Ment Sci* 1866–1867;12(July 1866):296 (Appointments). The *BMJ* announcement noted that Cleaton's appointment as a Commissioner in Lunacy was "in the room of S. Gaskell, Esq., resigned". For details of both Cleaton and Gaskell as Lunacy Commissioners, see *Biographies of Medical Lunacy Commissioners 1828–1912*. http://studymore.org.uk/6biom.htm (accessed 09/12/2023).

[122] According to Ashworth, 1975:75. Certainly at least twice, in 1868 (*Report*, 1869:7–12) and 1870 (*Report*, 1871:9–15).

3

The West Riding Pauper Lunatic Asylum 1866–1876

James Crichton-Browne[1] (Superintendent 1866–1876)[2]

When he was appointed to the superintendency of WRA in 1866 in succession to John Davies Cleaton, James Crichton-Browne (Fig. 3.1) evidently had plans, based on his prior training and practice,[3] for the development of the institution which were both structural and functional in nature. The latter, to be discussed in subsequent chapters, included: changes to the resident medical faculty (Part

---

[1] As for John Hughlings Jackson (see Chap. 7), Crichton-Browne is also a subject for what has been termed a "saga of the inconsistent hyphen" (this terminology is from Critchley and Critchley 1998:177–179, 181). He did not begin to hyphenate his name until the late 1870s, for example appearing as editor of and author in the *West Riding Lunatic Asylum Medical Reports* as "Crichton Browne" at least until 1876 (VI:170; VI:232 "under the care of Dr. Crichton-Browne"; see Table 6.1). However, at risk of being accused of anachronism, I have elected to retain the usage of "Crichton-Browne" here, and throughout, not least because, as pointed out by Oppenheim (1991:328n1), "most indexes and bibliographies today … alphabetize him under 'C'", a policy which is followed in the Bibliography here. Oppenheim also noted that "The *DNB 1931–1940* is a notable exception" and this remains the case in the 2004 *Oxford Dictionary of National Biography* (Volume 8:172–173; Neve, https://doi.org/10.1093/ref:odnb/32122). In the current Bibliography, some items are listed as "Crichton Browne" and others as "Crichton-Browne" in accordance with the exact publication details, rather than as a consequence of authorial inconsistency (or laziness). This "C" policy also disambiguates him from his father, William A.F. Browne (see Chap. 7), and his brother J.H. Balfour Browne (see Chap. 9).

[2] To my knowledge there is no full-length biography of Crichton-Browne, but snippets of autobiographical material may be found in Crichton-Browne (1926, 1927, 1930, 1932, 1937), and in Easterbrook (1937:18–26 and 1940:1–6). There are numerous shorter biographical pieces available, for example: Leyland (1888:II:27–34), Oppenheim (1991:54–78), Todd and Ashworth (1991:391–393, n.d.:115–150), Neve and Turner (1995), Rollin (2003), Neve, https://doi.org/10.1093/ref:odnb/32122, Jellinek (2005), Finn (2012:passim), Cavanaugh (2018), and Cambiaghi (2019).

[3] Biographical material on Crichton-Browne is presented in the Prosopography section in Chap. 5.

    33
A. J. Larner, *The West Riding Asylum and the Origins of British Neurology 1866-1876*, https://doi.org/10.1007/978-3-032-12591-0_3

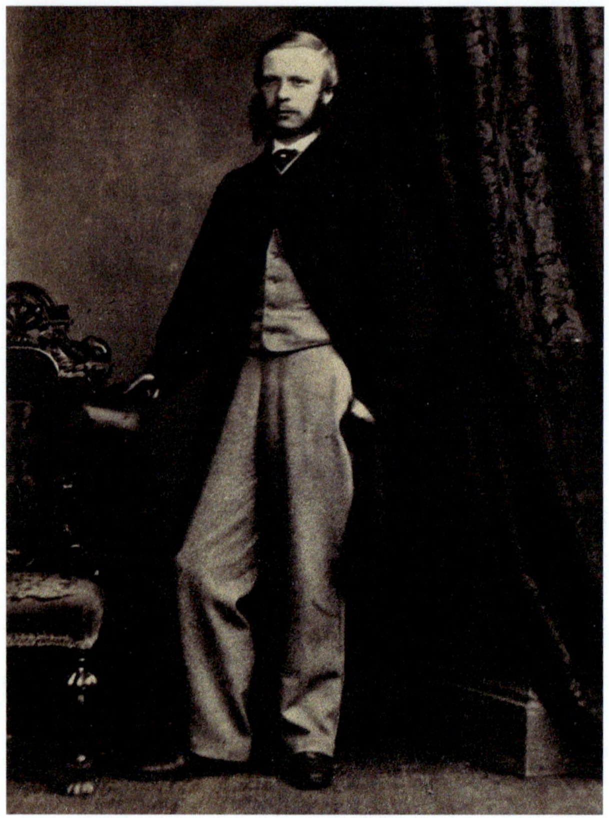

Fig. 3.1   James Crichton-Browne

II); inauguration of a house journal, the *West Riding Lunatic Asylum Medical Reports* (henceforward *WRLAMR*; Part III); and organisation of annual meetings, called medical *conversazione*, which aimed to raise the profile of the Asylum amongst practitioners in the West Riding and to communicate some of the clinical and research activities taking place there (Part IV). Here discussion is confined to the changes in infrastructure and administration initiated by Crichton-Browne, and thereafter to the nature of the establishment from the time of his arrival in 1866 and into the late 1860s and early 1870s.

As a consequence of the building programme supervised by Cleaton (detailed in Chap. 2), Crichton-Browne inherited very extensive facilities, as shown in the lithograph plan of the Asylum of 1862. Upwards of 1100 patients were now accommodated, but more space was still needed because of the apparent increase in the number of patients with insanity.[4] Hence "In

---

[4] Arlidge (1870).

1868 an old weaving-shed was converted into a large sick-ward and dormitory". Furthermore, "In the same year (1868) the important step was taken of acquiring Mount Pleasant House at Sheffield as a second centre for the treatment of the lunatics of the Riding".[5] By 1870:

> the new dining hall and bath-room for women patients, which have been fitted up temporarily as dayrooms and dormitories, were opened in November and are now fully occupied. … What will ultimately form the hall proper is now subdivided into two stories by a temporary floor, which will be removed after the completion of the South Yorkshire Asylum.[6]

Some of these changes were presumably in progress when the Asylum was visited by about 100 members of the British Medical Association, then in Leeds for their Annual Meeting, on Wednesday 28th July 1869.[7] After being taken through the various departments by Crichton-Browne, the members enjoyed a cold collation in the dining hall before adjourning to the lawn where "about 700 or 800 of the patients" were assembled to hear a promenade concert given by the Asylum Church choir.[8]

The BMA visit gave the *Lancet* an opportunity to note that "the asylum is for the most part an old building, constructed on the vicious plan of central corridors, with small rooms on each side, the corridors being lighted from the ends only, and from the rooms when the doors are thrown open. Anything more gloomy than the original state of these corridors, and of the rooms, could not well be conceived".[9] Changes had been effected by Crichton-Browne:

---

[5] Bolton (1928:609), who also pointed out that "This was the precursor of the South Yorkshire Asylum at Wadsley, which was opened in 1872". This was later known as Middlewood Hospital. Further institutions, also sharing the nomenclature of "West Riding Asylum" were opened at Menston (High Royds Hospital) in 1888, and at Huddersfield (Storthes Hall Hospital) in 1904. For historical material relating to Middlewood Hospital, see Thorpe (1972) (for F.T. Thorpe, a long-standing medical superintendent at Middlewood, see *Bulletin of the Royal College of Psychiatrists* 1984;8(12):244); for High Royds Hospital, see Bannister (2005), Davis (2013b), and (http://www.highroydshospital.com, accessed 22/10/2024); and for Storthes Hall Hospital, see Littlewood (2003) (I thank Mrs. Sarah Bates of Huddersfield for drawing my attention to and lending me this book, 25/01/2025).

[6] Bolton (1928:609); based on *Report* (1871:4, 18).

[7] The possibility of this visit being part of the Annual Meeting programme was noted in *BMJ* 1869;2:11 (3rd July; The Annual Meeting of the Association) and confirmed in *BMJ* 1869;2:123 (31st July; The Leeds Meeting), by which time the visit had already occurred.

[8] *BMJ* 1869;2:168 (7th August; Visit to the West Riding Asylum). *Yorkshire Post and Leeds Intelligencer* 29th July 1869, p.3 (Excursion to the West Riding Asylum). Perhaps this event was an inspiration, or even a trial run, for the subsequent WRA medical *conversazione*?

[9] *Lancet* 1869;2:312 (28th August; The West Riding Pauper Lunatic Asylum (Wakefield)). Also mentioned in passing in *Lancet* 1870;1:17.

By the use of some of the cheapest pigments and ornamentation, by the introduction of numerous pictures and common ornaments, and decorations of artificial flowers, made by the patients, the corridors and rooms are brightened, and have a comfortable aspect given to them to an extent almost incredible. ... The great result of these changes has been, to give a gratifying home-like aspect to all parts of the asylum ....[10]

These changes were also noted by the *Lancet* Commission on Lunatic Asylums in 1876, which:

alluded to what has been accomplished, with exceedingly small outlay, at the West Riding Asylum, Wakefield. Every bed has a tasteful covering, by the side of each there is a low chair with cushion, and a strip of carpet, while to every window there are curtains. The general effect is so comfortable, orderly, and tranquillising, that patients retire for the night with greater calmness, and sleep more peacefully, than they would amid surroundings like those too commonly found in county and borough asylums, and which reproduce the poverty without the comforts of *home*.[11]

However, according to Bolton, "During the period of office of Dr. Browne (1866–76) mechanical restraint was employed once or twice yearly".[12] Reporting on his unannounced visit to WRA sometime around August 1875, Charles Foller Folsom (1842–1907), secretary to the Massachusetts Board of Health and Medical Superintendent of the McLean Asylum at Somerville, Massachusetts, found not one of fourteen hundred patients undergoing mechanical restraint.[13]

Other improvements had been noted in the Commissioners' *Report* for the year 1871, such as the formation of a fully equipped Asylum Fire Brigade, the planting of 1500 trees in the airing courts, the extension of the farm to take more cows, and increased supplies of carpets, curtains, and furniture for the wards.[14] Turkish baths were erected in 1871, and in 1873 Field Head was opened as a convalescent home for female patients.[15]

---

[10] *Lancet* 1869;2:312 (28th August; The West Riding Pauper Lunatic Asylum (Wakefield)). Repeated verbatim in *Wakefield Free Press* 4th September 1869, p.5 (The West Riding Asylum).

[11] Anon. (1876:18) [italics in original].

[12] Bolton (1928:617). I presume this may be the origin of the comment by Walton (1981:191) that "At Wakefield, mechanical restraint was reintroduced in the late sixties", a dating which would coincide with Crichton-Browne's superintendency, and contrary to the policy of his predecessor, John Cleaton Davies.

[13] "F" in *Boston Med Surg J* 1875;93:316–319 (9th September: Letter from England), at 318. Reprinted in Folsom (1877:53–55). Also noted in *Medical Record* 1876;11:52.

[14] *Report* (1872:12). Also mentioned in Todd and Ashworth (n.d.:138).

[15] Bolton (1928:610). Fieldhead Hospital, opened 1972, now houses the Mental Health Museum containing artefacts from WRA. It was opened in September 1975 (previously known as the Stanley Royd Hospital Museum and the Stephen G. Beaumont Museum); see Ellis (2015).

By 1876 the *Lancet* was of the opinion that:

Perhaps the most striking example of the extent to which a badly-constructed asylum may be modified and rendered comfortable will be found at Wakefield, where, by refurnishing and refitting with a single eye to the comfort of the inmates, one of the most antiquated and ill-constructed of houses has been converted into one of the most commodious.[16]

Undoubtedly the administration of the Asylum demanded much of Crichton-Browne's time and energy.[17] For example, sanitation was a recurrent theme in his annual *Report*, an issue which had also troubled his predecessors. Filtering of drinking water remained a necessity for many years, even after provision of water from the Wakefield Waterworks Company in 1874.[18] Hence brewing of beer on site was not merely an indulgence but a requirement for safe adequate hydration.

According to White's *Directory* of 1866, the junior staff at the Asylum at this time consisted of Charles Etheridge[19] and George Southam.[20] These were presumably the junior staff in post as Cleaton departed and Crichton-Browne arrived. Indeed, writing the report of his first quarterly meeting on 25th October 1866, Crichton-Browne stated that:

In accordance with a proposal made by my predecessor Dr. Cleaton, I have great pleasure in recommending that Dr. Southam, the Medical Assistant in the Female Department, should in addition to his present office, be appointed Medical Assistant in the Hospital for Epidemic Diseases.

The Hospital has not yet been required during my period of superintendence, as the General health of the Asylum has been most satisfactory.[21]

---

[16] Anon. (1876:893).

[17] For Crichton-Browne's administrative achievements, see Todd and Ashworth (n.d.:132–149).

[18] Ashworth (1975:45–48).

[19] White (1866:827, 833). Also Scrimgeour (2015:331). The *Medical Directory* of 1864 (407) listed Charles Etheridge as "M.R.C.S. Eng. and L.S.A. 1863" at an address in Edmonton, Middlesex. In 1865 (344), to this was added "(*St. Thos.'s*); late of Cunard Roy. Mail Service." In 1866 (349), he was "Res. Asst. Med. Off. West Riding Asyl. Wakefield" and to his previous posts was added "late House Surg. Halifax Infirm". This entry persisted in 1867 (346), and 1868 (359) except that he was now "Sen. Res. Asst. Med. Off.", and by 1869 (376) he was "late Sen. Asst. Med. Off. W. Riding Asyl. Wakefield" and now working at Leighton Buzzard Union.

[20] The *Medical Directory* of 1866 (517) listed George Thomas Mitchell Southam as "Res. Asst. Med. Off. West Riding Lunat. Asyl. Wakefield—M.B. Lond. 1863; (*St. Barthol.*)". In 1867 (512), "M.R.C.S. Eng. and L.S.A. 1862" was added. By 1868 (529) he was at an address in Peterborough. White (1866), has three different sets of initials for Southam, all of which appear to differ from the *Medical Directory* entries: "G.F.W." (827); "G.T.Wm." (842); and "T.W." (851). Southam does not appear in Scrimgeour (2015).

[21] Medical Director's Journal 25th October 1866 (WYAS C85/1/13/1) [my transcriptions].

This was the "hospital for contagious diseases" completed during Cleaton's superintendency.

Southam appears to have remained in post until March 1867:

Dr. Southam, who resigned his appointment as Assistant Medical Officer at the January [1867] meeting, left the asylum upon the 5th of March and Mr. Charles Fox Oxley who was appointed in his place at the special meeting upon the 23rd of February entered upon his duties a few days afterwards.[22]

As for Etheridge, there is no information in Crichton-Browne's *Reports*, but in the Medical Director's Journal for 25th April 1867 one (cryptic) comment appears:

I have to bring before the Committee applications from Dr. Etheridge, the Assistant Medical Officer, from [?name uncertain] the Farm Bailiff ....[23]

The written text ends here without further explanation, but I presume these were applications for termination of employment.

Crichton-Browne was undoubtedly behind changes in the Asylum rules in 1866 which were pertinent to staffing. According to Bolton:

the peculiar powers of the consulting physicians are taken from them. One physician only is allowed for. He only attends when requested and only visits the asylum if required. If no physician is appointed the medical superintendent can call in to his assistance any physician practising in the neighbourhood. Rules for assistant medical officers and a dispenser appear, instead of the old rules for an unqualified house surgeon and apothecary.[24]

As for the Asylum's accommodation of patients, whilst the ground plan appearing in Wright's 1850 book (Chap. 2, Fig. 2.1) had indicated distinct male and female wards, it had not differentiated them to any further degree. Some indication of the uses to which the various buildings at WRA were put may be gleaned incidentally in later written records. For example, in his account of cases of othaematoma, dating from 1870, Patrick Nicol, one of the junior doctors at WRA (see Chap. 5), gave a table indicating the various wards in which he had examined patients, including: Ward 1 "Refractory ward"; 2

---

[22] Medical Director's Journal 25th April 1867 (WYAS C85/1/13/1) [my transcription; I thank Thomas Larner for helping me with this transcription, 22/11/2024].

[23] Medical Director's Journal 25th April 1867 (WYAS C85/1/13/1) [my transcription; uncertain].

[24] Bolton, 1928:590.

"Suicidal ward"; 4 and 14 "Undefined"; 18 "Weak, ailing, and demented patients"; 6 and 35 "non-working wards".[25] In 1872, Crichton-Browne showed a visitor to WRA, William Turner (see Chap. 9), "the ward for female mental defectives, where some thirty idiots and imbeciles were seated in chairs surrounded by toys, flowers and pictures and every comfort, and attended by nurses".[26] Other wards may have been devoted to those patients with frequent epileptic seizures and there was a dedicated infirmary for those with intercurrent illnesses.

However, it was the construction and fitting up of rooms for pathological and photographic purposes which were the most significant changes in terms of the facilities of the Asylum at this time, since these were instrumental in forwarding Crichton-Browne's ambition of establishing WRA as a centre for scientific research work on insanity.

Pathological Laboratory

The founding of a dedicated pathological department by Crichton-Browne is described in Bolton's history of WRA:

In 1870 he [Crichton-Browne] indicates the existence of a pathological department by speaking of the "erection of a new photographic studio in lieu of that removed from the courtyard of 35, with a small pathological museum attached." This building appears to have been erected adjacent to the pathological laboratory near the infectious hospital which was opened in 1866.[27]

However, in his *Report* for the year 1872, Crichton-Browne stated that:

To give full scope to the energies of such an Officer as a Pathologist, and to utilize to the highest advantage his labours, a Pathological Institute or detached building, containing a museum, laboratory, microscopic, photographic, and lecture rooms, is certainly requisite. I am confident that I am not over-estimating the practical sagacity and prudent liberality of the West Riding, in anticipating that such an Institute will, at no distant date, be provided in connexion with this great Hospital.[28]

---

[25] Nicol (1870b:198) (table). Whether these ward numbers correlated with those used by Wright 20 years earlier I am not able to say, although Wright's numbering went no further than 18 (Wright 1850:x, xi). As noted above, the large ward 20 for working-out patients was opened in 1866 (Bolton 1928:606).

[26] Crichton-Browne (1926:47).

[27] Bolton (1928:608).

[28] *Report* (1873:28) [capitals in original].

Hence the exact date of opening of the pathological laboratory at WRA is uncertain.[29]

The purposes of the pathological laboratory, department, or Institute, were multiple: not only to ensure postmortem examinations of all unclaimed pauper patients who died at WRA, and hence establish cause of death and provide illustrative specimens for the pathological museum which might subsequently be of teaching value, but also to forward scientific investigative studies of brain pathology in the various subtypes of insanity. In other words, Crichton-Browne's aims were to put this ancillary discipline on a more professional footing than had existed hitherto.

How was the pathological laboratory equipped? No account has been found but, based on the research work undertaken at WRA, as communicated through *WRLAMR* and other journals[30] and at the WRA medical *conversazione* and other meetings, a number of inferences may be made. For the postmortem work, mortuary slabs and appropriate instruments for opening the body would be required. For postmortem examination of the brain, vats for storage along with fluids for preserving and hardening the tissue would be necessary. To view brain sections, a microtome to cut sections (the freezing microtome only came later), appropriate staining materials,[31] and microscopes would be required, along with materials for hand drawing of microscopic appearances (photomicrography only came later). Any attempt at chemical analysis, for example of urine, would have required specific reagents. As for the cost of such a laboratory, a suggestion was made around this time that "The building or adaptation of a room, and properly fitting it with microscope and other requisite apparatus, would only amount to a few hundred pounds, and when these were once provided, the annual outlay for chemicals, etc., would form a very small item in the expenditure".[32]

---

[29] The photograph of the WRA pathological laboratory (WYAS C85/1413) was dated as "mid 1890s" by Wallis (2017a:128) and "*c.*1898" by Davis (2013a:25). These dates suggest the photograph may have been taken after the reconstruction of the pathology department to include a complete outfit of laboratories which was completed by 1895. The plan of 1888 shows the laboratory adjacent to the mortuary and postmortem room with the dark room in between (Davis 2013a:47). That a pathological laboratory was an innovation may be indicated by the account in Murphy (2004:17) that at Chester County Asylum a pathological laboratory was opened in 1900.

[30] Dedicated "Methods" sections were largely non-existent in journal publications at this time.

[31] Some clues as to the methods used for the preparation of microscopic slides may be gleaned from the doctoral thesis by Herbert Major (1875:4–6), which was written at WRA (see Chap. 5), probably based on the methods of Jacob Lockhart Clarke (1817–1880): partial hardening of brain tissue in "alcohol" (presumably ethanol) for 48 h, then potassium dichromate for 1 week, then chromic acid for 4 or 5 days; followed by staining with logwood (haematoxylin) rather than carmine; stained sections were then dehydrated in spirit, rendered transparent by oil of cloves, and mounted in Canada balsam dissolved in benzol (see Larner and Triarhou 2024a).

[32] Ward (1877).

For experimental animal work, in other words for physiological research, a host of other requirements would need to be met although not, at this stage, any legal stipulations, since the Cruelty to Animals Act, requiring licencing of experiments, registration of places where animal experiments were performed and their periodic inspection, *inter alia*, only became law in 1876.[33] Firstly, sources of animals (although this may have fallen to individual researchers to arrange) and their housing, although most animals were killed at the time of experimentation. Anaesthesia required provision of ether and/or chloroform, and experimental pharmacology depended upon the provision of therapeutics (again it may have fallen to individual researchers to source these, perhaps with the assistance of the Asylum pharmacist). Other pieces of equipment might be needed for dedicated experiments: for example, a demonstrating ophthalmoscope, calorimeters, and Ludwig's Strom-uhr (a method of determining the amount of blood passing through any vessel in a given time) are all mentioned in papers in *WRLAMR*. For the experiments undertaken by David Ferrier, which brought renown to the Asylum (see Chap. 7), very specific equipment was required:

> For the purposes of stimulation I employed one Stöhrer's cell (with carbon and zinc elements), and the induced current of the secondary coil of Du Bois Reymond's magneto-electrometer. This allows of tolerably exact graduation of the strength of the current by sliding the secondary coil along a measured scale. As a rule, the current was not stronger than could be borne without great discomfort on the tip of the tongue. (III:32)

Named after Dr. Emil Stöhrer of Dresden, the inventor of these machines, the "double-celled induction battery" was also used for the purpose of gauging "Electro-muscular contractility" in another study examining the "State of the pupil as an indication of certain physical phenomena in the insane" (VI:138; also VI:145, 147). Likewise, John Lowe used this instrument to examine electro-muscular contractility to faradisation in patients with general paralysis, epilepsy, mania, dementia, and locomotor ataxy, amongst others (III:196–215).

This was a time when the Asylum was heated by coal and lighted by oil gas; provision of electricity was not made until the end of the century.[34] Moreover, as regards funding, Crichton-Browne later made acknowledgement of "the instruments of precision that are so exceedingly costly, but that

---

[33] Ryan (1963).
[34] Ashworth (1975:17).

are so essentially requisite in modern physiological and pathological inquiries".[35]

In the context of a proposed research school or "Pathological Institute", it is perhaps surprising that no dedicated library seems to have been available, or contemplated, at WRA. The importance of such a resource was later made explicit by Thomas McDowall, the first person to be appointed to the role of Pathologist and Assistant Medical Officer at WRA (Chap. 4):

> great libraries are almost inaccessible to a worker residing in the provinces, and it is only by means of much labour and searching that one can gradually accumulate a sufficient number of works on the subject to obtain a correct idea of the work done by former observers. Such a state of matters places the provincial worker at enormous disadvantages. (III:131)

One presumes that Crichton-Browne had his own personal library, but whether junior resident doctors or visiting clinicians were granted access is not known, although the former group were, at least according to the 1871 national census returns, members of Crichton-Browne's household.[36] It is perhaps possible that journals were housed in the laboratory, or perhaps it was anticipated that, since there were relatively few journals relevant to asylum medicine at this time (i.e. the *Journal of Psychological Medicine and Mental Pathology* and the *Journal of Mental Science*), interested practitioners would have personal subscriptions (likewise to the *Lancet* and the *British Medical Journal*). Nearly 50 years later, another asylum doctor stated that:

> It was difficult for men who were away from the great centres of learning to get hold of the literature on the subject and to learn what was being done else-

---

[35] Crichton-Browne (1878–1879:369). Star (1989:32; cited by Finn 2012:63) observed that "the lunatic asylums occasionally provided a place to do basic research. Though resources were not lavish, at least the equipment and subjects for experiments were available. The West Riding Pauper Lunatic Asylum provided such opportunities". I would suggest that WRA was the only asylum to provide such equipment, rather than simply large numbers of subjects, at this time. Star's comments were prefaced by the statement that "The doctors who administered lunatic asylums in the late nineteenth century had considerable discretion. There were few standard forms of treatment, and there were even small sums of money for research (Viets 1938)." However, I find no reference to money or funding in Viets (1938).

[36] Many of the resident staff seem to have had access to the standard textbook of the day, Bucknill and Hack Tuke's *A Manual of Psychological Medicine* (first published 1858) since it was cited or quoted by several of them: Crichton Browne (I:8n), Bywater Ward (I:162), Nicol (I:201), Major (II:44; IV:231), Sutherland (II:65), Bevan Lewis (V:95, 97), Newcombe (V:207), Merson (VI:107).

where. … the scientific journals were not within their reach, and as a rule, any journal they wished to see must be provided out of their own pocket.[37]

A library was included in the reconstruction of the WRA pathology department in 1895 which included a complete outfit of laboratories.[38]

Photographic Studio

Photography as a new modality for the study of the insane, both inside and outside the asylum, was increasingly used in the second half of the nineteenth century.[39] This was based in part on the presumption that photography permitted an empirical mode of study. By the time of Crichton-Browne's arrival at WRA, this was not a new phenomenon, as since the 1850s it had been advocated by John Conolly (1794–1866)[40] and pursued by Hugh Welch Diamond (1809–1886), the Superintendent of Surrey County Asylum, who had popularised the idea. Another pioneer in medical photography, of whom Crichton-Browne may have been aware, was Guillaume Duchenne de Boulogne (1806–1875) whose monograph *Mécanisme de la physionomie humaine* was first published in 1862, possibly coincident with Crichton-Browne's period of postgraduate training in Paris (see Chap. 5).[41] Journals based on medical photography were inaugurated, perhaps most notably in this context Jean-Martin Charcot's (1825–1893) first journal devoted to neurology, the *Iconographie photographique de la Salpêtrière* (although this did not appear until 1876).[42] In this context, Crichton-Browne's desire to have a

---

[37] Rows (1914:655). Quoted in Shephard (1996:437). For Rows' contacts with the neurological profession, see Larner (2024a). Even in the 1960s "most psychiatric units and mental hospitals had totally inadequate libraries" according to Bewley (2008:62).

[38] Wallis (2017a:80 and n92), citing "WYAS C85/1/12/6 Annual reports [*sic*] of the Medical Superintendent (1894–1904). *Report of the Sub-Committee and of the Medical Superintendent of the West Riding Pauper Lunatic Asylum, Wakefield, for the year 1895.* (Wakefield: West Yorkshire Printing Co. Ltd., 1896). Report of the Medical Superintendent, 11." (not seen by me). The AMOAHI and its successor, the Medico-Psychological Association, reportedly aspired to a library from 1863, but it appears that no significant collection accrued until the 1890s when Daniel Hack Tuke bequeathed his library to the Association (Bewley 2008:140–142).

[39] There is an extensive literature on photography of the insane including, but not limited to, Gilman (1976, 1982), Didi-Huberman (1982), and Rawling (2017, 2021).

[40] Conolly published thirteen articles on "The Physiognomy of Insanity" in the *Medical Times and Gazette* in 1858–1859. See Gilman (1976:25–72).

[41] Crichton-Browne might also have learned of Duchenne's photographic work from his colleague Clifford Allbutt (see Chap. 7) who had undertaken postgraduate study with Duchenne in 1860–1861 (Reynolds and Broussolle 2018).

[42] Goetz et al. (1995:95) (their Table 3.1).

dedicated photographic studio with dark room, and to appoint a dedicated photographer (see Chap. 4), is readily understood.

It has been established that photography of asylum patients served various purposes.[43] At WRA during this era, these seem to have been principally educational.[44] Two photographs of patients were used in *WRLAMR*, in Crichton-Browne's papers on acute dementia (IV:265–290, between pages 264 and 265) and chronic mania (V:284–292, between pages 284 and 285). Lowe, discussing response of the facial muscles to an electric stimulus, stated that "I had some photographs taken illustrating the action of several of them under it" (III:208). Photographs of patients were also exhibited at medical meetings, both at the WRA *conversazione* and elsewhere. They were reported to be displayed at all five of the annual WRA medical *conversazione* held between 1871 and 1875 (see Chap. 8).[45] Externally, at a meeting of the Royal Medical and Chirurgical Society in London held in June 1872, Henry Sutherland, a former WRA Clinical Clerk (see Chap. 5), "exhibited, for Dr. Crichton Browne, a collection of Photographs of cases of Mental Alienation, Chronic and Recurrent Mania, Imbecility, Idiocy, and General Paralysis of the Insane".[46]

The use of photographs of patients from WRA by Charles Darwin is well attested to.[47] A selection of photographs, around 40 in total, was sent by Crichton-Browne to Darwin whilst he was pursuing his research for *The expression of the emotions in man and animals*, although in the event none was used in the final (1872) publication.[48] That this involvement of Darwin was generally known is suggested by John Milner Fothergill's comment in his paper in *WRLAMR* on "Cerebral anaemia" in which he wrote that "If a vol-

---

[43] Dahlquist and Kinderman (2023).

[44] Wallis (2017a:21–59) addressed the use of photography at WRA in a later period of the nineteenth century. I am not aware of any photographs of tissue specimens, gross or microscopic, at WRA from the period under study here.

[45] For 1871: WYAS C85/1362. For 1872: *BMJ* 1872;2:474–475 (26th October; Medical Conversazione at the West Riding Asylum); *Medical Press and Circular* 1872;14:360 (23rd October; Conversazione and lecture by Professor Turner). For 1873: *Leeds Mercury* 27th November 1873, p.7 (Medical Conversazione at the West Riding Asylum). For 1874: *Medical Times and Gazette* 1874;2:609–610 (28th November; Annual Conversazione at the West Riding Asylum); Ashworth (1975:70). For 1875: *Medical Times and Gazette* 1875;2:603 (27th November; Conversazione at the West Riding Asylum). On his single attendance at a WRA medical *conversazione*, in 1873, Lowe manned the table displaying scientific and surgical instruments rather than photographs (see Chap. 8).

[46] *BMJ* 1872;1:646 (15th June; The Royal Medical and Chirurgical Society) [capitals in original]. Although the source of the photographs was not stated, I presume it was WRA since they were "exhibited, for Dr. Crichton Browne". Incidentally, there are references to two other conversazione on this same page of the *BMJ*, held at the College of Physicians and at University College, London.

[47] For example: Gilman (1982), Browne (1985), and Edwards (2014).

[48] Photographs sent to Darwin with Crichton-Browne's letter of 3rd April 1871 may be seen at Darwin Correspondence Project, "Letter no. 7658," https://www.darwinproject.ac.uk/letter/?docId=letters/DCP-LETT-7658.xml (accessed 22/09/24).

ume of portraits … were submitted to Mr Darwin, that gentleman would experience no difficulty in recognising in the features of some of them the characteristics of the depressing emotions" (IV:132–133). This work by Darwin was also noted by other *WRLAMR* authors (VI:137 and 146n1).[49]

Establishment

The West Riding Asylum was a community comprised of many individuals with multiple roles. Whilst for the purposes of this work the focus is predominantly on the medical practitioners working at or otherwise associated with the institution, this approach, which might reasonably be deemed Whiggish, risks neglecting other personnel at the Asylum: the attendants and nurses who delivered day-to-day patient care; the many other ancillary workers who provided indirect care, for example through the maintenance of the fabric and fittings of the estate, provision of food and clothing; and of course the patients themselves, the *raison d'etre* for the entire enterprise. Crichton-Browne later reported that "I had a staff of 200 nurses and attendants under my control, a large farm, a butcher's shop, a bakery and a brewery, weaving sheds".[50] Hence a broader, if brief, description of "the lunacy profession and its staff"[51] is attempted here as contextualisation.

Attendants and Nurses

Attendants and nurses were the first-hand deliverers of care to the Asylum's patients. In a disciplinarian system, with a small staff, and a large number of involuntary inmates, they played key roles in patient management.[52] Their work was undeniably demanding: poorly paid, with long working hours (night attendants were on duty for nine hours: VI:121),[53] in sometimes under-staffed wards, with a requirement to live in the asylum. Thus, the recruitment and retention of good staff were recurrent issues.[54]

---

[49] A number of photographs of patients taken at WRA during this period may be viewed online at the Wellcome Collection (https://wellcomecollection.org)

[50] Burdett (1891:183).

[51] This terminology is taken from Russell (1988).

[52] They remained so: see Goffman (1961:315).

[53] Jones (1993:118) reported that attendants at WRA spent on average of 70 hours per week on duty.

[54] General accounts of asylum nursing may be found in Walk (1961), Carpenter (1980), Russell (1988:306–311), Nolan (1996), and Bewley (2008:109–121).

Visiting WRA in 1875, Folsom noted that "these attendants are carefully selected in the first place, and all unfitted for the work are unsparingly weeded out" with a staff:patient ratio of 1:8.[55]

The recruiting net was cast far and wide, although most appointments were assuredly from the local community. Adverts appeared not only in the local press but also in organs such as *The Army and Navy Gazette*, since military experience, particularly its discipline, was deemed a good attribute for an attendant. More specialised skills were also called for: a "Wanted" advert in February 1872 sought a violin player, a clarionet player, a French horn player, an oboe player, and a bassoon player "who will be required to act as Attendants", salary to commence at £25 a-year, and advance £2 annually up to £37, with board, lodging and washing, and a suit of clothes every eight months. A similar "Wanted" advert in July 1872 sought an oboe player, a French horn player, and an euphonium player "who will be required to act as Attendants".[56] The gender pay differential was clearly illustrated by an advert for "Women Attendants" placed by Superintendent Cleaton in December 1865 which offered "wages to commence at £13 and advance £1 a year up to £18; with board, lodging and washing, and two dresses annually. Candidates must be active and intelligent women, not exceeding 32 years of age, and able to read and write".[57]

A study of attendants and nurses working at WRA during the period 1852 to 1889 noted the poor pay and high staff turnover, with just over 50% of male attendants and at least one-third of nurses leaving within one year, and although some staff gave many years of service few completed the 15 years required to qualify for a pension.[58] Russell reported that "91 out of the 567 male attendants employed at the West Riding Lunatic Asylum between 1860 and 1880 were sacked by the superintendent for reasons varying from 'dishonesty' to being found 'drunk'".[59] The possibility of pensions for attendants,

---

[55] Folsom (1877:54).

[56] *The Army and Navy Gazette*, 3rd February 1872, p.76; 13th July 1872, p.445.

[57] *Wakefield Free Press*, 16th December 1865, p.4 (West Riding Asylum). These salaries may be compared with those of the Assistant Medical Officers (see Chap. 4).

[58] Sheehan (1998). Finn (2012:69) stated that "attendants typically lasted no more than twelve months" but cited no source(s). In 1890, Joseph Wiglesworth, Medical Superintendent at Rainhill Asylum, stated that "I think I may say that something like 70 per cent. of the attendants and nurses have not seen more than two years' service" (*J Ment Sci* 1889–1890;35:447).

[59] Russell (1988:309) (citing "Register of Attendants, SRHM [Stanley Royd Hospital Museum]"). Nolan (1996:177–178) ascribed these data thus: "Robertson (1861) noted that at the West Riding Asylum one Medical Superintendent dismissed 91 of the workforce of 567 attendants during his term of office for reasons ranging from dishonesty to being drunk on duty". Nolan's citation was: "Robertson, C.L. (1861) Some results of night nursing at the Sussex Lunatic Asylum. *Journal of Mental Science*, **30**, 352". Even if this citation were correct, it would make no sense if the figures covered the period from 1860 to 1880.

if they served for a minimum of 10 years, was floated in the early 1870s,[60] perhaps as an inducement to staff retention.

What training did attendants and nurses receive in order to perform their duties successfully? Probably very little, or none at all—perfunctory, on-the-job advice from an experienced staff member was probably the norm. Certainly there seems to have been no dedicated training, as adverted to in a letter from "An Asylum Chaplain" published in the *Journal of Mental Science* in July 1870, suggesting "the Medico-Psychological Association authorise some qualified persons to write a simple catechism, embodying what is required of an efficient attendant".[61] As President of the Medico-Psychological Association (MPA) in 1871, Henry Maudsley did not go that far, but suggested something to raise their status by organising an office to register those who had proved their merit, thinking this a better method to raise standards than a pay rise.[62] However, it was not until 1884 that the MPA issued a *Handbook for the Instruction of Attendants on the Insane*.[63] A better approach might have been expected at WRA since Crichton-Browne's father, William Browne (see Chap. 7), was reportedly the first to provide classes to educate asylum staff.[64]

There was a strict hierarchy for both attendants and nurses. The arrangement of husband and wife serving as medical superintendent and matron respectively which occurred during the superintendencies of Ellis and Corsellis was thereafter terminated, and a Matron, Zillah Paige, appointed at the same time as John Septimus Alderson became superintendent (1853). Paige's resignation on the grounds of ill-health in 1866, shortly after the arrival of Crichton-Browne, coincided with a change in the Asylum rules such that the Matron's power of hiring and firing all female servants was removed, and the

---

The paper I find is: "Roberston CL. Some results of night nursing; being a record of the wet and dirty cases in the Sussex Lunatic Asylum, Hayward's Heath, during the first six months of 1861. *J Ment Sci* 1861–1862;7(October 1861):391–398" and, as might be anticipated from its title, this paper makes no mention of the West Riding Asylum. Nolan did not reference Russell (1988), in his bibliography but did have Russell's (1983) thesis which is the ultimate source of the data (Russell 1983:313).

[60] Howden (1871, 1872–1873).

[61] *J Ment Sci* 1870–1871;16(July 1870):310–311 (Attendants in asylums).

[62] Maudsley (1871–1872:328). Walk (1990:19). On the contrary, Joseph Wiglesworth in 1890 thought that "the only thing that will keep attendants in the asylum is the increase of pay, and unless we get an increase of pay we shall not get any more satisfactory results than we have in the past" (*J Ment Sci* 1889–1890;35:447).

[63] *J Ment Sci* 1885–1886;31(April 1885):149 (Instruction of Attendants).

[64] Hack Tuke (1892:860) stated that "Dr. Browne, at the Crichton Institution, Dumfries, in 1854, made the first attempt 'to educate the attendants upon the insane' by a course of thirty lectures to his staff". I am not aware of any evidence that Crichton-Browne instituted similar teaching for attendants at WRA.

requirement to nurse sick male patients was deleted.[65] Thereafter the counterpart to the chief male attendant was the chief female officer.

Traditionally the roles were strictly gendered: male attendants cared for the male patients, and female nurses (or "Women Attendants") cared for the female patients.

One reform introduced in the Crichton-Browne era was the deployment of female nurses on male wards at WRA:

> How to provide suitable and trustworthy attendants is certainly the great problem of the day in the management of our lunatic asylums, and anything which may assist even in its partial solution is deserving of consideration. Such an auxiliary [*sic*] seems to be found in the appointment of female nurses to male wards, an arrangement which tends to inspire the male attendants with gentleness and self-command, and confers great benefits upon the patients. One such appointment has taken place here during the last year. A female nurse, the wife of an attendant, was placed in April [1867], in one of the largest male wards, containing 70 epileptic and suicidal patients. Her presence in the midst of these lunatics … has been productive of the most excellent and pleasing effects, which have transcended even the sanguine anticipations that led to her appointment.[66]

This innovation was noted in the medical journals.[67]

Attendants and nurses had multiple roles in the care of the Asylum patients but only occasional glimpses of their work are forthcoming from the published records.[68] A few examples recorded in papers published in *WRLAMR* are presented here. As they were involved in the day-to-day care of patients, attendants and nurses could sometimes make clinical observations:

> The nurse states that she often hears her conversing with them [her children]. (I:244).
> the attendant said he was relieved of all trouble with them. (II:262).

---

[65] Bolton (1928:589). From our vantage point of history, we may wonder if this was in fact an example of constructive dismissal.

[66] *Report* (1868:26). Cited at I:139. Also mentioned in *J Ment Sci* 1868–1869;14(July 1868):203–205 (Female nursing in asylums).

[67] *BMJ* 1868;1:405 (25th April; The County Asylums). *BMJ* 1868;2:63 (18th July; A reform in nursing) credited both Henry Maudsley (see Chap. 2) and Crichton-Browne with this innovation, although Maudsley had surely abandoned county (as opposed to private) asylum work by this time. His contribution was merely a comment in his *Physiology and pathology of mind*, cited in *J Ment Sci* 1868–1869;14(July 1868):203–205 (Female nursing in asylums), at 203.

[68] Digby (1985:140–170) characterised the asylum attendant as "a hidden dimension".

On January 26th, 1876, the night-attendant found his [patient's] rupture down and irreducible.[69]

Based on a patient's behaviour:

the nurse, taught by experience, knew that convulsions and unconsciousness would supervene in about two hours from that time. (III:163).

As "instruments of the physician's will",[70] attendants and nurses might be involved in assisting with clinical procedures, ranging from persuading patients to eat food (I:212) to assisting with artificial feeding:

he is placed in the supine position upon a bed, and held by a sufficient number of assistants, and that without any risk of bruising or inflicting any injury. (I:214)[71]

The administration of medications might fall to the responsibility of an attendant:

With the purpose of further testing the nitrite of amyl, the night attendants, who are in charge of certain dormitories in which epileptics sleep, and who watch them constantly to prevent any cases of suffocation by rolling on to the face during a fit, were provided with bottles containing a little of it, and were instructed to employ it whenever they knew with absolute certainty in any case that a fit was beginning, noting in their report books the effects of the inhalations. One of these attendants has had occasion to employ it twice, and his reports in his own words are as follows: … (III:164)

Administering injections to recalcitrant patients might also require attendant input:

As to the mode of injection, if the patient be inclined to resist and be in bed, this is easily accomplished in any case with the assistance of two attendants, one of

---

[69] *BMJ* 1876;2:430–431 (30th September; West Riding Lunatic Asylum. Cases of disease and extravasation into the cerebellum. (Under the care of Dr. Major.)); quotation at 430. Another example of an attendant's contribution is found at VI:74.

[70] This wording is from Maudsley (1871–1872:328).

[71] Also in the context of artificial feeding, see Sutherland (1872): "At the West Riding Lunatic Asylum, where there were sometimes as many as four patients to be fed by artificial means three times a day, endeavours were always made first to induce them to take their food naturally, feeding themselves. If that failed, an attendant would try to feed them, as one would feed a child or sick person, with a spoon. Sometimes an attendant's wife would persuade a male patient to take his food; and vice versa, the physician would often succeed with a female patient when the nurse had failed."

whom presses the shoulders of the patient, while laid on his back, firmly on the bed, while the other holds the arm to be injected across the body in a semiflexed position, and restrains his other hand. Should the patient not be in bed, if the patient's arm be passed round the waist of an attendant standing close to him, and be held in that position, the injection will still be easily accomplished. (I:154–155)

The work of attendants and nurses could also be dangerous. During the time period under study, in 1871, one attendant at WRA, Thomas Lomas, was killed when attacked by a patient, George Lawton.[72] In another incident, a "patient had almost succeeded in smashing the head of an attendant with a water-bucket" (VI:80). Also during this time period, in 1873, one of the Commissioners in Lunacy, Robert Wilfred Skeffington Lutwidge (the uncle of Lewis Carroll—Charles Lutwidge Dodgson), died of injuries received at the hands of a patient during an inspection visit at Fisherton House Asylum in Salisbury. In his official capacity, Lutwidge had visited WRA in March 1870 and November 1871, so may well have been known to staff members as well as to Crichton-Browne.[73] So shocking was this distant event that it was even reported in the local Yorkshire press.[74] Lutwidge's death also provoked comment in the *Journal of Mental Science*:

> An event of this kind is well calculated to make us appreciate more justly than we perhaps commonly do the trials, the endurance, and the unwelcome work of those attendants upon the insane who are in constant intercourse with them, and from whom we demand a long-suffering and a gentleness that are more than human.[75]

Conversely, mistreatment of patients by attendants and nurses was not unknown, including beatings and ill-treatment which might occasion dismissal and court proceedings.[76] In 1869 two attendants at

---

[72] *Report* (1872:6, 22–23). Also, see Anon. (1873:470). If referring to the Lawton case, Finn (2012:2) seemed to date this event as 1872. Lawton's story, including accounts of the murder which appeared in the popular press, may be found in Scrimgeour (2015:341–350). Murder of a patient by another patient might also occur, as in the case of William Burran, reported in *BMJ* 1865;2:693 (30th December); also discussed by Scrimgeour (2015:331–334) who noted that the last case note on Burran was entered by Charles Etheridge: "Murdered on 28th November, 1865 by Jonathan Waite, another patient" (at 331).

[73] *Report* (1871:9–15) and *Report* (1872:7–14). For more on Lutwidge, see Larner (2025c).

[74] For example *Leeds Mercury* 26th May 1873, p.3 (Dangers of Lunacy Inspectors) and, after the fatal outcome, *Yorkshire Post and Leeds Intelligencer* 30th May 1873, p.4.

[75] *J Ment Sci* 1873–1874;19 (July 1873):264–265 (The late Mr. Lutwidge). In 1884, Ernest Birt, Assistant Medical Officer at WRA, survived an attack by a patient who tried to stab him in the neck (Wallis 2017a:106).

[76] For example, *BMJ* 1867;1:98 (26th January; Alleged cruelty to a lunatic).

Lancaster Asylum were convicted of the manslaughter of their patient and sentenced to seven years penal servitude.[77] The original design of WRA included a "crow's nest" at both intersections of the H-shaped building permitting surveillance ("espionage" was Tuke's word) of all staff, a mechanism which was thought to be one means to counter the risk of such happenings.[78]

A further "occupational hazard" for attendants and nurses, perhaps unique to WRA as a research-oriented institution, was to become the subjects of experimental procedures.[79] Mr. Benjamin Beaumont, chief male attendant, appointed in 1863,[80] was injected three times by Wilkie Burman (see Chap. 5) as part of his investigations of conia, derived from hemlock, (II:16), and other "attendants" may also have been injected (II:16,17). An attendant is also mentioned as assisting in one of the animal experiments undertaken by William Benham (IV:309).[81]

Other Staff Members

A large number of ancillary or general staff was also required to keep an establishment of up to 1500 people,[82] patients and staff, running smoothly, for example: Clerk and Steward of the Asylum; Assistant Clerk; Clerk of works; storekeeper; assistant; housekeeper; in addition to the chief male attendant and the chief female officer. Servants were required to supervise patient labour such as cooking, baking, brewing, gardening, engineering, and domestic tasks such as laundry, clothes making (seamstress, tailor), and cleaning. The fabric and fittings were attended to by carpenters, joiners and painters. The Asylum also had its own farm, requiring a "Farm Man" and assistants, likewise gardeners. Only occasionally do the names of these workers surface: for example, with respect to the decorations of the Hall for the medical *conversazione* we

---

[77] Walton (1981:186–187) and Digby (1985:308n4).

[78] Ashworth (1975:17).

[79] Although this might be assumed under the Asylum *Regulations and Orders* (1873:20) which obliged Nurses to "carefully assist in any scientific investigation that it may be desired to carry out" by the Medical Officers or Clinical Clerks.

[80] Todd and Ashworth (n.d.:106).

[81] The "Sane men in ordinary health" tested by Lowe (III:203) might perhaps have been attendants, either at South Yorkshire Asylum or at WRA; the initials do not match those of any of the resident WRA medical staff.

[82] I counted 1390 entries for WRA in the 1871 Census records. This would not include any non-resident members of staff.

hear of Cashburn, head gardener; Norbury, foreman carpenter; Crossland, foreman painter (1874); and Norbury as joiner (1875).[83]

A requirement of the 1845 County Asylums Act was the appointment of an asylum chaplain in priest's orders, to attend to the spiritual needs of patients and staff. Furthermore, the Visiting Magistrates at WRA required their Chaplain to keep a diary to be made available for their perusal each quarter. The Reverend T.B. Clarkson faithfully did so during the 26 years that he served as WRA Chaplain (1843–1869), a source of much interesting information, but regrettably no such later diaries, covering the period examined in this study, exist.[84] Clarkson's chaplaincy encompassed the opening of the new Asylum Church, dedicated to St Faith, in 1861 and its consecration in 1867 by the Bishop of Ripon. At this time, Wakefield was part of the Diocese of Ripon, only becoming a separate Diocese of Wakefield in 1888 when its parish church was elevated to cathedral status (Cathedral Church of All Saints).[85]

Patients

To my knowledge there is no first had account from a patient cared for at WRA during the time period under consideration in this work.[86] Hence to present a "patient account" one would need to "read against the grain" of the available professional discourses, which necessarily present a "gentleman's history" of the institution and its practices, emanating as they do from a relatively homogeneous medical faculty (absolutely so in terms of gender, relatively so in terms of class) which exerted a profoundly asymmetrical power

---

[83] *Wakefield and West Riding Herald with which is incorporated the Wakefield Journal & Examiner* 21st November 1874, p.5, col.6 (Medical Conversazione at the Asylum); *Leeds Mercury* 20th November 1875, p.3, col.6 (Medical Conversazione at Wakefield Asylum).

[84] Ashworth (1975:42). White's *Directory* (1870:533) listed "Rev. John E. Boyce, M.A." as Asylum chaplain.

[85] With the closure of the Stanely Royd Hospital, the Asylum Church was closed in 1996, fell into disrepair, and was subsequently destroyed by a fire on 18th June 2012. Wakefield is now in the Diocese of Leeds.

[86] See, for example, a talk entitled "Object voices" by Cara Sutherland ("former Director of the Mental Health Museum") to the Wakefield Historical Society, 11th April 2018: "There is an absence of first hand patient accounts". (www.wakefieldhistoricalsociety.org.uk/whs-events/lecture-programme/lecture-notes-2017-2018) (accessed 07/01/2024). I take these "lecture notes" to be a second-hand transcription, as they contain a number of errors, e.g. "James Crichton-Brown [*sic*], director from 1866–1876, created a journal 'Conversassiones' [*sic*] (later The Brain Journal [*sic*])." However, I believe the comment on first-hand patient accounts to be correct. More generally, there is nothing of relevance in Peterson (1982). The nearest contemporary account "from the inside" is, to my knowledge, that of Herman Charles Merivale, writing as "A Sane Patient", in *My experiences in a lunatic asylum*, published in 1879, specifically from Ticehurst in Sussex, a private asylum.

relationship over their charges.[87] This approach can no more give us authentic "voices from the asylum" than do the extant photographs taken by Crichton-Browne and his staff.[88] Hence any ambition to write a history from below, or bottom-up history,[89] cannot be fulfilled. Moreover, such is the framing of the current work, focused as it is on issues of professional development, that the patients are inevitably decentred, peripheral, marginalised, seen only by means of a "through-view", indeed almost incidentally to the account presented.

Hence the patients at WRA are seen through the eyes of the predominant class, as reported in the pages of the Asylum case books and in the medical journals, in particular the Asylum's house journal, the *WRLAMR* (Part III). In many of the papers in *WRLAMR* patient details appear, such as initials, age, and date of admission, sometimes occupation and place of origin, and occasionally photographs, all of which would permit identification by reference to the original asylum case books (now held at West Yorkshire Archive Service; www.wyjs.org.uk). Some of the life stories of WRA patients, all too often overlooked, have been investigated by these means, both at Wakefield[90] (some for mostly earlier[91] or later periods[92]) and at Menston (for a later period[93]).

Crichton-Browne's reference, in a letter to Darwin, to "the mass of interesting material" at WRA concealed the flesh-and-blood lives of the patients under his care, some resident in the Asylum for decades, and many without hope of clinical recovery. One gets some feel for this ennui in reading his annual *Reports*. For example, speaking of cases of suicide and the far more frequent attempts at suicide by patients, Crichton-Browne speaks of "The amount of mental dejection and weariness of life prevailing amongst the inmates".[94] Two members of the resident medical staff, Nicol & Dove, gave the following account of "the conditions under which the inmates in such institutions live":

---

[87] I take these insights from Parenti (2003:10, 41, 206). (I thank Dr. Guleed Adan for bringing this book to my attention, September 2023.) Celia Davies was of the opinion that "much can be achieved by interrogating elite records from a rank-and-file point of view" (Carpenter 1980:123). Despite the apparent homogeneity of the medical faculty, some interesting differences will become apparent when comparing the prosopography of the resident medical staff, presented in Chap. 5, with that of the visiting and/or contributing clinicians presented in Chap. 7.

[88] The quoted phrase is taken from the title of Davis (2013b), although his work was focused on patients at Menston Asylum (High Royds Hospital) and from a slightly later time period.

[89] This terminology is from Thompson (1966) and Porter (1985).

[90] Levine-Clark (2000, 2004).

[91] Scrimgeour (2015).

[92] Wallis (2017a).

[93] Davis (2013b).

[94] *Report* (1868:20).

There are certain conditions in asylum life that are in favour of the vital energies. The diet is good, and exercise is more or less enforced. But the diet is monotonous, a circumstance which undoubtedly takes away from the benefit derived from it, and, for those that have mind enough left, it is not received with the zest of that earned by the sweat of the brow, but with the depressing feeling that it is the "rates" that pay for it. The exercise is undoubtedly a genuine benefit in some forms, such as those of work in which the patient takes an interest, of dances, of country walks and other excursions that are often hailed with delight. On the other hand, the formal striding about in the airing court seems, though still much better than nothing, but a small advantage compared with that which the word "exercise" suggests to a sane man. Then a separate advantage, and one of an unmixed sort in the degree that it is sympathisingly and judiciously carried out, is the influence of sane, educated, reflective minds among the superior officers, on the wandering degraded natures under their care. As a modification to this must, it is to be feared, be put an influence of an opposite tendency from some inferior officers in every asylum, though this is, as all hope, small and diminishing.

In some asylums the state of the atmosphere in which the patients are immersed may be put as a favorable, in others as an unfavorable, condition. The same may be said as regards temperature; the relation between this and ventilation is one the proper maintenance of which is most difficult of attainment.

Among the unfavorable conditions operating probably more or less in every asylum is first the crowding together of the patients, by which during the night (in many cases), and during considerable parts of the day, or the whole day in bad weather, some of the respired air must have already given up its virtues at the pulmonary capillaries of many patients. Secondly, there is in very many cases the sense of confinement itself, the depressing effect of which nobody practically conversant with the insane will be inclined to deny. Thirdly, along with this goes the sense of subordination to discipline, and to discipline which, unfortunately but unavoidably, often seems to the patient of a most unreasonable kind. (I:246–247).

Most patients at WRA were of working-class origin, and hence paupers (or at risk of pauperism): "the patients in this asylum, drawn as a rule from colliery and manufacturing districts" (III:130). However, as with all such "Pauper" asylums, some patients capable of paying fees were admitted (for example, the architect James Walker who drew the plan of WRA in 1862; see Chap. 2), helping to defray some of the substantial costs to the ratepayers for the maintenance of the paupers. The weekly maintenance rates for pauper lunatics at WRA in 1872 and 1873 were reportedly 9 s 1d and 9 s 11¾d respectively, slightly below the national average.[95]

---

[95] *J Ment Sci* 1874–1875:20(April 1874):165.

Crichton-Browne later referred to "the coarse and somewhat degrading associations of pauper establishments" as one of the arguments in favour of the establishment of a "middle class asylum" in order to "save much suffering and distress to a number of educated and refined persons who had been accustomed to comfort and retirement in their private homes".[96]

It is not difficult to believe that many of the patients at WRA did not want to be there, and longed for release, however unfeasible that may have been.[97] Crichton-Browne's attempts to brighten the Asylum environment, to give it a "home-like aspect", have already been mentioned. The provision of employment and entertainment were other ways to render patients' lives more bearable, as well as serving as methods of treatment. Patient employment also generated income for the Asylum, as recorded in the annual *Report* balance sheets.

Patient employment had been a feature at WRA from the time of William Ellis, for example "doing the laundry, repairing clothes and uniforms, acting as farm labourers on the asylum farm, or performing various menial tasks around the institution".[98]

Such ergotherapy, as it later became known, is occasionally evident in *WRLAMR*, for example reference to the "Tailor's shop" (II:24).

Entertainments and amusements were also integral to the operation of WRA. In October 1866, Crichton-Browne reported that:

> A few of the officers and attendants have formed an amateur theatrical company and are preparing a few farces by which to beguile the tedium and monotony of the winter evenings as is now done in most county asylums.[99]

In his *Report* for 1870 Crichton-Browne stated that:

> Ample provision continues to be made for recreation and amusements. In addition to the Saturday evening weekly dances, at which upwards of 400 patients

---

[96] *The Wakefield Free Press and West-Riding Advertiser*, 6th December 1873, p3, col. 2 (A middle class asylum for the West Riding); *BMJ* 1873;2:678–679 (6th December; Middle-Class Lunatic Asylum for Yorkshire).

[97] Although Vera Brittain stated of Winifred Holtby's (1936) novel *South Riding* that the "West Riding … forms no part of her 'English Landscape'" (Holtby 1936:517), nevertheless the desire expressed by one of the patients at the fictional "South Riding Mental Hospital" (possibly modelled on the Hull Borough Asylum at Cottingham, close to where Holtby's parents lived from 1919, and where John Merson [see Chap. 5] was superintendent from the 1880s) to be released because "I'm not mad" (Holtby 1936:334) is a complaint very likely to have been heard from patients at WRA, as at other asylums, and as attempts to escape may indicate. For Holtby on mental health in *South Riding*, see Larner (2024b, 2025d).

[98] Scull (1979:201).

[99] Medical Director's Journal 25th October 1866 (WYAS C85/1/13/1) [my transcription].

are generally present, there have, since the last visit [of the Commissioners], been about 20 associated entertainments, including seven dramatic and other performances, and two promenade concerts, and which have been usually attended by upwards of 500 patients of both sexes.[100]

An annual fancy dress ball and musical events at WRA dated to the Cleaton era.

Following his father William Browne's innovation of introducing private theatricals at the Crichton Royal Institution in Dumfries in 1843,[101] Crichton-Browne also inaugurated private theatricals at WRA, handbills for which were printed under the spoof heading of "Theatre Royal, Stanley-cum-Wrenthorpe" (the township outside Wakefield where the Asylum was sited). Members of the Asylum junior medical staff often took parts in the productions, sometimes parodying their own characters.[102]

Perhaps the most remarkable entertainment to take place at WRA was the performance of *Pygmalion and Galatea* on Friday 2nd April 1875 with the author, W.S. Gilbert (of "Gilbert and Sullivan" fame), playing one of the lead roles. Mrs. Emily Crichton-Browne was also in the cast (as "Daphne, Chrysos' wife", according to the programme), one of the very few times that she appears in the historical record.[103] Her husband's account was that "Six hundred patients and one hundred nurses and attendants witnessed it" and that he and his guest, Ernest Hart, editor of the *British Medical Journal* (see Chap. 9), "found that it had been generally highly appreciated and understood".[104]

---

[100] *Report* (1871:11–12).

[101] Crichton-Browne called this "the first theatrical performance ever given in a lunatic asylum" (Easterbrook 1937:23, 1940:4). Williams (1989:23–24) includes the playbill.

[102] WYAS C85/1362 contains many examples. Golding (2021), discussed theatrical events at WRA.

[103] The 1871 Census is another.

[104] Crichton-Browne (1926:149–151). The event is described in Crowther (2013), which also cited reports of the event published in *The Manchester Examiner and Times* of 5th April 1875 and *The Times* of 6th April 1875 (I thank Andrew Crowther for kindly sending me a copy of his fascinating paper, 02/09/2023). There were also brief notices in the medical press: *Lancet* 1875;1:521 (10th April; Modern treatment of lunacy) and *BMJ* 1875;1:488-489 (10th April; The West Riding Lunatic Asylum), although they differed in their estimates of the numbers attending: the *Lancet* stated "over a thousand lunatics" whereas the *BMJ* said "Nearly a thousand of the lunatic inmates were present". *Medical Times and Gazette* 1875;1:421 (17th April; The drama in lunacy treatment) said "More than 700 insane patients listened with breathless interest". A copy of this latter report may be found in WYAS C85/1382, two columns pasted onto a sheet of blue notepaper headed "West Riding Asylum, Wakefield". This report dated the performance as taking place "on Friday last" which would be 16th April, surely an error if reports had appeared elsewhere as early as 5th April, but this may explain why Todd and Ashworth (n.d.:147) date the performance as "April 16, 1875" and Finn (2012:3n11) dated it as 17th April 1875. A copy of the programme, dated "Friday, 2nd April, 1875", may be seen at the Wellcome Collection (MS 8915), along with Ernest Hart's letter (see Chap. 9).

Discussion

For the first 50 years of its existence, the West Riding Asylum at Wakefield probably differed very little from the other county asylums built after the enabling Act of 1808. Like them, it was essentially a custodial, if no longer a punitive, institution, gradually silting up with increasing numbers of patients and requiring repeated expansion of the building stock.[105] An increasing percentage of the patients, often characterised as "inmates", were chronic cases amenable to neither cure nor relief of their ailments sufficient to permit discharge. The problems addressed by successive superintendents and visiting physicians at WRA were akin to those faced by the same functionaries at asylums elsewhere.

County asylums were neither conceived nor constructed with the idea of research into the causes and treatment of insanity in mind. The Commissioners in Lunacy, in their desire for uniformity of practice, baulked at any hint of innovation, effectively discouraging any notion of research studies into the pathology and treatment of insanity, reflective of the conservatism and essentially lay perspective of Lord Shaftesbury, the head of the Commission.[106] Being located by design (after Samuel Tuke) far from urban medical schools and hospitals, county asylums in general and WRA in particular had not developed any expertise or tradition in experimental or research methods, and conversely the clinicians working in the medical schools and hospitals had no particular interest in the insane.

How to transform an institutional, administrative, bureaucratic profession into a research-based scientific culture was to attempt to square the circle between segregation and integration. The question, the dilemma, which faced Crichton-Browne, in his desire for a scientific approach to "insanity", indeed for any clinician optimistic about the possibilities of medical as opposed to moral treatment, was which course would prove to be the easier: "to bring the problem of mental disorder into the controllable confines of the elite laboratory or to relocate the scientist within the remote world of the asylum".[107] As has been described, Crichton-Browne's solution was, in essence, to bring the laboratory to the asylum.[108]

---

[105] Digby (1983:219): "English asylums … were becoming increasingly custodial during the second half of the nineteenth century." However, she viewed the transition as from curative to custodial in character.

[106] I acknowledge my indebtness here to Hervey (1985) (especially 104, 110–111, 118). As an example, "Bucknill believed the medical commissioners failed to represent the interests of scientific medicine".

[107] The quotation is from Pressman (1998:45) and related to a different time (1930s) and place (USA) yet seems equally applicable here.

[108] A case of "Build it, and they will come"? Ultimately his hope was to convert asylums into clinical schools (see Crichton Browne 1878–1879).

It took a determined effort to develop the necessary infrastructure for this purpose at WRA, requiring persuasion of the purse-holders, the Committee of Visitors, to exercise their "practical sagacity and prudent liberality" in order to fund the necessary changes. This was a "long game" which even Crichton-Browne, a man blessed with the "most conciliating manner", took between four to six years of superintendency to achieve. To what extent, if any, the expansion of the infrastructure of British physiology which occurred around 1870, largely as a consequence of the requirement of degree granting bodies (Royal College of Surgeons, University of London) that "practical physiology" should be taught to medical students,[109] played in the development of the laboratory at WRA is not known. Although this novel infrastructure at WRA might be seen simply as part of the "scientific enterprise in Late Victorian Society", medical students were not an integral part of the "lunacy profession and its staff" (see Chap. 4) so this influence was unlikely to have been relevant.[110]

Even the most state-of-the-art laboratory, as of 1872, was worthless without the appropriate personnel to exploit its resources. Presumably one of the hopes which animated Crichton-Browne in his endeavours was that, by this means, clinicians interested in the possibilities of research might be attracted to the Asylum to avail themselves not only of its laboratory facilities but also its extensive clinical population. Accordingly, it is to the WRA resident faculty that attention is now turned.

---

[109] Geison (1978, esp. 149–156).
[110] Crichton-Browne's comment (1878–1879:369) about "modern physiological and pathological inquiries" was retrospective.

Part II

Faculty

It remained an isolated specialty, with only superficial ties with the rest of the medical enterprise.[1]

---

[1] Scull (1979:176).

4

"The Lunacy Profession and Its Staff" at the West Riding Asylum 1866–1876

Resident Clinical Staff of the West Riding Asylum 1866–1876

Whilst an appropriately equipped institutional base is necessary for its emergence (see Part I), a profession is ultimately composed of its practitioners who share a common interest in a body of specialised knowledge which relates to the core purpose of the profession. Medical specialisation requires a large and integrated community of doctors devoted to advancing knowledge through rigorous empirical clinical and experimental research. This chapter examines the resident clinical staffing of the West Riding Asylum in the period 1866 to 1876.

Medical Superintendent/Director; Deputy Superintendent

In a letter dated 22nd September 1868 which was published in the *Journal of Mental Science* in January 1869, James Crichton-Browne outlined the various medical positions at the West Riding Asylum at Wakefield (henceforward WRA)[1]:

---

[1] Crichton Browne (1868–1869). The publication in fact reads "Chrichton [*sic*] Browne" (at 600) but I have regularised this spelling for the purposes of the Bibliography to avoid any potential confusion.

The medical staff of this Asylum consists of a Medical Director, two Assistant Medical Officers – one acting in the male and one in the female department – and two Clinical Clerks – one acting under the direction of each of the Medical Assistants.[2]

The nature of the resident faculty of asylum doctors[3] at WRA during Crichton-Browne's superintendency is explored here to indicate some of the similarities and differences from the staffing at other comparable county asylums.[4]

At the apex of the asylum clinical faculty was the Medical Superintendent, also sometimes known as the Director. Initially there had been no obligation that an asylum Superintendent or Director should hold a medical degree, as visiting physicians and surgeons supplied any clinical input required. However, medically qualified Superintendents gradually became the norm, and indeed this was always the case at WRA. Medical Superintendency was the position most often aspired to by trainees dedicated to the field of asylum medicine.

The role of Medical Superintendent had come into being with the development of the asylum system as a consequence of the permissive, discretionary County Asylums Act of 1808, under the auspices of which WRA was built.

The Lunacy Act of 1845 (8&9 Vict. c.100) stipulated that County Asylums must have a resident physician[5] and this was reflected in the *Rules for the management of the Pauper Lunatic Asylum, for the West Riding of the County of York* published in 1847, specific to the "Resident Medical Officer or Director":

23. He shall be a Member of the Royal College of Surgeons of London, Edinburgh or Dublin, and shall be the principal resident Officer and Superintendent of the Asylum, and act as Treasurer.[6]

---

[2] Crichton Browne (1868–1869:599).

[3] Various terms were used for the clinicians working in asylums, including mad doctors, alienists, alienist physicians, medical psychologists ("psychiatrist" was not in use at this time), but I have opted here for the purely descriptive, and non-judgmental, "asylum doctors". An American journal titled *The Alienist and Neurologist* was published between 1880 and 1920 (Lipson et al. 2002).

[4] Russell (1988:303–312) has written on the "employment structure" (303) of the "lunacy profession" with special reference to the WRA at Wakefield in the second half of the nineteenth century but his chapter largely covers the period after Crichton-Browne's superintendency, although there is obviously overlap of roles, though not of specific personnel.

[5] The Madhouse Act 1828 (9 Geo. 4. c.41) had required a resident medical officer in establishments with over 100 patients (Hervey 1985:100).

[6] This was the rule which apparently, according to Bolton (1928:605), prevented John Chapman from being appointed WRA Superintendent in 1858 (see Chap. 2).

28. He shall never absent himself for more than one night, without the previous written consent of two of the Committee of Visitors; nor for any longer period than a week, without the permission of the Board of Visitors ...

29. He shall see every patient at least once in each day, and shall give up the whole of his time to the duties of his office, and shall not attend to or engage in any professional or other business or employment except that of the Asylum.[7]

Initially visiting physicians from the asylum locality were intimately involved in clinical decision making within the asylum, but in 1853 the Commissioners in Lunacy stipulated more exactly the role of the Medical Superintendent:

He[8] should have paramount Authority in the Asylum, and be precluded from private Practice, and should devote his whole Time and Energies to the Duties of his Office. ...The Commissioners think it the preferable Arrangement that there should not be any Visiting Physician or other Medical Visitor with a Salary, but that in lieu thereof the resident Medical Superintendent should have the power to call in Medical or Surgical Advice.[9]

Hence the full responsibility of the asylum lay on the shoulders of the Medical Superintendent, not simply the clinical care of the patients but the supervision of the junior staff and the general upkeep of the whole establishment. Accordingly, there was a perception that Medical Superintendents were overburdened with non-medical duties, as reflected in the Annual Reports prepared by Medical Superintendents as required by the Commissioners.[10]

The Medical Superintendent has been characterised as the "arbiter of a rigid social system that embraced every aspect of asylum life",[11] a power considered

---

[7] *Rules* (1847:9–11). Finn (2012:67) stated that no layman was ever given control at WRA but that this only became stipulated in law in 1866, citing "*Rules and Regulations for the Management of the Pauper Lunatic Asylum, for the West Riding of the County of York* (1866) No. 21". I have not seen this document, but Finn's quotation reads similarly to the 1847 *Rules*, presumably updating or superseding them.

[8] Asylum medicine, like medicine generally at this time, was an exclusively male profession. Not until the end of the century does one read of "Ladies as Medical Superintendents of Asylums", for example *Medical Press and Circular* 1894;58:655 (19th December; Notes on current topics). The first woman to serve as a doctor on the staff of WRA was Margaret Dobson, appointed in January 1906 (Todd and Ashworth n.d., 230).

[9] Cited by Renvoize (1991:30) [capitals in original].

[10] See any of Crichton-Browne's Reports as Superintendent (*Report* 1868, 1869, 1871, 1872, 1873, 1874). These are for the years 1867, 1868, 1870, 1871, 1872, and 1873 respectively. Like Finn (2012:185n579) I have not found Reports for the years 1869 or 1874, either at WYAS or at the Wellcome Collection.

[11] Russell (1988:304).

"feudal" in its extent.[12] However, superintendents were in reality "merely the salaried employees of individual asylum committees" which had "control over the key area of finance".[13] Hence "The superintendent's power to choose a medical officer was his alone (though officially the appointment was made by the local Committee of Visitors)".[14] These bodies, composed of local magistrates and perhaps a dignitary from the aristocracy or the local Member of Parliament, needed to be handled with tact if a superintendent was to have his way, particularly if changes costing money, such as new building or staffing, was requested. Crichton-Browne apparently excelled in these diplomatic skills.[15] Some years later (1891) he summarised the situation of the Superintendent thus:

> The duties devolving upon the medical superintendent are so numerous – he is called upon to attend to the choice of the staff; he is responsible for the farm, for the commissariat, and for the clothing, and these and other functions interfere very much with his medical duties. Then, as a matter of practical experience, the medical superintendents of England have found that the committees of magistrates, who are their masters, are very much better able to appreciate the way in which they carry on the farm and attend to the finances or the general administration of the establishment than the way in which they do their medical work. This latter the justices are scarcely capable of judging of, ...[16]

James Crichton-Browne's appointment as Medical Superintendent at WRA at the ripe age of 25 was not atypical.[17] For example, John Charles Bucknill (for whom, see Chap. 9) was appointed Medical Superintendent at the Devon County Lunatic Asylum at Exminster in 1844 at the age of 26[18]; Frederick Needham at York Asylum in 1858 at the age of 23[19]; Henry Maudsley (for whom, see Chap. 2) was appointed at Manchester

---

[12] Breathnach (1996).

[13] Scull (1979:174).

[14] Russell (1988:304).

[15] If one accepts the identity of Crichton-Browne as "Horniblow", as portrayed in the 13th September 1873 issue of Dickens's journal *All the year round* (as I do: Larner 2025e; see also www.wakefieldasylum. co.uk/people-and-events/all-year-round-the-suspicions-of-mr-ashworth, last accessed 11/12/2024), he was described there as having the "blandest and most conciliating manner" (Anon. 1873:470).

[16] Burdett (1891:182).

[17] Crichton-Browne had previously been appointed Medical Superintendent at Newcastle-upon-Tyne in 1865 (Leyland 1888:II:28), and this was the post he held at the time of election to WRA (*Lancet* 1866;2:140 (4th August; Medical Appointments)).

[18] Scull et al. (1996:191).

[19] Adams (2025:118–119).

Royal Lunatic Asylum at Cheadle in 1859 at the age of 24[20]; and Thomas Clouston was appointed at the Cumberland and Westmoreland Asylum in Carlisle in 1863 at the age of 23.[21] Whilst such early appointments might reflect the stellar qualities of those appointed, and hence be based exclusively on merit, there were suspicions that abilities alone were not always the determining factor, the moreso as other clinicians languished for many years in the junior grades awaiting promotion, since Medical Superintendent posts rarely became vacant. As a consequence, the Medical Superintendent might be younger, and hence less experienced as an asylum doctor, than members of his "junior" staff. Although there is no reason to doubt Crichton-Browne's abilities, his family name could not have hindered his advancement (for details of his father, William A. F. Browne, see Chap. 7).[22]

All powerful as the Medical Superintendent's role might appear to have been, bringing as it did a good salary, housing, and full board, nevertheless by the time of Crichton-Browne's appointment concerns were being expressed. In 1854 the *Lancet* had spoken of "a class of medical men – an almost peculiar class – the medical superintendants [*sic*] of the public asylums",[23] and in 1869 Thomas Laycock (1812–1876), one of Crichton-Browne's mentors and then President of the Medico-Psychological Association, suggested that the public "look upon asylums as places of detention, and on the Medical Superintendents as little better than jailers".[24]

Nevertheless, Crichton-Browne made changes to the Asylum rules which might be construed as steps to consolidate and indeed strengthen his position, perhaps in the pursuance of the "paramount Authority" previously suggested by the Commissioners in Lunacy. Specifically, the number of consulting physicians to the Asylum was reduced from two to one (i.e. Dr. T.G. Wright; for whom, see Chap. 2).

One physician only is allowed for. He only attends when requested and only visits the asylum if required. If no physician is appointed the medical

---

[20] Scull et al. (1996:230).

[21] Beveridge (1991:363) and James (1996:370).

[22] The fact that W.A.F. Browne was President of the Medico-Psychological Association in 1866 may, or may not, have been pertinent to Crichton-Browne's appointment at WRA. Patronage and nepotism were acknowledged to play a significant role in the appointment of asylum medical personnel in the Irish district asylum system in the nineteenth century (Malcolm 2003:322).

[23] *Lancet* 1854;1:367. Incorrectly referenced by Turner (1991:6) as "*Lancet* 1864;1:376".

[24] Laycock (1869–1870:332).

superintendent can call in to his assistance any physician practising in the neighbourhood.[25]

Furthermore, "Rules for assistant medical officers and a dispenser appear, instead of the old rules for an unqualified house surgeon and apothecary".[26] The requirement that the Director must be accompanied by the Matron or her deputy when visiting the female wards of the Asylum proved irksome to Crichton-Browne; it was perceived that he was instrumental, perhaps by removing the Matron's role in hiring and firing all female servants,[27] in the resignation of Zillah Paige, Matron since 1853, on the grounds of ill-health in 1866.

As for research or publication, after 1845 the national Lunacy Commissioners had effectively discouraged public asylum superintendents from undertaking research projects that might distract them from their administrative duties. This was an era when Medical Directors or Superintendents of asylums were, generally, valued more as administrators rather than as doctors.[28]

A position of Deputy Superintendent was also recognised at WRA, at least this designation is accorded to various staff members over the period under examination (Mitchell in 1868, Burman in 1872–3, Major in 1874, and Merson in 1876). A vacancy specifically for "Deputy Superintendent" at WRA was advertised in the *BMJ* in 1872.[29] The *Journal of Mental Science* had previously advocated for use of the term "Deputy Medical Superintendent" to denote an AMO acting in charge of an asylum in the absence of the Medical Superintendent.[30]

Assistant Medical Officer

In addition to the Medical Superintendent, pauper asylums generally employed one or more Assistant Medical Officers (AMOs). The 1853 publication of the Commissioners in Lunacy had suggested that:

---

[25] Crichton-Browne was perhaps aware of the conflict between a previous Visiting Physician, Caleb Crowther, and at least two of his predecessors as WRA Medical Superintendent, Ellis and Corsellis (see Chap. 2).

[26] Bolton (1928:590).

[27] Bolton (1928:589).

[28] For example, John Davies Cleaton at WRA (Bolton 1928:606); John Merson at Hull Borough Asylum (Bickford and Bickford 1983:88).

[29] *BMJ* 1872;1:329 (23rd March; Medical Vacancies), when the previous Deputy Medical Superintendent, Samuel Mitchell, was appointed Medical Superintendent at the South Yorkshire Asylum.

[30] Anon. (1868–1869:380) [capitals in original].

… In the event of the Asylum becoming full … it may be advisable to appoint an Assistant Medical Officer.[31]

These were junior clinicians, subordinate to the Medical Superintendent, who were sometimes (but not always) intent on building a career for themselves in asylum medicine, and who handled the day-to-day management of the patients.

The lot of AMOs in asylum medicine was acknowledged to be not a happy one, for multiple reasons: low salary; requirement to live in, leading to social isolation and, potentially, sharing the stigma of the insane; lack of opportunities for research; and prohibition from marrying.[32] Because teaching and training in insanity was not obligatory for medical students, AMOs often had to "learn their duties after they are appointed".[33] Moreover, whilst some superintendent appointments appeared to be "fast-tracked" (e.g. Crichton-Browne), for many AMOs promotion was uncertain, some appointments lasting for years with the consequence that AMOs sometimes found themselves subordinate to a medical superintendent who might be younger and less clinically experienced than themselves. Furthermore, if for any reason the medical superintendent was absent, the AMO found himself in charge.[34] As Crichton-Browne later observed:

> it used to be not an uncommon thing, in county asylums, for a young medical assistant, fresh from the schools, who had perhaps never seen a case of insanity in his life, to be put into one department, and given entire charge of it – many hundreds of cases being put completely under his medical guidance, while his chief, the superintendent, devoted himself to building or farming, and sometimes did not visit the wards for long periods together.[35]

Crichton-Browne's letter to the *Journal of Mental Science* in 1868 had been written as a response to ongoing discussion in its pages concerning the education, position, and pay of AMOs, the perceived low standard of whom was

---

[31] Cited by Renvoize (1991:30) [capitals in original].

[32] House physicians at the National Hospital for the Paralysed and Epileptic at Queen Square, London, were obliged to endure similar limitations in the late nineteenth century, according to Shorvon and Compston (2019:109).

[33] *BMJ* 1875;2:52–53 (10th July; The study of insanity).

[34] See Chap. 2 for the situation at Wakefield Asylum in 1857 when the superintendent, John Alderson, was ill, and a member of the junior staff, either John Chapman or Henry Maudsley, was in effect acting superintendent. If it was Maudsley, he did so with no prior experience of asylum work, unlike Chapman (hence this seems implausible to me).

[35] Burdett (1891:182).

felt to be related, in part at least, to their insufficient emolument ("the mere honorarium of from £80 to £100 per annum").[36] Thomas Laycock had contributed to this debate, noting that:

> the position, pay, and prospects of assistant medical officers of asylums are such that an appointment of that kind is not worth their notice, in comparison with advantages offered to a successful career in other departments of practice … An appointment of £70 or £80 per annum may be taken for a year or two, but this even is hardly thought worth the skill of the class of men I refer to; not intending to follow up the specialty they think it a waste of time.[37]

According to Crichton-Browne's letter, at WRA "the salary of the Senior Medical Assistant for the time being is £125, with the usual allowances, and that of the Junior, £100".[38] Hence, at WRA the AMO salary was at the upper end of the commonly encountered rates. Moreover, it was Crichton-Browne's hope that:

> When the additions now in progress here, which will raise the number of lunatics to 1300, are completed, I mean to suggest to the Committee of Visitors some modifications of the present arrangements. I shall propose that the salary of the Senior Assistants be raised permanently to £150 per annum, that of the Junior remaining where it is at £100.[39]

Advertisements for AMO posts at WRA appeared in the Medical Vacancies column of the *British Medical Journal* (henceforward *BMJ*) from time to time,[40] later in combination with that of "Pathologist".[41] These advertisements appear to be less frequent than those for Clinical Clerk or Clinical Assistant posts (*vide infra*), presumably because AMOs were often previous clinical clerks or assistants who, as a consequence of their work at WRA, had proved themselves suitable for internal promotion to AMO.

---

[36] *J Ment Sci* 1868–1869;13:354–355 (October 1867); Anon. (1868–1869:380).

[37] Laycock (1867–1868).

[38] Crichton Browne (1868–1869:599).

[39] Ibid., 600.

[40] *BMJ* 1871;1:574 (27th May; Medical Vacancies), when the previous AMO, George Thompson, was appointed Medical Superintendent of Bristol Lunatic Asylum. *BMJ* 1873;2:563 (8th November; Medical Vacancies), presumably because of Wilkie Burman's appointment as Medical Superintendent of the Wilts County Asylum. Also *BMJ* 1873;2:591 (15th November; Medical Vacancies).

[41] *BMJ* 1874;1:255 (21st February; Medical Vacancies) specified "Assistant Medical Officer and Pathologist"; ditto *BMJ* 1874;2:726 (5th December: Medical Vacancies), *BMJ* 1874;2:758 (12th December; Medical Vacancies), and *BMJ* 1874;2:798 (19th December; Medical Vacancies).

In addition to their clinical duties, AMOs at WRA during Crichton-Browne's superintendency contributed to the house journal, the *West Riding Lunatic Asylum Medical Reports* (henceforward *WRLAMR*, for which see Part III) and to the annual public medical *conversazione* (Part IV). It is possible that AMOs were encouraged to join the Medico-Psychological Association (MPA), the professional body for asylum doctors which had emerged from the Association of Medical Officers of Asylums and Hospitals for the Insane (AMOAHI); certainly numbers of them did so during or shortly after their time at WRA.[42] Crichton-Browne also saw the AMOs as having a therapeutic role as part of the workings of moral treatment: "The Medical Officers are really dispensing medicines when chatting with their patients",[43] although how two or three AMOs could chat meaningfully with any but a tiny handful of the ever-increasing Asylum patient population is unclear.

Concerns about the role of AMOs persisted long after Crichton-Browne had left WRA. Whilst the original practice had been to employ only one assistant per asylum, by 1888 the appointment of several men in different positions had become so commonplace that the MPA set up a committee to represent this "large and growing body" of men, the findings of which differed little from those expressed in the late 1860s.[44]

Clinical Clerk, Clinical Assistant

The third component of the resident medical staff at WRA comprised the Clinical Clerks or Clinical Assistants. According to Crichton-Browne,

the Clinical Clerks receive no salary, but only furnished apartments, board, &c., and instruction in mental and nervous diseases, in return for their services. After eighteen months' experience of them, I am strongly impressed with the value of these Clinical Clerks, and should not now like to be without them. They are of great service, not merely in keeping the case books, but in widening and extending that general and unremitting supervision which I believe to be so important in a large establishment like this, and in helping on the medical work in various ways. It is almost impossible for me to describe to you the vivifying influence which these ardent young men, fresh from the schools, exert upon the more confirmed

---

[42] For the history of the Medico-Psychological Association and its forerunner, the Association of Medical Officers of Asylums and Hospitals for the Insane, see Outterson Wood (1896), Walk and Walker (1961), Renvoize (1991), and Bewley (2008:10–70).

[43] *Report* (1872:30).

[44] Dodds et al. (1890). Indeed, little had apparently changed by 1918 (Anon. 1918).

Asylum Medical Officers. They rub off the rust of routine, and create a necessity for vigorous reading. They afford, too, wonderful facilities for carrying out scientific investigations and careful treatment, while they are themselves undergoing the best preparation for subsequent Asylum appointments, and even for general practice. One of my present assistants commenced here as Clinical Clerk. The important point is that the Clinical Clerks should be wisely and cautiously chosen, as it would not do to introduce young practitioners indiscriminately into an institution of this kind. Judicious selection, however, together with paramount and summary authority over them left in the hands of the Medical Superintendent, ought to obviate every danger and difficulty. I hold each of my Medical Assistants responsible for the good conduct of his particular clerk, and have never any trouble. They all work quietly and discreetly, and harmoniously together.[45]

Evidently, then, there was much more to say about Clinical Clerks, also known (later) as Clinical Assistants, than Assistant Medical Officers, as the former represented a staffing innovation introduced at WRA by Crichton-Browne,[46] whereas AMO posts were common to all asylums. As early as 1867, he made a plea for "the appointment of a competent pathologist and a few clinical clerks to each of our large asylums, in order to secure complete and reliable post mortem examinations and careful medical records of cases".[47]

In his 1868 letter to the *Journal of Mental Science*, Crichton-Browne proposed:

that £50 a-year be allowed to each of the Clinical Clerks. I feel persuaded that even this small sum will enable me to command a very superior class of men, will render those appointed more contented, and will induce them to remain with me for twelve months.

He added:

By the way, the best Clinical Clerk who has joined me is a graduate of the Edinburgh University, with first-class honours. When he was appointed I had a Cambridge man as an applicant, and the next vacancy I have promised to an F.R.C.S. Eng., by examination.[48]

---

[45] Crichton Browne (1868–1869:599–600).

[46] Crichton-Browne attributed the idea of introducing the role of clinical clerks to Dr. Rhys Williams, of Bethlem Hospital (*Report* 1869:28). Also noted by Sloffer (2023:27) who erred with "'Report for 1868,' p.29".

[47] Cited in *BMJ* 1867;2:186–187 (31st August; Lunatic Asylum reports), quote at 186. I have not seen a copy of Crichton-Browne's 1866 Report.

[48] Crichton Browne (1868–1869:600). I presume the Edinburgh graduate referred to was Samuel Mitchell (see Chap. 5). To my knowledge, none of the resident staff employed during Crichton-Browne's superintendency held the "F.R.C.S. Eng.", an advanced qualification, although several had the "M.R.C.S. Eng.", a basic qualification.

Perhaps in view of the novelty of this type of appointment, Crichton-Browne appended to his letter in the *Journal of Mental Science*:

Regulations as to Clinical Clerks.

1. They shall be appointed by the Medical Director, for periods of three or six months, or longer duration under special circumstances, and shall be subject to summary removal by him on account of misconduct or neglect.
2. They shall devote their whole time to the duties of their office, and shall not engage in any other occupation.
3. They shall be under the control and authority of the Medical Director, and subject to his supervision, shall receive instructions from the Assistant Medical Officers as to the performance of their duties.
4. They shall accompany the Medical Officers on their ordinary visits to the wards of their respective departments, and shall take careful notes of their observations on the various cases and the treatment ordered, for insertion in the case book.
5. They shall also visit the wards of their respective departments at other times when directed by the Medical Officers to do so, with the view of obtaining additional information respecting the cases under treatment.
6. They shall aid the Assistant Medical Officers generally in the discharge of their duties, but shall pay special attention to the condition of the case books, in which they shall keep careful records of all the cases under treatment, being more particularly full and explicit regarding those which are of recent origin, which are undergoing modifications in their character, which are being subjected to active treatment, or which are complicated by accidents or dangerous propensities.
7. They shall attend in the waiting rooms of their respective departments on the admission of new patients, shall note their condition, and endeavour to obtain from the relatives or friends, or Poor Law Officers accompanying them, reliable information as to their antecedent history.
8. They shall attend all post mortem examinations and assist in their performance, or take notes of the pathological conditions revealed, according as they may receive instructions from the senior Medical Officer present.
9. They shall assist in any surgical operations or scientific investigations that may be in progress in the Asylum during the period of their residence there, and in the absence of the dispenser shall compound the medicines for the wards, under the supervision of the Assistant Medical Officers.
10. They shall exert what moral influence they can with the patients for their benefit, and shall endeavour to promote their employment and recreation.

11. They shall immediately report to the Medical Director any instance of misconduct or neglect on the part of a subordinate officer, attendant, nurse, or servant, that may come to their knowledge.
12. They shall not leave the Asylum together, and shall only absent themselves at any time with the sanction of the Medical Director, and for such period as he may permit.[49]

In addition to their clinical duties, clinical clerks and assistants contributed to *WRLAMR* and to the medical *conversazione*. Like the AMOs, they may have been encouraged to join the MPA if contemplating a career in asylum medicine.

Although it is possible that the Clinical Clerk posts were filled informally, candidates being made known to Crichton-Browne by word of mouth, advertisements for clinical clerk or clinical assistant posts appeared in the medical press from time to time (most often the *BMJ* and the *Medical Times and Gazette*).[50] It has been suggested that Crichton-Browne hired "mostly from Edinburgh (Laycock's course) and London (Sankey's course)".[51]

---

[49] Crichton Browne (1868–1869:600–601).

[50] For example: *BMJ* 1869;2:361 (25th September; Medical Vacancies) clinical clerk vacancy ("applications after 28th Sept"); *BMJ* 1870;1:455 (30th April; Medical Vacancies) clinical clerk vacancy ("applications, 30th" [*sic*]); *BMJ* 1870;2:347 (24th September; Medical Vacancies) clinical clerk vacancy ("applications before 30th inst."); *BMJ* 1872;1:29 (6th January; Medical Vacancies) clinical assistant vacancy; *BMJ* 1872;2:179 (10th August; Medical Vacancies) clinical assistant vacancy; *BMJ* 1872;2:456 (19th October; Medical Vacancies) clinical assistant vacancy; *BMJ* 1873;1:105 (25th January; Medical Vacancies) and *Medical Times and Gazette* 1873;1:104 and 129 (25th January and 1st February; Vacancies) clinical assistant vacancy; *BMJ* 1873;1:452 (19th April; Medical Vacancies) clinical assistant vacancy; *BMJ* 1873;1:481 (26th April; Medical Vacancies) clinical assistant vacancy; *Medical Times and Gazette* 1873;1:456 (26th April; Vacancies) clinical assistant vacancy ("Applications with testimonials to J. Crichton Browne, M.D., Medical Director, on or before April 26."); *BMJ* 1873;2:50 (12th July; Medical Vacancies) clinical assistant vacancy; *Medical Times and Gazette* 1874;1:550 (16th May; Vacancies) clinical assistant vacancy ("Junior Practitioner or Senior Student, to Act as Clinical Assistant."); *BMJ* 1874;1:668 (16th May; Medical Vacancies) clinical assistant vacancy ("Applications, 23rd instant, to J. Crichton Browne, M.D., Medical Director."), ditto *BMJ* 1874;1:699 (23rd May; Medical Vacancies); *Medical Times and Gazette* 1874;2:676 and 703 (12th and 19th December; Vacancies) clinical assistant vacancy .

[51] Suggested by Finn (2012:73n249), presumably meaning W.H.O. Sankey at University College London. The evidence for this hiring policy seems to me weak; from the former source I count only two recruits (Herbert Major, Robert Lawson; although others, such as McDowall, may have passed through Laycock's Edinburgh class); from the latter only one (J.W.F. Watson). A case might also be made for Crichton-Browne's propensity to hire, or associate WRA with, the sons of famous medical fathers (Sutherland, Tyler Smith, H.R.O. Sankey).

Other Appointments

Pathologist

As previously noted, included in his 1867 plea for clinical clerks, Crichton-Browne had also expressed a desire for the appointment of a "competent pathologist … to secure complete and reliable post mortems".[52] The changes to infrastructure that he had initiated at WRA, with the foundation of a dedicated pathological laboratory (see Chap. 3), indicated his seriousness in forwarding this ambition.

This aspiration was finally achieved in 1872 when "a third permanent Assistant Medical Officer and Pathologist was appointed".[53] Perhaps there were misgivings amongst the Committee of Visitors about this appointment, as Crichton-Browne explained to them in his *Report* for 1872 that:

> The appointment of a Pathologist, which you have thus sanctioned is, I believe, a somewhat momentous step in the march of scientific progress in the Lunatic Asylums of this country. As far as I am aware, no other Asylum is yet provided with such an officer, but there can be little doubt that the example here set will be followed before long in other Counties, with the result of rapidly expanding our knowledge of brain disease, and of the means by which it may be averted or controlled. It is proposed that our Pathologist should perform all post-mortem examinations, should have care of the Museum which we are endeavouring to form, should undertake any special enquiries or experiments that may be deemed desirable by the Medical Director, and should by microscopic and chemical research seek to elucidate some of the dark points which are still so numerous as to make a Cimmerian gloom of cerebral pathology. It is proposed also that in order to keep up his clinical acquaintance with disease, and to extend that medical inspection of the wards to which paramount importance is attached, he should make an evening visit, accompanied by the Clinical Clerks, and should guide their observations.[54]

Evidently then, this post was envisaged as part clinical and part laboratory appointment ("Assistant Medical Officer and Pathologist"), a combination which may have been more palatable to the funders than an exclusively laboratory role. Certainly, this was the title used in an 1873 paper by the first

---

[52] Cited in *BMJ* 1867;2:186 (31st August; Lunatic Asylum reports).

[53] *Report* (1873:27).

[54] *Report* (1873:27–28).

appointee, Thomas William McDowall,[55] suggesting that the pathologist role was subsidiary, rather than substantive (and hence unlike the trained and certified position of pathologists we are familiar with today). In McDowall's only paper in *WRLAMR* (III:129–152) these roles were reversed ("Pathologist, and Assistant Medical Officer, West Riding Asylum"), and this was the case with the notification of appointment of some his successors, such as John Lowe. Joint "Assistant Medical Officer and Pathologist" posts at WRA were advertised in the *BMJ* from 1874.[56] Following McDowall, others appointed to this joint role were Lowe (1873), John Merson (1873), William Benham (1874), Robert Lawson (1874 or 1875), and William Bevan-Lewis (1876). Despite his extensive pathological research, Herbert Major does not at any time appear to have been designated as "Pathologist"; his initial appointment at WRA (1871) predated the inauguration of the joint post.

Dispenser/Pharmacist

> Mr. BRACEY has been appointed Dispenser in the room of Mr. EVANS, who has secured a better situation, and promises to justify the strong recommendations which led to his selection.[57]

The position of dispenser at the Asylum had been advertised in April 1870[58] and presumably George William Bracey[59] was the successful candidate. He had an important role at the Asylum in future years, sourcing and dispensing medications not only for everyday treatment but also for the many therapeutic trials which Crichton-Browne was keen to pursue through the agency of his medical subordinates. A large variety of medications was used at WRA, as evidenced in the pages of *WRLAMR*, for both clinical and experimental purposes (see Chap. 6 for further details on some of these medications). These included bromide (usually of potassium), morphia, ergot of rye, chloral hydrate, conia/conium, hyoscyamine, amyl nitrite, nicotine, and strychnia. Bracey was able to advise on the best method for making suppositories (VI:124).

---

[55] McDowall (1873:161).

[56] For example, *BMJ* 1874;1:255 (21st February; Medical Vacancies); *BMJ* 1874;2:726 (5th December: Medical Vacancies); *BMJ* 1874;2:758 (12th December; Medical Vacancies); *BMJ* 1874;2:798 (19th December; Medical Vacancies).

[57] *Report* (1871:27) [capitals in original].

[58] *Medical Times and Gazette* 1870;1:456 (23rd April).

[59] He is listed as "G.W.B. Bracey" at II:308, along with the "Resident Medical Officers" of the Asylum.

Whether drugs for animal or human experiment, such as chloroform and nitrous oxide, came through the pharmacy or were sourced by individual researchers is not always clear. Burman seems to have been very industrious in exploring different sources of conia (II:1–40) and Benham obtained nicotine from a supplier in London (IV:307). Alcohol was also used for (allegedly) therapeutic purposes but it is likely this came via the kitchen rather than the pharmacy.[60]

Bracey made other contributions to the life of the Asylum. He presided over stalls displaying drugs and medicinal preparations at the medical *conversazione* (see Chap. 8), in 1874 with C.E. Watson and in 1875 with J.H. Arbuckle.[61] He also appeared in some of the theatrical entertainments staged at WRA (Chap. 3), for example "Lady of Lyons" and the farce "Fortunes Frolic" (?27th May 1870), "Illustrious Stranger" (10th November 1871), "Robin Hood" (17th November 1874), "The Waterman" and "Ganem, Slave of Love" (25th February 1876), and as "Sister Anne" in "Blue Beard" (20th March 1877).[62] He was described as "stage manager" after the Crichton-Browne era.[63] "Mr. Bracey", presumably the same man, favoured the audience with a song at a Concert held at WRA, "Once again" by Sullivan (20th March 1873).[64] He was also the Asylum photographer.

Photographer

Crichton-Browne was interested in the possibilities of photography, still a relatively new technology in clinical practice at the time of his superintendency at WRA.[65] As previously shown (Chap. 3), he was instrumental in the setting up of a photographic studio with a dark room at WRA around 1870. Here George Bracey, the asylum's dispenser, took an active role. In 1874, Crichton-Browne observed that:

---

[60] According to the balance sheets in the annual *Reports*, "Wine, Spirits, and Porter" fell under the costs of "Surgery and Dispensary" whilst malt and hops came under "Provisions". Ashworth (1975:31) stated that beer for the patients and staff was brewed on the premises, and certainly a "brew-house" is found on the ground plan of Wright (1850:x). Beer was probably safer to drink than the Asylum water supply, a topic of recurrent concern in the *Reports* of successive medical superintendents.

[61] For 1874: *Medical Times and Gazette* 1874;2:609 (28th November; Annual Conversazione at the West Riding Asylum). For 1875: *BMJ* 1875;2:680.

[62] WYAS C85/1382.

[63] Golding (2021:150).

[64] WYAS C85/1382. Ditto 14th March 1884.

[65] Gilman (1982:179) called Crichton-Browne "an amateur photographer of considerable talent". Certainly, he was sending photographs to Darwin before Bracey's appointment at WRA.

> Our Dispenser, MR. BRACEY, an industrious and valuable Officer, has devoted much time and attention to the work of the Photographic Studio,[66]

Examples of Bracey as photographer may be found in *WRLAMR* (e.g. IV:276). It is possible that he was later joined in photographic work by Henry Clarke (for whom, see Chap. 7).

Non-resident Faculty

Visiting Clinicians and External Collaborators

In addition to the resident staff, a number of clinicians whose primary affiliations were elsewhere either visited WRA and/or contributed to *WRLAMR*, or were in some way associated with the Asylum, during the years 1866 to 1876. Indeed, this involvement of outside expertise was held to be one of the particular achievements of Crichton-Browne, as noted at the time of his departure from WRA:

> Special reference was made to the praiseworthy manner in which Dr. Browne had at all times been ready to throw open the asylum to medical men and others, so as to enable them to form correct ideas regarding the humane treatment of insanity, and to share in the observations made within its walls.[67]

Retrospectively, Crichton-Browne himself emphasized the need for collaborative research to maintain contact between asylum doctors and scientific medicine, even to the extent of converting asylums into clinical schools.[68]

The purposes of such openness to visitors were potentially many. Although the public asylums had some of the facilities necessary for the scientific study of mental illness, and WRA particularly so through the efforts of Crichton-Browne (see Chap. 3), there was an obvious lack of asylum doctors scientifically trained for the task of advancing the discipline beyond the merely custodial. Those visitors to WRA with scientific interests might encourage or foster collaboration, develop the research ethic amongst the resident staff, and thus produce trained medical men imbued with a scientific spirit which might then be disseminated through their subsequent appointments to other county

---

[66] *Report* (1874:28–29) [capitals in original].

[67] *BMJ* 1876;1:516 (22nd April; Dr. Crichton Browne).

[68] Crichton-Browne (1878–1879).

asylums. In other words, visitors might effectively bring the laboratory to the asylum. Outsiders might thus enrich the clinical community beyond the resources of the resident staff, with a consequent reduction in social and intellectual isolation of the latter and the attendant risk of stigma. Additionally, all of these considerations would of course raise the profile of WRA (and, by extension, of Crichton-Browne) and so encourage further applications for resident posts and collaborations with other clinicians and scientists interested in the workings of the brain.[69]

These associations and/or collaborations could be either with clinicians based locally (e.g. Dr. Allbutt from Leeds; Dr. Rabagliati from Bradford; Dr. Henry Clarke from Wakefield Jail) or from further afield, such as established experts visiting from London (e.g. Ferrier, Milner Fothergill, Lauder Brunton, Lennox Browne).[70] These visiting clinicians and external collaborators will be considered in detail in Part III.

Medical Students

Although not part of the faculty, other than in an honorary sense, medical students did have the opportunity to attend WRA during the Crichton-Browne superintendency. No profession or medical specialty can survive without attracting new recruits to the discipline, and the student years are an opportunity to enthuse the potential doctors of the future. Perhaps mindful of the influence on his own career of Laycock's teaching during his student years in Edinburgh (see Chap. 5), Crichton-Browne offered in March 1868 to give six lectures on mental diseases at the Leeds School of Medicine and to hold a weekly clinic at WRA "with provision of luncheon for the students, provided they were select and not too numerous".[71] This represented another attempt by Crichton-Browne to bridge the gap between the urban medical school and the county asylum.

For some years, adverts for the Leeds School of Medicine in the *BMJ* carried the note that "The West Riding Lunatic Asylum at Wakefield is open to Students for the study of Mental Diseases" and, from 1871, that "a course of

---

[69] Over 30 years later, similar ideals were expressed by Henry Maudsley with respect to his projected hospital, namely that it would supply scientifically trained medical men to work in the asylums (Maudsley 1909:7; see also Walk 1990:26). converse of Crichton-Browne's policy and actions, to bring scientifically trained men to the asylum. I would suggest that in the short-term Crichton-Browne's policy prospered, whereas in the long run it was Maudsley's plan that triumphed.

[70] All these individuals are discussed in Chap. 7, which also includes the reasoning why John Hughlings Jackson has not been included in this list.

[71] Anning and Walls (1982:55). They erred with "Dr Crichton Brown", as also in their index (167).

lectures will be given during the summer".[72] A more extensive note appeared in the *Medical Times and Gazette* in September 1875 to the effect that:

> Dr. J. Crichton Browne, F.R.S.E., the Medical Director of the West Riding Lunatic Asylum, lectures on Mental Diseases during the summer session. The systematic lectures are given at the School, and the clinical lectures at the Asylum, which now accommodates 1500 patients. It is needless to point out how great and unusual an advantage is here presented to those inclined to make themselves conversant with the improvement made of late years in the treatment and management of the insane.[73]

Crichton-Browne's series of papers entitled "Clinical lectures on mental and cerebral diseases" published in the *BMJ* between 1871 and 1874 may possibly be the substance of these lectures.[74]

Crichton-Browne was a signatory of a petition in 1875 from "Lecturers on Insanity at the Medical Schools of the United Kingdom" which was "presented to the medical examining boards, praying that students of medicine may, if they so desire, substitute a three months' course of clinical instruction in the wards of a lunatic asylum for the same period of attendance in the medical wards of a general hospital".[75] However, training in the field of "mental disorders" was not obligatory for medical students until 1885, when the General Medical Council (GMC) "resolved that a certificate of a course of instruction should be required for the final MB and that the examination should embrace insanity".[76]

It would be interesting to know how many Leeds medical students availed themselves of the training opportunities afforded by WRA and/or Crichton-Browne's lectures. Although I have no definite information on these points, the last page of the second volume of *WRLAMR* gives a list of "Gentlemen attending Dr. Crichton Browne's lectures on mental diseases. Summer session, 1872" which runs to 20 names, four of whom (all either MD or Esq)

---

[72] *BMJ* 1868;2:292 (12th September); *BMJ* 1869;2:312 (11th September); *BMJ* 1870;2:313 (17th September); *BMJ* 1871;2:305 (9th September); *BMJ* 1872;2:310 (14th September); *BMJ* 1873;2:330 (13th September); *BMJ* 1874;2:355 (12th September); *BMJ* 1875;2:347 (11th September). The same wording was still being used after Crichton-Browne's departure: *BMJ* 1876;2:351 (9th September); *BMJ* 1877;2:356 (8th September).

[73] *Medical Times and Gazette* 1875;2:322 (11th September; West Riding Lunatic Asylum, Wakefield).

[74] Crichton Browne (1871d, f, 1872b, 1873, 1874a).

[75] *BMJ* 1875;2:52–53 (10th July; The study of insanity).

[76] Walk (1990:18). Also Crammer (1996:212). However, Finn (2012:74) stated that "it was 1893 before the General Medical Council made psychiatry a compulsory subject for students". Around 1885 the MPA was also forming an action committee with a view to setting up a certificate of efficiency in psychological medicine (Crammer 1996:220; Loughran 2017:33).

were placed above the remaining 16. In their history of the Leeds School of Medicine, Anning and Walls stated that in 1875 Crichton-Browne reported that "average attendance in the last five years had been eighteen – the largest class of psychological medicine in the United Kingdom".[77] This was at a time when the annual intake of new students at the Leeds School of Medicine was less than 50. Crichton-Browne later acknowledged that "The backwardness of students in availing themselves of the opportunities hitherto given them of attending in Asylum wards must, I think, be partly attributed to the desultory character of the teaching which has been there provided for them".[78] One presumes that Crichton-Browne's teaching was more dynamic in character.

---

[77] Anning and Walls (1982:55). In 1868, Laycock observed of his course in medical psychology and mental diseases in Edinburgh that "the attendance is … very small compared with the number of students" (Laycock 1867–1868:587).

[78] Crichton-Browne (1878–1879:368).

5

Prosopography: The Resident Clinical Faculty at WRA

The purpose of this chapter is to present an extended prosopography of some of the resident clinicians, the asylum doctors, who worked at the West Riding Asylum at Wakefield (WRA) in the period 1866–1876,[1] beginning with Crichton-Browne and then working through his Assistant Medical Officers (AMOs) and Clinical Clerks/Clinical Assistants, as far as these are known. It has been noted that the "subsequent careers of these young men have not been fully researched",[2] and whilst no claim to "full research" is espoused here, nonetheless some details are provided. It has also previously been noted that "We are lacking in detailed biographies of many of the leading members of the psychiatric profession in the 19th century".[3] Although this deficiency has been redressed for some of the leading members of the profession,[4] it is certainly the case that, to paraphrase, "We are lacking in biographies, detailed or otherwise, of many of the lesser members of the profession in the 19th century".

---

[1] It should be noted here that Russell's (1988) chapter entitled "The lunacy profession and its staff in the second half of the nineteenth century, with special reference to the West Riding Lunatic Asylum" does not mention any of the clinical personnel who worked at WRA in the period 1866–1876 with the sole exception of William Bevan-Lewis, and this only in his later capacity as superintendent (i.e. after 1884), hence there is no overlap between Russell's chapter and the material presented here. Ditto Russell (1983:263–319).

[2] Neve and Turner (1995:407); they also noted that "several did reach senior asylum positions", footnoting (n48) Herbert Major and Crochley Clapham. As will be shown, many others also reached senior asylum positions (see Table 5.2).

[3] Beveridge (1998:52).

[4] For example, see Scull et al. (1996).

A. J. Larner, *The West Riding Asylum and the Origins of British Neurology 1866-1876*,
https://doi.org/10.1007/978-3-032-12591-0_5

With the institution shaped to facilitate the pursuit of a scientific approach to insanity (see Chap. 3), the analysis of the resident faculty encompasses their associations with, contributions to, and clinical trajectory after leaving, the West Riding Asylum. This examination seeks to understand in what ways, if any, these clinicians, both individually and collectively, advanced the scientific knowledge which contributed to the origins of British neurology.

The data are taken from several sources:

- extracted from the annual *Report of the Committee of Visitors and of the Medical Superintendent of the West Riding Pauper Lunatic Asylum* (henceforward denoted *Report*, with the corresponding year of publication, which refers to activity at the Asylum in the previous calendar year);
- information gleaned from the Asylum house journal, the *West Riding Lunatic Asylum Medical Reports* (henceforward *WRLAMR*);
- information from appointments columns and publications in the contemporary medical literature, especially the *BMJ*, *Lancet*, *Medical Press and Circular*, *Medical Times and Gazette*, and the *Journal of Mental Science*.

The personal names used as headings for each subsection are those which appear in the *Reports* and/or *WRLAMR* although some of these are either incorrect or suspect (*viz.* "W.P. Ledgard"; "William Lawrence"; "J.W.F. Watson"; "G.W. Baroll"; "F. Wright"), as addressed in the individual subsections (and also in Table 5.1).

This exposition builds upon the work of Michael Finn who produced an alphabetical table of "all those known to have worked between 1866 and 1876 as either medical officers or clinical clerks" at WRA, a list of 33 men which he deemed "to form the starting point for a prosopography".[5] In addition to these 33, I have included two others known to Finn but not included in his table (C. Fryer, W.P. Ledgard), and identified four others (C.F. Oxley, J. Hay, F. Wright, J. Davy) whose names appear in the Medical Director's Journal or "Appointments" columns in medical journals indicating their employment in posts at WRA during this period, but who do not appear in *WRLAMR* or in any *Report* of the Superintendent. Details about these six individuals, and indeed some of the others, is at best limited. These data are presented in Table 5.1 in provisional chronological, rather than alphabetical, order. Not all of those working at WRA left a "footprint" in terms of publications (only 26

---

[5] Finn (2012:181–184) table; quotes at 180 and 185 respectively. Sloffer's thesis reportedly "develops a prosopography of the members of the medical staff of the West Riding Pauper Lunatic Asylum" (2023:16) but rather than "Examining the contributions and career arcs of all these players" (Idem) in fact omitted any such details on the vast majority of the individuals to be examined here.

Table 5.1 Provisional "dating profile" of Assistant Medical Officers/Clinical Clerks/Clinical Assistants working at WRA, 1866–1876

Name	Qualifications[a]	Posts, dates at WRA	MPA	Papers in *WRLAMR* (Part III)	Attendance at *conversazione* (Part IV)[b]
OXLEY, Charles Fox	MRCS Eng 1864 LRCP Edin 1868	1867	–	–	–
FRYER, Charles Sherburn	LKQCP Irel & LM 1866 FLS	CC 1867	–	–	–
LEDGARD, "W.P." [?William Edward Ledgard]	MRCS Eng 1868, LRCP Edin & LM 1870	CC 1867	–	–	–
THOMPSON, George	MRCS Eng 1867 LRCP Lond 1868 LSA 1869	CC 1867 AMO 1867	1869	I:58–70 II:302–306	–
MITCHELL, Samuel	CM 1865 MD Edin 1867	AMO 1867 DMS 1868	1869	I:27–57 II:73–96	?1872 (variable documentation)
ALDRIDGE, Charles	LRCP Lond 1868 MB (Aberd) & CM 1872 MD (Aberd) 1876	CC 1868 AMO 1868	1869	I:71–128 II:223–253 IV:291–304	1872
BURMAN, James Wilkie	MB Edin 1868 LRCS Edin 1868 MD Edin 1871	CC 1868 AMO 1871 DMS 1872	1869	I:129–151 II:1–40 III:216–257	1872, 1873
MAYHEW, Charles Henry	LRCP Lond 1869 MRCS Eng 1869	CC 1869	–	I:252–260	–
WARD, John Bywater	MRCS Eng 1866 BA 1867 MB Cantab 1868 LSA 1868 MD Cantab 1872	CC 1869	1871	I:152–163	–

(continued)

Table 5.1 (continued)

Name	Qualifications[a]	Posts, dates at WRA	MPA	Papers in *WRLAMR* (Part III)	Attendance at *conversazione* (Part IV)[b]
PEDLER, George Henry	LSA 1868 MRCS Eng 1869 LRCP Lond 1871	CC 1869	1873	I:164–177 II:137–156	–
NICOL, Patrick	MA Aberd 1866 MB & CM (Aberd) 1869 MD (Aberd) 1871	CA 1869 AMO 1870	1870?	I:178–208 I:233–251 II:177–202	(invited 1872)
LAWRENCE, "William" [?Alexander Lawrence]	MA Aberd 1866 MB & CM (Aberd) 1869 MD (Aberd) 1872	CC 1870	1870?1872?	I:209–217	–
HAY, J.	MB CM, MRCS Eng	CC 1870	–	–	–
FOX, Edward Churchill Pigott	MB CM Edin 1868	CA 1870	1877	I:261–265	–
SUTHERLAND, Henry	BA Cantab 1867 MA MB Oxon 1869 MRCP Lond 1870 MD Oxon 1872	CC 1871 Acting AMO 1871	1870	I:218–232 II:53–72 III:299–314 VI:108–119	–
DOVE, William Watson	LRCP Edin 1870 MRCS Eng 1870	CC 1871	1871	I:233–251	–
WATSON, "John W. F." [?John Wilcocks Watson]	LSA 1871 MRCS Eng 1873	CC 1871	–	–	–

MAJOR, Herbert Coddington	MB Edin & CM 1871 MD Edin 1875	CA 1871 AMO 1872 MS 1876	1872	II:41–52 II:157–176 III:97–112 IV:223–239 V:160–170 VI:1–10	1872, 1873, 1874, 1875
LOWE, John	MB Edin & CM 1871	CA 1871 AMO + P 1873	1872	III:196–215	1873
COURTENAY, Edward Mazière	AB TCD MB MCh 1871	CA 1872	1872; Hon 1891	II:254–277	–
McDOWALL, Thomas William	MD Edin 1866 LRCS Edin 1870	AMO + P 1872	1870[c] Hon 1932	III:129–152	1873
WOODS, Oscar T.	BA TCD 1868 LM Rot Hosp Dub 1868 MB 1869 LRCSI 1869 MD Dub 1875	CC 1872	1873	–	1872
CLAPHAM, W. Crochley S.	MRCS Eng 1871 LRCP Lond 1872	CC 1872	1878	III:285–298 VI:11–26 VI:150–169	–
WOOD, W. Bryan	–	CC 1872	–	–	1872
BAROLL, G.W. [?George William Barroll]	LRCP Ed 1867 MRCS Eng LSA 1867	CA 1873	–	–	–

(continued)

Table 5.1 (continued)

Name	Qualifications[a]	Posts, dates at WRA	MPA	Papers in *WRLAMR* (Part III)	Attendance at *conversazione* (Part IV)[b]
GALTON, John Charles	MA Oxon 1866 MRCS Eng 1866 FLS	CA 1873	–	III:258–272	–
LEVINGE, Edward George	AB MB Dub 1873 LRCSI 1873	CA 1873	1874	–	–
SMITH, Ernest Louis Tyler	BA Cantab 1870 LRCP Edin 1874 MB Edin 1875	CA 1873	–	–	1873
WRIGHT, F. [?Frederick Wade Wright]	MRCS Eng 1872 MB Aberd & CM 1875	CA 1873	–	–	–
WATSON, C.E.	–	CA 1873	–	–	1873, 1874
NEWCOMBE, Charles Frederick	MB Aberd & CM 1873 MD Aberd 1878	CA 1873–4	1876	V:198–226	–
LAWSON, Robert	MB Edin & CM LM 1871	CA 1874 AMO + P 1874–5	Yes[d]	IV:240–264 V:40–84 VI:65–84 VI:120–149	1874, 1875
MERSON, John	MA Aberd 1866 MB CM (Aberd) 1870 MD Aberd 1874	AMO + P 1873 DMS 1876	1877	IV:63–93 V:1–23 VI:85–107	1873, 1875
BENHAM, William T.	MB and CM 1871 MRCS Eng 1871 LSA 1871 MD Aberd 1873	AMO + P 1874	1872	IV:152–178 IV:305–317	1874 ("T.W. Benham")

DAVY, J. [?John Davy]	MB CM (Aberd) 1874	CA 1875	–	–	–
LEWIS, William Bevan	LRCP Lond 1868 MRCS Eng 1868 LSA 1868 FRMS	CA 1875 AMO + P 1876 MS 1884	1879	V:85–104 VI:43–64 VI:120–149	1875
ARBUCKLE, John Hunter	MB CM (Glasg) 1870 MD Glasg 1872	CA 1875	–	V:130–148	1875
WALLIS, John Augustus Michael	LRCSI 1866 LRCP Edin and LM 1867 MB CM Aberd 1875 MD Aberd 1883	AMO 1874	1876	V:257–270	1874
PLAXTON, Joseph William	MRCS Eng 1869 LSA 1869	AMO 1877	1877	–	–

aQualifications are as per entries in the *Medical Directory* 1867–1876 (rather than *WRLAMR* publications, which may differ); if no *Medical Directory* entry has been found (e.g. Hay), qualifications are as per details in notification of appointment in the medical press
bOnly *conversazione* attendances with documentary confirmation are included (i.e. minimum attendance); no details on 1871 attendees available at the time of writing
cMcDowall's obituary notice in the *Journal of Mental Science* [1937;83(January 1937):xl] says an Ordinary Member since 1876
dFor Lawson, Finn (2012:182) stated "[Yes]", square brackets not explained, but I have not found Lawson's name on any of the Annual Lists of MPA members. Perhaps the rapidity of his promotion to Commissioner status precluded his election to MPA membership?
Abbreviations
Posts: *AMO* assistant medical officer, *AMO + P* assistant medical officer and pathologist, *CC* clinical clerk, *CA* clinical assistant, *DMS* deputy medical superintendent, *MS* medical superintendent
MPA member of the Medico-Psychological Association
WRLAMR West Riding Lunatic Asylum Medical Reports

of these 39 individuals published in *WRLAMR*), perhaps because the opportunity did not arise and/or they were not aiming for a career in asylum medicine. At least one reportedly retired through ill health (J.W.F. Watson).

These biographical sketches do not claim to be exhaustive but aim to give specific details for each individual, where available, on the subjects of:

- Location of medical training;
- Appointment to and duration of service at WRA;
- Specific information on work undertaken at WRA and publications (if any) related to that work;
- For those subsequently leaving WRA (the vast majority), brief details of career trajectory, including significant publications and appointments.

Those clinicians who visited WRA, probably by invitation, for the purposes of clinical or experimental work oriented to research rather than day-to-day clinical care, and/or who contributed papers to the *WRLAMR*, but who were not appointed to the institution as resident staff, are considered in Chap. 7. The degree of interaction between these clinicians and the resident staff is open to question, but some examples are apparent.[6]

Those clinicians whose connection with WRA appears solely in relation to the medical *conversazione*, mostly for the purpose of delivering invited lectures, are considered in Chap. 9 (along with some other visitors deemed significant). Other than listening to their presentations, and possibly inspiring their ongoing work, there is unlikely to have been any interaction between the resident staff, other than the Medical Superintendent, and these visiting clinicians.

Some comment should be made here about the nature, purpose, value, and shortcomings of prosopography.[7] Evidently the proposal of such an extended prosopography risks, if not mandates, the accusation of Whiggishness, ignoring as it does the non-clinical staff (attendants and nurses) and other personnel required for the running of such a huge establishment (including service industries outside the walls), as well as, most importantly, the patients themselves for whose benefit the institution existed.[8] However, as the overarching aim of this study is the examination of the origins of neurology as a profession,

---

[6] For example, as discussed below, Allbutt worked with Major; Ferrier worked with Galton and McDowall, and was possibly known to Lawson. Further consideration of interactions between resident and visiting staff is given in Chap. 10 (Faculty section).

[7] A more extended account of my ruminations on the subject of prosopography appears in Larner (2025f).

[8] These groups are considered in Chap. 3.

it is those individuals with clinical and/or scientific backgrounds and qualifications who require further examination. This provides an opportunity to examine, where known, the social origins, training, and subsequent career trajectories of individuals in this specific employment group, searching for any commonalities. As pointed out by Felix Goodbody, "prosopography is suited to the study of local medical networks".[9]

Whilst the order in which these individuals is discussed might follow various methods (e.g. alphabetical; by date of birth; importance to posterity, presumed or otherwise), the chosen approach is roughly chronological, based on information (where available) about date of appointment to WRA, and/or dates of work undertaken at WRA, and/or, in the absence of any other information, dates of publication in the WRA house journal, the *WRLAMR* (for discussion of this journal *per se*, see Part III). This approach has been chosen to emphasize possible overlap of, and hence possible influences on, and/or dialogue and collaborations between, different individuals, factors which may be deemed of importance to the development of a sense of profession rather than simply individual advancement.[10]

James Crichton-Browne (1840[11]–1938)[12]

In the *Lancet* issue of 7th July 1866, the following announcement was made:

J.D. CLEATON, M.R.C.S., Resident Medical Superintendent of the West Riding Lunatic Asylum at Wakefield, has been appointed a Commissioner in Lunacy.[13]

---

[9] Goodbody (2020:36).

[10] Wallis (2017a:127) suggested that dialogue between researchers may not have been the case at WRA after Crichton-Browne's departure.

[11] Peculiarly the 1871 census listed Crichton-Browne's estimated birth date as 1841, presumably because of his listed age of 30. He was born on 29th November 1840. Perhaps this was the source for Bewley's claim (2008:35) that Crichton-Browne was "born in 1841".

[12] No attempt is made here to document Crichton-Browne's whole career trajectory, merely those aspects deemed pertinent to his clinical and research contributions during his time as the superintendent at WRA (1866–1876), a relatively brief period in his long and distinguished career. For his contributions to administrative and social life of WRA, and references to existing biographical material, see Chap. 3.

[13] *Lancet* 1866;2:27 (7th July; Medical Appointments) [capitals in original]. Also *BMJ* 1866;1:30 (7th July; Medical News) which noted that Cleaton's appointment as a Commissioner in Lunacy was "in the room of S. Gaskell, Esq., resigned". Ditto *J Ment Sci* 1866–1867;12(July 1866):296 (Appointments). For Samuel Gaskell, see Scull et al. (1996:161–186) and Larner (2016) (reprinted in adapted form in Larner 2023a:69–76).

This appointment opened up a vacancy, as noted in the issue of the same journal the following week, 14th July.[14] The post was soon filled, as the *Lancet* of 4th August 1866 reported:

> J.C. BROWNE, M.D., M.R.C.S.E., Medical Superintendent of the Newcastle-on-Tyne Borough Lunatic Asylum, has been elected Medical Superintendent and Director of the West Riding of Yorkshire Lunatic Asylum, vice J.D. Heaton [*sic*], Esq. appointed Commissioner in Lunacy.[15]

At the age of 25, James Crichton-Browne was on his way to Wakefield Asylum.[16]

When, nearly ten years later, in December 1875, Crichton-Browne was appointed to the Visitorship of Chancery Lunatics, so presaging the end of his time at Wakefield, the rapporteur in the *Medical Times and Gazette* commented that he had "studied lunacy practically almost from his childhood".[17] As the son of the noted asylum doctor, William Browne (1805–1885),[18] James had grown up at the Crichton Royal Institution in Dumfries in south west Scotland,[19] and had added the surname of the deceased benefactor, Dr. James

---

[14] *Lancet* 1866;2:55 (14th July; Medical Vacancies).

[15] *Lancet* 1866;2:140 (4th August; Medical Appointments) [capitals in original]. Crichton-Browne's election to the superintendency was also reported in *Medical Times and Gazette* 1866;2:158 (11th August; Medical News) and *J Ment Sci* 1866–1867;12(October 1866):455 (Appointments). Finn (2012:52n174) stated that the "appointment was sanctioned on 24 July" referring to this volume of the *Journal of Mental Science* but I do not find this date mentioned in the Appointments section or elsewhere therein. I have found no mention of Crichton-Browne's appointment in the *BMJ*, despite the earlier reference to Cleaton's onward appointment. Indeed, Cleaton was still recorded as "Medical Superintendent of the West Riding Asylum, Wakefield" in the list of BMA members for Yorkshire published in November 1867 (*BMJ* 1867;2:400), more than a year after Crichton-Browne's appointment, and also in November 1868 (*BMJ* 1868;2:562). Crichton-Browne's name was not included in either of these lists but it appeared in November 1869 (*BMJ* 1869;2:510) and thereafter: *BMJ* 1870;2:506; *BMJ* 1871;2:778; *BMJ* 1873;1:511; *BMJ* 1874;2:45 ("Browne J.C."); *BMJ* 1875;2:4 (18th December; British Medical Association). Presumably the BMA membership lists were not regularly updated.

[16] Crichton-Browne's appointment may have been made a few days before the *Lancet* announcement, as in April 1868 the *Lancet* reported that "Since July, 1866, the Asylum has been under the superintendence of Dr. J. Crichton Browne" (*Lancet* 1868;1:510). Viets (1938:477) erred in saying that Crichton-Browne took up the superintendency at Wakefield in 1871, possibly as a consequence of mixing up the date of inauguration of *WRLAMR* (the subject of Viets's paper) with the date of Crichton-Browne's appointment to WRA. Walmsley (2003:21) was also in error when stating that Crichton-Browne was appointed superintendent in 1868, likewise Breathnach (1996) who gave his dates of tenure as superintendent as "1864–1876".

[17] *Medical Times and Gazette* 1875;2:683 (18th December; The Visitorship of Chancery Lunatics). Leyland (1888:II:28) suggested that in deciding to pursue a career in asylum medicine Crichton-Browne "yielded, as it were, to hereditary predisposition".

[18] See Chap. 7 for biographical material on W.A.F. Browne.

[19] Crichton-Browne published "Some early Crichton memories" in Easterbrook (1937:18–26; reprinted in Easterbrook, 1940:1–6).

Crichton (1765–1823), whose bequest had enabled his widow, Elizabeth (1779–1862), to fund the foundation of the asylum.[20] This institution gave the opportunity to William Browne to enact at Dumfries the ideals outlined in his influential work of 1837, *What asylums were, are, and ought to be: being the substance of five lectures delivered before the managers of the Montrose Royal Lunatic Asylum.*[21] Whether or not this unusual locus of upbringing proved advantageous to Crichton-Browne's subsequent career, and orientation towards research, may be debated,[22] but certainly this was the route he chose to pursue after his medical qualification from Edinburgh (MB CM 1861, LRCS Ed 1861).

Crichton-Browne's years of medical training in Edinburgh between 1857 and 1862[23] coincided with the period during which Thomas Laycock (1812–1876) was teaching at the University.[24] As Chair of the Practice of Physic at Edinburgh University from 1855, Laycock had initiated instruction in medical psychology and mental diseases and was one of Crichton-Browne's teachers. This teaching may have prompted Crichton-Browne's address as Senior President to the Royal Medical Society of Edinburgh on "The history and progress of psychological medicine" which was published in the *Journal*

---

[20] For the history of Crichton Royal Institution, see Easterbrook (1937, 1940) (he became Physician Superintendent there in 1908, and also wrote an appreciation of Crichton-Browne: Easterbrook 1938); Tait (1972) and Williams (1989). The plan of the asylum at Dumfries was apparently based on Watson and Pritchett's published designs for the West Riding Asylum at Wakefield, although the history of Crichton Royal Hospital by Morag Williams reported the architect to have been William Burn of Edinburgh (Williams 1989:14). According to Williams (1989:21), Elizabeth Crichton was Godmother to James Crichton-Browne.

[21] Browne (1837). As a consequence of this work, Browne was "head-hunted" by Mrs. Crichton for the institution she had commissioned in Dumfries.

[22] The Swedish visual neurophysiologist and Nobel Laureate Torsten N. Wiesel (b.1924) had a similar upbringing, in the 1920s and 1930s, living in the "mental hospitals" where his father was a psychiatrist (Hubel and Wiesel 2005:25–26). In this context, an incidental comment made by Erving Goffman (1922–1982), based on his field work in an American psychiatric hospital in the late 1950s, may be pertinent: "children of resident doctors were the only non-patient category I found that did not evince obvious caste distance from patients; why I do not know." (Goffman 1961:192n68). If true, this might explain any affinity for working with patients with mental disorders manifested by Crichton-Browne. One might also note here a comment of Daniel Hack Tuke who worked as a steward at the York Retreat from 1847 for two years before studying medicine: "Actual residence in an asylum is almost essential to a thorough understanding of the life, nightly as well as daily, of the inmates" (Ireland 1895:381; cited by Renvoize 1991:51). Other examples may be furnished by James Foulis Duncan (1812–1895), MPA President in 1875 (Duncan 1875–1876:338), and John Cade (1912–1980), the Australian psychiatrist who discovered the utility of lithium in mania, who grew up in the grounds of the mental hospitals where his father was superintendent (Cade 1999).

[23] This was Crichton-Browne's own dating, as found in his penultimate "notebook" (Crichton-Browne 1937:31). I thank Dr. Tom Hughes of Rhiwbina, Cardiff, for lending me his grandfather's copy of this book (December 2024). Crichton-Browne's graduation in 1862 is confirmed in *Alphabetical list of graduates of the University of Edinburgh …*, 1889:25.

[24] Biographical material on Laycock may be found in James (1996).

of Mental Science whilst he was still a medical student.[25] Laycock was also a friend of William Browne.[26] Like him, Laycock had visited the Paris hospitals in the 1830s. Both through his teaching and his writings, such as *Mind and Brain* (1860), Laycock may have stimulated Crichton-Browne's interests. Certainly, in later years Crichton-Browne attributed much of his success to Laycock's teaching,[27] writing in 1926:

> Looking back on my medical training in the sixties of the last century in the University of Edinburgh where there was at that time an unusually brilliant galaxy of medical professors … I should unhesitatingly fix on Laycock as the most original and inspiring of them all.[28]

After achieving his initial medical qualifications (MD 1862, LSA 1863), and during his training in asylum medicine (he joined the Association of Medical Officers of Asylums and Hospitals for the Insane, AMOAHI, in 1863[29]), Crichton-Browne had visited Paris,[30] thus following in the footsteps of his father, William, who had visited Esquirol, Pinel's successor, in the summer and autumn of 1832.[31] Although there are few existing details of Crichton-Browne's time in Paris,[32] this visit apparently occurred around 1862–3.[33] It would seem inconceivable that Crichton-Browne would not have visited the Salpêtrière during his sojourn in Paris, as this was one of the scenes, along with the Bicêtre, of Pinel's (mythical) release of the insane from their chains.

---

[25] Crichton Browne (1860–1861).

[26] William Browne lectured "before Professor Laycock's class of Medical Pyschology [*sic*], at their visit to the Inverness District Asylum, July, 1865" (Browne 1865–1866:336). As late as 1873, he again lectured to "Laycock's class of psychological medicine" (Browne 1873).

[27] *J Ment Sci* 1869–1870;15(October 1869):470–471 (Psychological news). Batty Tuke (1874:109) described Laycock as Crichton-Browne's "master".

[28] Crichton-Browne (1926:36) (also at 45: "the most interesting and inspiring of all my teachers"); likewise "My revered teacher" (Crichton-Browne 1937:245).

[29] James (1996:368).

[30] Crichton-Browne (1926:239–240) wrote that "When I was studying in Paris in 1863 an epidemic of smallpox was raging there, and there were many cases in the La Charité Hospital, which I was attending". It seems he was not alone there, noting "my friend, Dr. Pyle, who had been with me in Paris" (279).

[31] William Browne's visit to the Bicêtre is mentioned, but undated, in *Edinb Med J* 1860;5(11):1050–1051 (Royal College of Surgeons—Conversazione), specifically at 1051.

[32] That he learned French during this period may be suggested by a later publication in that language (Crichton Browne 1876).

[33] According to Neve (https://doi.org/10.1093/ref:odnb/32122), Crichton-Browne "qualified LSA London 1863, before visiting a number of medical schools and asylums in Paris". With respect to the exact dating, it may be noted that he published a paper on "mania ephemera" from his appointment as an "Assistant Physician, Derby County Asylum" in January 1863 (Crichton Browne 1863).

After appointments as Assistant Physician to Derby County Asylum (in 1862, presumably predating his visit to Paris)[34] and as the Medical Superintendent at Newcastle-upon-Tyne Asylum (1865–6),[35] Crichton-Browne became the incumbent at WRA. In the following ten years, he would attract to Wakefield numbers of young men to undertake clinical duties and to publish clinical and experimental research findings, found a journal, the *West Riding Lunatic Asylum Medical Reports*, through which much of this research was disseminated (see Part III), and inaugurate annual clinical meetings, termed medical *conversazione*, at which new and developing ideas in mental health were discussed (see Part IV).

Once appointed at Wakefield, what prompted Crichton-Browne to pursue what might now be considered a "research agenda" at WRA, rather than confining his energies to administration of the asylum, a demanding enough requirement, as superintendents did elsewhere? The question is apt in light of the 1845 national Lunacy Commissioners instruction discouraging public asylum superintendents from undertaking research projects.[36] Possibly one stimulus was his father's view, stated in his Presidential address to the Medico-Psychological Association (MPA) in 1866, that "Such a view [of prescribing, and over-prescribing, for the mental condition] does not exclude enlightened therapeutical treatment. … If our knowledge of the physical changes upon which the different forms of alienation depend was more extensive and sound, the limits and effects of remedies might be as much relied upon as in other maladies".[37]

Crichton-Browne was evidently aware of the possibilities for research presented by the large number of patients under his care at WRA. In his initial *Report* from the Asylum (for the year 1866, published 1867), as reported in the *BMJ*, he noted the "Unparalleled opportunity which our large lunatic asylums offer for the study of nervous and mental diseases" in light of which, and the apparent increase in the numbers of patients with insanity, he made his plea for the appointment of a competent pathologist and clinical clerks (see Chap. 4).[38]

---

[34] Crichton Browne, 1862–1863 emanated from his appointment at Derby. Two articles signed "J.C.B." in the same volume of the *Journal of Mental Science* may well also be his: *J Ment Sci* 1862–1863;8(July 1862):262–275 (Kleptomania); *J Ment Sci* 1862–1863;8(July 1862):308 (The Scotch Lunacy Bill).

[35] *J Ment Sci* 1865–1866;11(July 1865):295 (Appointments).

[36] I find no call or recommendation, let alone exordium, to undertake research in the chapter of William Browne's book entitled "What asylums ought to be" (Browne 1837:176–231).

[37] Browne (1866–1867:312). Cited in Harrington Tuke (1873:448).

[38] *BMJ* 1867;2:186–187 (31st August; Lunatic Asylum reports); quotes at 186. Finn (2012:56 and n184), citing "'Report of the Medical Superintendent', Wakefield, 24th January 1867 (WYAS, C85/1/12/2) p.23" (not seen by me), quoted "the unparalleled facilities which they [asylums] offer for

In the Medical Superintendent's *Report* for 1867 (dated as 29th January 1868), his first full year in the post, Crichton-Browne expressed the "regret that our Asylum medical officers have not more time to investigate the action of drugs" for controlling or curing mental derangements.[39] These concerns may have been prompted by, or at least echoed or endorsed, Laycock's comments published in the *Journal of Mental Science* in January 1868:

> It is a matter of general complaint how little our public asylums contribute to the theory and practice of medicine in that special department, and the solid reason has been as often advanced as the complaint, namely, that the superintendents are overworked. Now, an educated assistant would be able to co-operate effectively in this duty of our superintendents, to the great advancement of mental science.[40]

Writing to Charles Darwin (1809–1882) on 1st June 1869, Crichton-Browne noted "the mass of interesting material which is as it were going to waste … in this huge hospital for want of accurate observation & which might be of immense value".[41] Darwin had originally approached Crichton-Browne, at the suggestion of Henry Maudsley (see Chap. 2), for information on facial expressions in the insane as part of the research for his book *The expression of the emotions in man and animals*, subsequently published in 1872.[42]

It is possible that Crichton-Browne's visit to Paris was significant in this context. Its timing, 1862–3, was coincident with the period when Jean-Martin Charcot (1825–1893) and Edmé Félix Alfred Vulpian (1826–1887) had both been appointed to chief of service positions at the Salpêtrière and were beginning their work with the large patient numbers accommodated

------

the study of nervous and mental diseases have not yet been taken advantage of as fully as could be desired".

[39] *Report* (1868:23).

[40] Laycock (1867–1868:588).

[41] Darwin Correspondence Project, "Letter no. 6769,"

https://www.darwinproject.ac.uk/letter/?docId=letters/DCP-LETT-6769.xml (accessed 10/04/2023). For details of the correspondence between Darwin and Crichton-Browne, see Pearn (2010). Also Edwards (2014), https://publicdomainreview.org/essay/the-naturalist-and-the-neurologist-on-charles-darwin-and-james-crichton-browne (accessed 21/11/2024). Crichton-Browne's observation was not unique: at the Annual Meeting of AMOAHI on 22nd June 1854, as reported in the first volume of the *Asylum Journal* (1853–1855;1:88), Bucknill had noted that the "case books of asylums contained an unworked mine of golden wealth".

[42] Crichton-Browne supplied around 40 photographs to Darwin but none was eventually used in the book. Darwin's autobiography has nothing to say about this matter, devoting as it does only a single paragraph to *The expression of the emotions in man and animals* (Barlow 1958:131). The book was later cited in *WRLAMR* (by Lawson & Bevan Lewis, VI:137, 146n1). *Contra* Wallis (2017a:10), I very much doubt that Darwin ever visited WRA.

there, for the purposes of clinical assessment and subsequent pathological examination, the clinico-anatomical method. Whether these developments influenced Crichton-Browne is uncertain, since the psychiatric and neurological services at the Salpêtrière were quite separate.[43] However, it was the view of the historian Janet Oppenheim that Crichton-Browne's "choice of Paris influenced the rest of his career, for clinical observation in hospital or asylum wards and the performance of autopsies, on the French model, became Crichton-Browne's basic approach to psychological medicine".[44] Charcot's predilection for the founding of new medical journals might also have influenced Crichton-Browne in commencing *WRLAMR*.[45]

Crichton-Browne had made only limited attempts to exploit the mass of clinical material at his disposal at WRA prior to 1870, at least in terms of publications,[46] presumably for want of time to do more,[47] although he had permitted and/or invited others to see patients at the Asylum for the purposes of their own research, such as Clifford Allbutt from Leeds (see Chap. 7) and Lawson Tait (*vide infra*).[48] The perceived inadequacy of Crichton-Browne's output of publications was possibly both the cause and effect of his drive to make structural and administrative changes at WRA in the years 1866–1870 (detailed in Chap. 3). Notably, further publications from Crichton-Browne

---

[43] Goetz et al. (1995:208).

[44] Oppenheim (1991:61–62).

[45] Professor Andrew Lees (personal communication, 28/07/2025) has pointed out to me that Charcot attended the BMA meeting in Leeds in 1869 (discussed in Chap. 3), as documented in *BMJ* 1869;2:279–280 (4th September; Members present at the Leeds Meeting), an event which included an invitation from Crichton-Browne to visit the nearby West Riding Asylum at Wakefield, which took place on Wednesday 28th July 1869. I have not been able to discover whether or not Charcot availed himself of this opportunity to visit; no list of the visitors was included in either *BMJ* 1869;2:168 (7th August; Visit to the West Riding Asylum) or *Lancet* 1869;2:312 (28th August; The West Riding Pauper Lunatic Asylum (Wakefield)).

[46] I have found only one pertinent publication, and this was merely a case under his care (*Lancet* 1868;1:720–721 (6th June; Provincial Hospital Reports. West Riding Pauper Lunatic Asylum.)), although he also made some comments based on his clinical experience at WRA, regarding general paralysis of the insane, at the Medico-Psychological Association meeting in January 1871 (*J Ment Sci* 1871–1872;17(April 1871):147–149). Although the primary affiliation listed in Crichton Browne (1867), is "West York County Lunatic Asylum" the paper is in fact based on lectures delivered in Newcastle in the summer of 1866. It is possible that his course of lectures offered to medical students attending WRA from 1871 (Crichton Browne 1871d, f, 1872b, 1873, 1874a) may be based on clinical material seen during his initial years at WRA. Despite his limited publication record, he was nevertheless elected FRSE in 1870.

[47] He informed Darwin in June 1870 that "As a rule I *toil* daily from 8. a.m. to 11. pm. contending all the while with bad health & great anxiety." [italics in original]. Darwin Correspondence Project, "Letter no. 7220,"

https://www.darwinproject.ac.uk/letter/?docId=letters/DCP-LETT-72200.xml   (accessed 11/12/2024).

[48] He had also communicated two cases to Henry Maudsley, as mentioned in the latter's Gulstonian Lectures of 1870 (Maudsley 1870a:47, 49). Also Maudsley (1870b:610).

himself did follow once the AMO/Clinical Clerk system was well-established and the *WRLAMR* had been founded. These publications were not confined to *WRLAMR* (although he was its most prolific contributor), and included not only further instalments in a series of lectures on mental and cerebral diseases[49] and occasional case reports and series[50] but also review articles[51] and even laboratory based experimental research (nearly 100 experiments).[52] Unsurprisingly, some of his therapeutic interests were later researched and published on by junior Asylum staff (e.g. ergot of rye by Churchill Fox; conium by Burman; chloral hydrate by Wallis; *vide infra*). Further cases "Under the care of Dr. Crichton Browne" also appeared in the journals, presumably based on information in the WRA case books written by the AMOs and Clinical Assistants.[53]

Crichton-Browne's clinical work sometimes extended beyond the walls of the Asylum. On at least one occasion he visited a patient at the direction of the Commissioners in Lunacy, according to a report of the case heard at the York Assizes.[54] He also supported moves for the establishment of a "Middle-Class Lunatic Asylum for Yorkshire".[55]

Despite the relative geographical isolation of the Asylum from the town of Wakefield, Crichton-Browne did take some part in municipal affairs. For example, he contributed to Netten Radcliffe's Report, issued by the Medical Department of the Privy Council, on the sanitary state of Wakefield.[56] He reportedly promised to attend the inaugural meeting of the 1870–71 session of the Wakefield Mechanics' Institute,[57] and lectured in the 1870–1871 session ("Observations on Obsequies").[58] As for local scientific endeavours, however, he does not appear to have attended the Wakefield Microscopic

---

[49] Crichton Browne (1871d, f, 1872b, 1873, 1874a). The second of the two parts of his 1873 paper in the *BMJ* was immediately followed by Ferrier's first report ("Preliminary Notice") of his researches on cerebral localisation based on his experimental work at WRA (Ferrier 1873a; to be discussed in Chap. 7).

[50] Crichton Browne (1871a, b, c, e, 1872a, 1874b, c).

[51] Crichton Browne (1873–1874, 1875–1876b).

[52] Crichton Browne (1875a).

[53] *BMJ* 1875;1:345 (13th March; West Riding Asylum. Obstruction of the bowel by a biliary calculus. (Under the care of Dr. Crichton Browne.)); *BMJ* 1875;1:774 (12th June; West Riding Asylum. Case of apoplexy of the cerebellum. (Under the care of Dr. Crichton Browne.)).

[54] *BMJ* 1873;1:378 (5th April; Profit and wilful negligence).

[55] *BMJ* 1873;2:678–679 (6th December; Middle-Class Lunatic Asylum for Yorkshire); *The Wakefield Free Press and West-Riding Advertiser*, 6th December 1873, p3, col. 2 (A middle class asylum for the West Riding).

[56] Anon., 1870. He was not mentioned in *Lancet* 1870;1:59 (8th January; The sanitary state of Wakefield), nor *BMJ* 1870;1:65–66 (15th January; The sanitary state of Wakefield). See also Marland (1987:343).

[57] *Wakefield and West Riding Herald*, 30th September 1870, p.2. *Wakefield Free Press*, 1st October 1870, p.4; and 8th October 1870, p.4. Dr. "Thos. G. Wright" was also amongst those promising to attend.

[58] Marland (1987:338).

Society, founded in 1854 but effectively moribund by 1871, even though one of the four remaining members was Dr. T.G. Wright, visiting physician to the Asylum (see Chap. 2).[59]

Crichton-Browne also appeared on the broader medical scene, for example as Lecturer on Mental Diseases to the Leeds School of Medicine. As well as the MPA and the British Medical Association (BMA), he was also active in what one might call the associative aspect of clinical medicine through his attendance at other medical societies (e.g. The Leeds and West Riding Medico-Chirurgical Society[60]; the Medical Society of London[61]) and clubs (e.g. Edinburgh University Club[62]). He was an indefatigable correspondent to the *BMJ*, although rarely published, on topical matters.[63]

When, in 1875, John Charles Bucknill resigned as the Chancery Visitor in Lunacy, Crichton-Browne's name was (first) amongst those several candidates mentioned as potential successors.[64] In fact he had been temporarily appointed whilst the incumbent, Bucknill, was on sick leave, as noted in the *Lancet*'s announcement of his official appointment to the Visitorship of Chancery Lunatics in December 1875.[65] Hence, according to the *BMJ* announcement, "The appointment had been foreseen".[66]

Crichton-Browne's departure from Wakefield was prolonged affair. After the announcement, a memorial was presented to him by "Dr Merson, Deputy Medical Director" on behalf of the WRA staff on 23rd March 1876.[67] There were further presentations at a banquet held at the Bull Hotel in Wakefield on

---

[59] Ibid., 307, 337.

[60] *BMJ* 1872;2:640 (7th December; Formation of a Medical Society for the West Riding); *BMJ* 1873;1:622–623 (31st May; The Leeds and West Riding Medico-Chirurgical Society); *BMJ* 1874;1:690 (23rd May; Leeds and West Riding Medico-Chirurgical Society). He was on the Committee in 1873 and 1874, as was Allbutt.

[61] *BMJ* 1875;1:618 (8th May; The Medical Society of London).

[62] *BMJ* 1869;2:217 (21st August; Edinburgh University Club); *BMJ* 1874;1:722 (30th May; Manchester Edinburgh University Club).

[63] For example, *BMJ* 1874;2:158–159 (1st August); *BMJ* 1875;1:757 (5th June).

[64] *BMJ* 1875;2:710 (4th December).

[65] *Lancet* 1875;2:896 (18th December; Medical Appointments).

[66] *BMJ* 1875;2:760 (18th December; Lunacy Appointment). The appointment was also noted in *Medical Times and Gazette* 1875;2:683 (18th December; The Visitorship of Chancery Lunatics) which was reprinted in *Wakefield and West Riding Herald*, 24th December 1875, p.4 (Dr. Crichton Browne's resignation); *J Ment Sci* 1875–1876;21(January 1876):633 (Appointments); *Yorkshire Post and Leeds Intelligencer*, 13th December 1875, p.3 (Visitor of Lunatics); *Leeds Mercury*, 17th December 1875, p.3 (Dr. Crichton Browne).

[67] *Medical Times and Gazette* 1876;1:365–366 (1st April; Dr Crichton Browne). Also *Medical Press and Circular* 1876;21:283 (5th April; Dr. Crichton Browne); *BMJ* 1876;1:449 (8th April; The West Riding Asylum).

18th April.[68] On 10th May, there was a "meeting of the past medical officers and others associated with the West Riding Asylum, … held at 6, Trevor-terrace".[69] Subscribers to the testimonial gift presented at the latter included many former WRA resident medical staff including Aldridge, Burman, Clapham, Courtenay, Dove, Fox, Galton, Lawrence, Lawson, Lowe, Major, Mayhew, Merson, Mitchell, Newcombe, Pedler, Sutherland, Wallis, Bywater Ward, "Dr. J. Ferra Watson", Woods and Wright (all discussed below); as well as a number of other clinicians who had been associated with WRA either through publication in *WRLAMR* and/or visiting to see patients or undertake experimental work: Lennox Browne, Lauder Brunton, Ferrier, Milner Fothergill, "Hughlings-Jackson" [*sic*, with hyphen], and Octavius Sankey (see Chap. 7 for details of all these individuals).[70] For good measure, the *Medical Times and Gazette* chipped in with an editorial, adulatory of Crichton-Browne's work at WRA.[71] One wonders if Crichton-Browne was more absent than present from WRA in late 1875 and 1876.[72]

In the years immediately after his departure from WRA, Crichton-Browne became president of the MPA (1878); although his presidential address (his name now hyphenated) made no specific reference to WRA, his statement that "every asylum takes its complexion from its medical head"[73] may have been a wistful look back to those years. With the cessation of publication of his brain-child, the *WRLAMR*, he went on to become one of the founders of a new journal, *Brain: a journal of neurology* (1878), along with John Charles Bucknill, David Ferrier, and John Hughlings Jackson. He continued to

---

[68] *Medical Times and Gazette* 1876;1:445–446 (22nd April). Further details of the dinner may be found in *BMJ* 1876;1:516 (22nd April; Dr. Crichton Browne); *Medical Press and Circular* 1876;21:348 (26th April; The West Riding Asylum); and *Lancet* 1876;1:647 (29th April). It was also reported in the local press: *Leeds Mercury*, 19th April 1876, p.8 (Dinner and presentation to Dr. Crichton Browne), and *Yorkshire Post and Leeds Intelligencer*, 19th April 1876, p.3 (Presentations to Dr. Crichton Browne). The latter gave some details of those present, including many with WRA connections: Lawson, Major, W. Wood, W.D. Wood, and T.G. Wright from Wakefield; Allbutt from Leeds; and Rabagliati from Bradford. Crichton-Browne of course gave an address: *BMJ* 1876;1:604–605 (13th May; Science Fellowships).

[69] *Lancet* 1876;1:726 (13th May; Medical News). I presume this was in London, as the address is that of George Henry Pedler (*vide infra*). Trevor Terrace was part of the Trevor Estate development in Knightsbridge: https://www.british-history.ac.uk/survey-london/vol45/pp97-102 (accessed 29/09/2024).

[70] *Medical Times and Gazette* 1876;1:529–530 (13th May; Presentation to Dr. Crichton Browne).

[71] *Medical Times and Gazette* 1876;1:524–525 (13th May; Lunacy and science).

[72] I wonder if an illness is also a possibility. In "A Reminiscence", Crichton-Browne (1926:305–306) reports "a dangerous illness" in which an old song heard at the age of five is recalled "thirty years after-wards". If these dates are correct (a big supposition), the illness would have occurred when Crichton-Browne was 35, which locates it somewhere between November 1875 and November 1876. His final entry in the WRA Medical Director's Journal was on 27th January 1876 (Finn 2012:165–166 and n539).

[73] Crichton-Browne (1878–1879:352).

publish therein, using data gathered at WRA.[74] His connection with neurology was also evident in his appointment as the inaugural vice-president of the Neurological Society of London when this organisation was founded in 1886, with Hughlings Jackson as President (see Chap. 10 for discussion of Crichton-Browne and neurology). He was elected FRS in 1883, proposed by John Charles Bucknill and seconded (posthumously!) by Charles Darwin.[75] He was knighted in 1886, was President of the Neurological Society of London in 1888, and of the Medical Society of London in 1895. He remained active into his later years, publishing several books of reminiscences.[76] He died in 1938 at the age of 97, at the time the oldest and longest serving FRS.[77]

Evidently, Crichton-Browne was a man of extraordinary energy, indeed there is something Dickensian about the exhausting multiplicity of his interests and his breadth of vision. He had the happy facility to implement his plans successfully, not least through his sociable nature and his ability to influence those around him to share and support his aspirations. However, he did on occasion overpromise and underdeliver. For example, a mooted series of "Monographs on mental diseases" never materialised,[78] likewise his plan to place on record further cases of the success of nitrite of amyl in status epilepticus (III:174) for which there was reported to be insufficient space in *WRLAMR*.[79] Another, later project which appears never to have reached fruition, was a "MANUAL OF LUNATIC HOSPITAL MANAGEMENT AND HYGIENE. By J. CRICHTON BROWNE, M.D., F.R.S.C.E. [*sic*]", advertised as a new work in preparation in the end papers of the final volume of *WRLAMR*.[80]

Central to realising Crichton-Browne's scientific ambitions for WRA was the appointment of resident staff who could fulfil not only clinical roles but also undertake research work at the Asylum, under his direction, of a standard suitable for dissemination through journal publications and meeting

---

[74] His paper "On the weight of the brain and its component parts in the insane" (*Brain* 1879–1880;2(1):42–67) was later credited with being one of the first to find "that the right hemisphere is longer, wider, and generally larger, as well as heavier, than the left" (McGilchrist 2019:33, 466n2).

[75] Easterbrook (1938:297).

[76] Crichton-Browne (1926, 1927, 1930, 1931, 1932, 1937, 1938) (the last not seen by me).

[77] Obituaries: *BMJ* 1938;1:311–312 (5th February); Easterbrook (1938) and Holmes (1939).

[78] *BMJ* 1874;1:210 (14th February; Monographs on Mental Diseases). See Chap. 6, section on "Origins and aims of *WRLAMR*" for further details.

[79] "The space at my disposal will not permit me to report three other cases, in which the status epilepticus was beneficially influenced by nitrite of amyl inhalation. At some future time I shall place these on record, and shall describe my further experience with this agent in the treatment of epilepsy" (III:174).

[80] Capitals in original. Presumably as Visitor of Chancery Lunatics as of December 1875 he was too busy to deliver the book or had perhaps become too distanced from the subject of "lunatic hospital management and hygiene".

presentations. Those individuals appointed during the Crichton-Browne years, 1866 to 1876, both AMOs and Clinical Clerks/Assistants, will now be considered (Table 5.1).

Charles Fox Oxley, Charles Fryer and W. P. Ledgard

Junior staff would obviously have been in post at WRA at the time of Crichton-Browne's arrival in 1866. Although definitive detail is lacking, the junior doctors in post at WRA at this time were most probably Charles Etheridge and George Thomas Mitchell Southam (see Chap. 3). Southam departed on 5th March 1867, and Etheridge possibly in April. In the Medical Director's Journal, Crichton-Browne noted that:

> Mr. Charles Fox Oxley who was appointed in his [Southam's] place at the special meeting upon the 23rd of February [1867] entered upon his duties a few days afterwards.[81]

Charles Fox Oxley thus appears to have been Crichton-Browne's first appointment at WRA.[82] As of 1869, "Oxley, Chas. Fox" appears in the *Medical Directory*, and as of 1872 his "late" posts included "Asst. Surg. Wakefield Lunat. Asyl.".[83]

Oxley's role may have been only temporary, a stopgap following Southam's departure, since in April of 1867, Crichton-Browne appointed his first Clinical Clerks:

> In accordance with the authority granted to me at the special meeting above mentioned, I have inquired for gentlemen, properly qualified to fill the office of Clinical Clerk, & have now to recommend that Dr. Charles Fryer, & Dr. W.P. Ledgard, whose testimonials I submit, should be appointed Clinical Clerks

---

[81] Medical Director's Journal 25th April 1867 (WYAS C85/1/13/1) [my transcription].

[82] However, I have not encountered Oxley's name in any other publication related to WRA that I have seen. He was not included in Finn's list (2012:181–184) of those working as either medical officers or clinical clerks at WRA between 1866 and 1876.

[83] The *Medical Directory* of 1869 (140) listed Oxley as "(*Address unknown*)—L.R.C.P. Edin. 1866; M.R.C.S. Eng. 1864; (*Univ. Edin.* and *Westm.*)" [italics in original]. In the *Medical Directory* of 1872 (526) he was listed as "Res. Med. Off. Toxteth-park Fev. Hosp. Liverpool – L.R.C.P. Edin. 1866; M.R.C.S. Eng. 1864; (*Univ. Edin.* and *Westm.*); late House Phys. Westm. Hosp.; Asst. Surg. Wakefield Lunat. Asyl., and Surg. Roy. Mail S.S. Co.".

for a period of three months, subject to immediate removal in case of misconduct or inefficiency, without salary but with board & lodging supplied to them.[84]

In the *Journal of Mental Science* issue for July 1867, the Appointments section noted:

Dr. Fryer, F.L.S., &c., late Senior Resident Medical Officer at St. Mary's Hospital, Manchester, has been appointed Physician's Assistant to the West Riding of York Lunatic Asylum.[85]

Charles Fryer appeared in the *Medical Directory* from 1867 onwards.[86] He trained in Manchester (Owens College and Lock Hospital), his entry from 1869 onwards noting not only his Fellowship of the Linnean Society (FLS), a large number of prizes (and their monetary amounts), and publications in the *Naturalist* in the 1850s, but also his appointment as "late Res. Phys. Asst. W. R. York Co. Lunatic Asyl.".

No "W.P. Ledgard" has been identified in the *Medical Directory*, but as of 1869 there is a "Ledgard, William Edwd." with addresses in Gateshead and then Ripon but no mention of any previous appointments. In view of the dates of his qualifications (MRCS Eng 1868, LRCP Edin & LM 1870) from St George's and the University of Durham, I think it possible that he may have been the "W.P. Ledgard" referred to by Crichton-Browne.

In the *Report* for 1867 (published 1868) the Chairman noted that "The two Assistant Medical Officers having during the present year, sent in their resignation with a view to professional promotion; Dr. SAMUEL MITCHELL, and Mr. GEORGE THOMPSON, Surgeon, have been appointed in their stead.".[87]

---

[84] Medical Director's Journal 25th April 1867 (WYAS C85/1/13/1) [my transcription]. Also cited in part by Finn (2012:72). Finn did not include either Fryer or Ledgard in his list (2012:181–184) of those working as either medical officers or clinical clerks at WRA between 1866 and 1876 although he acknowledged elsewhere (2012:122) that they were the first two clinical clerks in Wakefield.

[85] *J Ment Sci* 1867–1868;13(July 1867):284 (Appointments). *Lancet* 1867;1:687 (1st June; Medical Appointments [Orton]) noted Fryer's resignation from St Mary's Hospital, Manchester; his appointment there as Assistant House-Surgeon had been noted in *Lancet* 1866;2:567 (17th November; Medical Appointments).

[86] From 1876 he appears as Charles Sherburn Fryer. Whether or not related, he was appointed Medical Officer for the Sherburn District of the Scarborough Union in early 1875 according to *Medical Press and Circular* 1875;19:176 (24th February; Appointments).

[87] *Report* (1868:8) [capitals in original]. I find no mention of either Mitchell or Thompson in the Medical Director's Journal for the Quarterly Meeting of 25th July 1867 (WYAS C85/1/13/2); although signed by Crichton-Browne, this entry is not in his handwriting (and hence easier to read!). An example of Crichton-Browne's handwriting may be seen in Finn (2012:129, Fig. 3.10).

In the *Report* for the year 1868 (published in 1869), the Commissioners in Lunacy noted "In other parts of the medical records we observe arrears which we attribute to the shortcomings of the former Assistant-Surgeons, who have recently been succeeded by Dr. Mitchell and Mr. Thompson",[88] but no names were mentioned so it is not clear whether or not Fryer and/or Ledgard were those over whom a cloud of suspicion hung. If so, it is difficult to imagine how, in an era when personal recommendation was key to appointments, "their resignation with a view to professional promotion" as recorded in the previous year's *Report* could possibly materialise, unless their misdemeanours had gone unnoticed up to that time.[89] The designation of the presumed miscreants as "former Assistant-Surgeons", rather than Clinical Clerks, may possibly inculpate Oxley, Etheridge, or Southam.

Neither Fryer not Ledgard published in *WRLAMR*, perhaps being appointed too early and for too brief a period for that possibility to arise. Neither published in the *Journal of Mental Science*, although Fryer did publish a case report in the *Medical Press and Circular* in 1870.[90]

George Thompson (Born?1842[91])

In the *Lancet* issue dated 10th August 1867, the following note appeared:

> G. THOMPSON, M.R.C.S., has been appointed Resident Clinical Clerk in the West Riding Lunatic Asylum, Wakefield.[92]

Three weeks later the *Lancet* carried the following note:

> - THOMPSON, M.R.C.S.E, has been appointed Physicians' Assistant at the West Riding Asylum, Wakefield, vice Dr. Fryer, whose term of office has expired.[93]

At the end of the year, 14th December, a third announcement appeared:

---

[88] *Report* (1869:12).

[89] One of the Lunacy Commissioners who produced this report was Cleaton, Crichton-Browne's immediate predecessor as Medical Superintendent at WRA (see Chap. 2).

[90] Fryer (1870).

[91] "Estimated birth year" in the 1871 census.

[92] *Lancet* 1867;2:184 (10th August; Medical Appointments) [capitals in original]. Also *J Ment Sci* 1867;13(October 1867):434 (Appointments).

[93] *Lancet* 1867;2:283 (31st August; Medical Appointments). [capitals in original].

G. THOMPSON, M.R.C.S.E, has been promoted from the Office of Clinical Clerk to that of Assistant Medical Officer to the West Riding Lunatic Asylum, Wakefield.[94]

Both a native and a graduate of Leeds, Thompson was thus appointed AMO at the same time as Samuel Mitchell (*vide infra*).

According to the *Report* for the year 1867, these AMO appointments were made in October and duties commenced on 1st November: "These gentlemen have already displayed great energy and capacity, and promise to become most valuable members of the staff" according to Crichton-Browne's report.[95]

At the Quarterly Meeting on 30th January 1868, Crichton-Browne wrote that:

> The Medical Assistants appointed at the last Meeting entered upon their duties on the 1st of November and have, up to this time, proved themselves most efficient and agreeable officers. I have to request the Committee to confirm the appointment of Mr. George Thompson, the Junior assistant who has been on probation for 3 months.[96]

Evidence of this "energy and capacity" may be deemed to include Thompson's ophthalmological observations in a dying patient which were later published by Aldridge (I:73), and the notes "furnished by Mr. Geo. Thompson, Assistant Medical Officer, Male Department" which formed the basis of a report of a patient "under the care of Dr. Crichton Browne", a case of poisoning by the chloride of ammonium, which was published in the *Lancet* in 1868.[97] Thompson became a Licentiate of the Royal College of Physicians in the same year[98] and was elected to membership of the MPA in 1869.[99]

Aside from his purely clinical work at WRA, from around 1868 (I:58) George Thompson pioneered the use of the sphygmograph at the Asylum, a medical device which transcribed a patient's arterial pulse pressure on to

---

[94] *Lancet* 1867;2:754 (14th December; Medical Appointments) [capitals in original].

[95] *Report* (1868:25).

[96] Medical Director's Journal 30th January 1868 (WYAS C85/1/13/2) [my transcription]. I find no mention of either Thompson or Mitchell in the Medical Director's Journal for the prior Quarterly Meeting, 31st October 1867.

[97] *Lancet* 1868;1:720–721 (6th June; Provincial Hospital Reports. West Riding Pauper Lunatic Asylum. (Under the care of Dr. Crichton Browne.)); quote at 721.

[98] *Lancet* 1868;2:135 (25th July; Medical News).

[99] *J Ment Sci* 1869–1870;15(October 1869):464 (Psychological News. New members).

paper.[100] Thompson published two papers on the sphygmograph in *WRLAMR*, "The sphygmograph in lunatic asylum practice" (I:58–70) and "The sphygmograph in epilepsy" (II:302–306).

The first described the sphygmographic findings in patients with general paralysis of the insane, and Thompson's belief was that tracings could be used to confirm the clinical diagnosis (e.g. I:65).[101] In the latter paper, he suggested that a particular trace form was "the type while the epileptic 'status' exists" (II:305). His tracings in this clinical context were referred to by a later WRA clinician, Newcombe (V:218).

Thompson worked at Wakefield until 1871.[102] Having "with great discretion and assiduity, discharged the duties of Assistant Medical Officer here for a period of nearly four years",[103] he was then appointed Medical Superintendent of the Bristol Lunatic Asylum, Stapleton.[104] Indeed by the time of his two publications in *WRLAMR* he was listed as "Medical Superintendent of the Bristol City and County Lunatic-Asylum; late Assistant Medical Officer, and formerly Clinical Assistant, at the West Riding Asylum, Wakefield", and at least one patient in his second *WRLAMR* paper was from Bristol (and possibly all three of them).

After his move to the Bristol Lunatic Asylum, Thompson published in the *Journal of Mental Science*[105] but never in *Brain*. In the first of these papers, "On the physiology of general paralysis of the insane", Thompson reported of his two *WRLAMR* publications that "Both papers had been hastily prepared, though they really represented an amount of patient labour such as probably I shall never undertake again. The later one had also the disadvantage of being so cut and mutilated for want of space that, when finished, I hardly recognised my own work".[106] Thompson's paper drew a response from Crichton-

---

[100] For an account of the sphygmograph in asylum practice, see Wallis (2017b). Further discussion of sphygmography at WRA in this period is deferred to Chap. 6.

[101] A view possibly shared by Aldridge (*vide infra*), who says of one of his patients (II:228): "his pulse tracing was found to be that so characteristic of general paralysis of the insane."

[102] Thompson is listed in the 1871 census (taken Sunday 2nd April 1871) as "Medical Officer", aged 29, and a member of Crichton-Browne's household. White's *Directory* (1870:533) listed him as "house surgeon".

[103] *Report* (1872:32).

[104] *Lancet* 1871;1:730 (27th May; Medical Appointments); *Medical Times and Gazette* 1871;1:620 (27th May; Medical News); *Medical Press and Circular* 1871;11:478 (31st May; Appointments); *J Ment Sci* 1871–1872;17(July 1871):308 (Appointments).

[105] Finn (2012:183) reported two publications by George Thompson in the *Journal of Mental Science*, but I find four in all, published between 1874 and 1875 (Thompson 1873–1874, 1874–1875a, b, 1875–1876).

[106] Thompson (1874–1875b:579). Can the words "so cut and mutilated for want of space that, when finished, I hardly recognised my own work" be read as anything other than a criticism of Crichton-Browne as editor?

Browne, chastising Thompson for falling "into a grievous error in representing me as having confidence in the Calabar Bean as a *cure* for General Paralysis" rather than it having "a valuable power of modifying and arresting the progress" of the disease, and stating that his (Crichton-Browne's) report on two cases in the *BMJ* "were published in the form which they there assumed without my knowledge or sanction, and much to my regret".[107] As the *BMJ* paper in question[108] was a single author report by Crichton-Browne, his objections are a little hard to fathom, unless he had delegated the writing and handling of the paper to Thompson but without crediting his junior, and/or attending to what had been written (whoever the author might have been), a scenario that seems implausible to me. Certainly, Thompson had encountered patients treated with Calabar bean and recorded their sphygmographs whilst at WRA (I:67–70).

Thompson remained at the asylum in Bristol until he retired in 1890.[109] During his superintendency he ended use of the seclusion room and of the beer ration (1883) and pioneered the use of hyoscine in the treatment of mania, as reported in the *Lancet* in 1888.[110] This publication made no mention of the work at WRA in the 1870s on the related compound hyoscyamine, published by Robert Lawson[111] (*vide infra*).

Samuel Mitchell[112]

In the *Lancet* issue dated 14th December 1867, the following note appeared:

> S. MITCHELL, M.D., M.C., has been appointed Senior Assistant Medical Officer to the West Riding Asylum, Wakefield.[113]

However, as previously mentioned, in the *Report* for 1867 his appointment as AMO was made in October and commenced on 1st November, at the same

---

[107] Crichton Browne (1875–1876a) [capitals and italics in original]. See Thompson (1874–1875b:580), for his claim that Crichton-Browne's report is of cure.

[108] Thompson explicitly identified this paper as "in the 'British Medical Journal' for October 24th, 1874". Hence, in the current Bibliography, this is Crichton Browne (1874c).

[109] For some details of Thompson's career in Bristol, see Tobia (2017), where he is described as a "man of science" (250), as compared to his "humanitarian" predecessor.

[110] Thompson (1888).

[111] See V:40–84, IV:65–84, and Lawson (1876b).

[112] Biographical material on Mitchell may be found in Ashworth (1975:72).

[113] *Lancet* 1867;2:754 (14th December; Medical Appointments) [capitals in original].

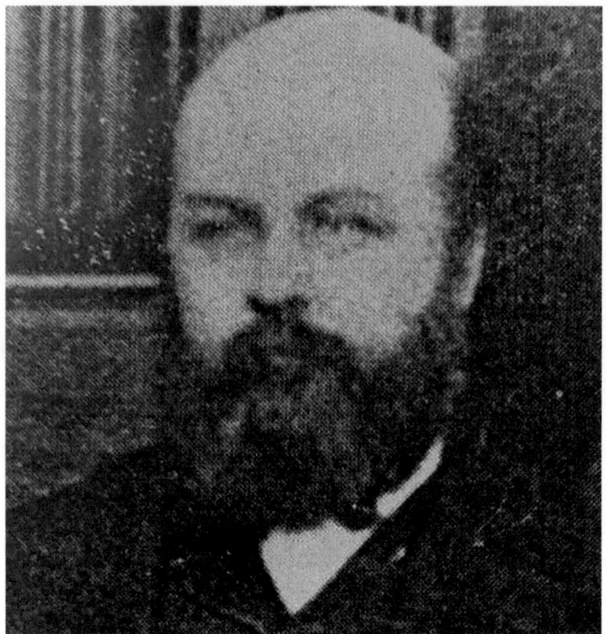

Fig. 5.1 Samuel Mitchell

time as George Thompson.[114] The fact that he was "Dr." whilst Thompson was still "Mr." suggests he was the senior in terms of his qualifications (he was listed in the *Medical Directory* as of 1868 with training in Edinburgh,[115] Paris, and Berlin). Indeed, Mitchell was promoted to "Deputy Superintendent" in late 1868, Charles Aldridge (*vide infra*) taking his place as AMO.[116]

The *Report* for 1868 noted that, as Senior Assistant Medical Officer, Mitchell (Fig. 5.1) had been placed in temporary charge of the "Auxiliary Establishment" opened at Mount Pleasant at Sheffield; "in whose judgment and discretion I have every confidence" reported Crichton-Browne, who visited weekly.[117] Mitchell was elected to membership of the MPA in 1869,[118] and in the autumn of 1870 spent four months on a visit to "Continental Asylums".[119] Having "most ably conducted the Mount Pleasant Branch of this

---

[114] *Report* (1868:25).

[115] *Alphabetical list of graduates of the University of Edinburgh ...*, 1889:63. MB CM, 1865; MD 1867.

[116] *Lancet* 1868;2:786 (12th December; Medical Appointments). Also *J Ment Sci* 1868–1869;14(January 1869):604 (Appointments).

[117] *Report* (1869:6, 17, 26 (quotation), 34). Also, Thorpe (1972:6).

[118] *J Ment Sci* 1869–1870;15(October 1869):464 (Psychological News. New members). The actual wording is "Mitchell, B.S." but the affiliation is correct.

[119] *Report* (1871:27).

Asylum in Sheffield for the four years of its existence" (1868–1872) he "had his merits recognised and rewarded, by his appointment to the important position of Medical Superintendent of the South Yorkshire Asylum" in 1872.[120] Many years later, Hack Tuke reported that "Wadsley was fortunate in securing the services of Dr. Mitchell".[121]

Mitchell published two papers in *WRLAMR*. Firstly, "Observations on the physiological action of nitrous oxide" (I:27–57), where he is listed as "Deputy Medical Director West Riding Asylum, and Physician to the Sheffield Hospital and Dispensary". Prompted by the attention nitrous oxide (N_2O) had received as an anaesthetic agent,[122] Mitchell set out to examine possible therapeutic uses by means of inhalation of the gas, experiments involving not only animals (rabbits) but also humans: he "administered it both to my friends and to certain patients suffering from melancholia" (I:44) as well as to himself (I:45–48).[123] The paper also included sphygmographic recordings made by George Thompson (I:49). A second paper followed, "Experiments to ascertain the effects of ether and nitrous oxide combined, to which are added some general observations on stimulants" (II:73–96), looking not only at these two substances but also at chloroform. After limited animal experiments (rabbits), Mitchell "proceeded to experiment on myself, and on such of my friends as were willing to join me in the investigation" (II:77).[124] Patients administered nitrous oxide by Mitchell were also examined by Aldridge (*vide infra*), and Mitchell's work was later cited by Harrington Tuke in his Presidential address to the MPA in 1873.[125]

---

[120] *Report* (1873:27). Also, Thorpe (1972:12).

[121] Hack Tuke (1889a:368, 1889b:11). Hack Tuke also referred to Mitchell in his work *on the provision for the insane poor in Yorkshire* (1889b:23, 24, 27, 29).

[122] On nitrous oxide see, for example, Snow (2008:11–20) and Stratmann (2003:11–15).

[123] This human work of Mitchell's was recalled many years later by Crichton-Browne (1895:73; see also 1927:33) in a lecture on dreamy states. He stated that Mitchell administered nitrous oxide to himself and to a "medical man"; indeed, Mitchell's account included mention of a "Dr. N–" (possibly Dr. Patrick Nicol?) who whilst under the influence of the drug "imagined that he had made a very important discovery" (I:44), which tallies with Crichton-Browne's account.

[124] Mitchell's account included a "Dr. E–" and a "Mr. J–" (II:78–79) but none of the WRA junior staff known to me have surnames beginning with either of these letters. If these initials refer to first names, the options, based on timing, might include E. Churchill Fox, J. Wilkie Burman, and J. Bywater Ward, but this is entirely guess work on my part. Of possible relevance, however, Mitchell was himself an experimental subject in the work of Burman (*vide infra*), who injected him with conia (II:16).

[125] Harrington Tuke (1873:448). At time of writing [2023], Mitchell's interest in nitrous oxide has a contemporary resonance, as increasing numbers of patients, usually young, who have symptoms following exposure to N_2O as a recreational drug, for example in "whippets", are currently seen in neurological practice, as a consequence of functional vitamin B_{12} deficiency causing demyelination of the spinal cord dorsal columns (Paris et al. 2023).

By the time of his second *WRLAMR* paper, Mitchell was listed as "Medical Superintendent, South Yorkshire Asylum, Late Assistant Medical Officer, West Riding Asylum". This promotion occurred around March 1872.[126] During the remainder of his career he published neither in the *Journal of Mental Science* nor subsequently in *Brain*. He resigned in 1888 on the grounds of ill-health, possibly related to the ever-increasing number of admissions to the Sheffield Asylum. However, after "a long sojourn abroad" his health was restored.[127] Joseph Shaw Bolton, a later WRA Superintendent, reported of Mitchell that "during the Great War in his old age [he] left his retirement to afford us valuable temporary help".[128]

Charles Aldridge[129] (1847–1919)

Born in Leeds, Charles Aldridge received his medical training there. He worked under Clifford Allbutt (for whom, see Chap. 7), then a physician in Leeds, as acknowledged in a publication in the *BMJ* dated 20th June 1868 in which Allbutt reported that:

> The following two cases of arthritis, granular(?) kidney and atheroma, and of polydipsia, lately occurred in my practice at the Leeds Infirmary. They were reported, with other cases, by Mr. Aldridge, the successful competitor for the Hardwicke prize in Clinical Medicine at this school. The notes were so carefully taken, that I have thought it worth while to send these two cases for publication. I have necessarily condensed Mr. Aldridge's notes very much, in order to save space. I have, for the same reason, been obliged almost to suppress his comments. I have not altered in any way the substance of his records, nor have I inserted anything of my own.[130]

Allbutt later described Aldridge as "my old pupil" and "my friend and former pupil … now one of the resident medical officers of the Wakefield Asylum";

---

[126] *BMJ* 1872;1:303 (16th March; Medical Appointments); *Medical Press and Circular* 1872;13:266 (20th March). In the announcement appearing in *J Ment Sci* 1872–1873;18(April 1872):152 (Appointments), Mitchell was described as "Medical Superintendent [*sic*], and formerly Assistant Medical Officer" at WRA, evidently an error of omission (should read "Deputy Medical Superintendent").

[127] Thorpe (1972:19).

[128] Bolton (1928:609). Thorpe (1972:19) reported that Mitchell was a locum tenens medical officer at Wakefield Asylum during the First World War, when he was presumably in his mid-70s

[129] Biographical material on Aldridge may be found in Todd and Ashworth (1991:399–400).

[130] *BMJ* 1868;1:610–611 (20th June; Leeds General Infirmary. Medical Cases). The first case included an ophthalmoscopic examination.

and in Allbutt's monograph on ophthalmoscopy Aldridge's drawing of the fundus of a patient seen by Allbutt on 23rd August 1866 was included.[131]

Aldridge became a Licentiate of the Royal College of Physicians of London in 1868, at the same time as George Thompson, the notice of this award locating him at "West Riding Asylum, Wakefield".[132] His appointment as AMO (to the Female Department) was noted in the *Lancet* in December of that year[133] and the presumption that he was a Clinical Clerk or Clinical Assistant prior to this is confirmed in a further note, of his promotion to AMO which appeared in the *Lancet* in January 1869.[134] He was elected to membership of the MPA in 1869.[135] Aldridge is listed in the 1871 national census (taken Sunday 2nd April 1871) as "Assistant Officer", aged 23, and a member of Crichton-Browne's household.

Aldridge's clinical work may be seen in a case report later published by Crichton-Browne who noted that, in his capacity of AMO to the Female Department, Aldridge was "called to see" a patient on 22nd August 1869.[136] Crichton-Browne also credited Aldridge with being the first to detect the earliest appearance of the rash associated with chloral hydrate treatment.[137] Aldridge also communicated details of a case of chronic mania managed with hypodermic injection of morphia to Bywater Ward (I:157).

Aside from these general clinical activities, Aldridge distinguished himself by taking up the cause of ophthalmoscopy at WRA,[138] the clinical application of which was thoroughly explored in three papers in *WRLAMR*. In this endeavour, he was following the previous work at WRA of Clifford Allbutt, an interest which is not surprising considering that Aldridge had worked for, and may even have been a protégé of, Allbutt in Leeds. A demonstration of the reflecting ophthalmoscope given by Brudenell Carter at the inaugural WRA medical *conversazione* in October 1871 (see Chap. 8) might have acted as a further stimulus to this work, but since Aldridge's first paper in *WRLAMR*,

---

[131] Allbutt (1871a:230, 278, 349) (Case 96).

[132] *Lancet* 1868;2:135 (25th July; Medical News). *BMJ* 1868;2:98 (25th July; Medical News) has "W.R. Asylum, Wakefield" for both Aldridge and Thompson. White's *Directory* (1870:533) listed both Aldridge and Thompson as "house surgeons".

[133] *Lancet* 1868;2:786 (12th December; Medical Appointments). Also *J Ment Sci* 1868–1869;14(January 1869):604 (Appointments).

[134] *Lancet* 1869;1:106 (16th January; Medical Appointments).

[135] *J Ment Sci* 1869–1870;15(October 1869):464 (Psychological News. New members).

[136] Crichton Browne (1871b:222).

[137] Crichton Browne (1871c:473).

[138] Ophthalmological observations were also made by other WRA junior staff: Thompson (I:73); Nicol (I:99), and Arbuckle (1876c). McDowall apparently intended to make ophthalmoscopic observations in his study of colour blindness (III:147 and 152) but none was reported in his paper.

detailing over 100 patients, was published in 1871 (I:71–128) his ophthalmological researches were evidently well advanced by the time Brudenell Carter gave his demonstration. Although this first paper acknowledged the previous work on ophthalmoscopy undertaken by Allbutt, and also by Hughlings Jackson (Chap. 7) and by John Ogle (1824–1905),[139] there is no acknowledgement of any specific input, training, or encouragement from Allbutt.

Aldridge made ophthalmological observations "in mental and cerebral diseases" (I:71–128), "in general paralysis, after the administration of certain toxic agents" (II:223–253), and "in acute dementia" (IV:291–304).[140] He observed the effects of potassium bromide and, more systematically, ergot of rye, nitrite of amyl, nitrous oxide and chloral hydrate (I:94–99), as well as belladonna and hyoscyamus on retinal appearances (II:223–253), the retinal circulation considered to be a proxy for the cerebral circulation. Allbutt noted in his monograph on ophthalmoscopy that Aldridge had examined the effect on the retina of bromide of potassium, ergot,[141] chloral, nitrite of amyl, and nitrous oxide, stating that Aldridge "is now publishing in the first volume of the West Riding Asylum 'Medical Reports' for 1871".[142] Aldridge's presentation of cases at the end of his first paper mirrored Allbutt's presentation of cases in an appendix to his monograph.

Aldridge also reported on 43 patients with general paralysis of the insane (see Chap. 6) undergoing ophthalmological assessment but "in two cases only was there any sign of syphilis" (II:227). He referred to Allbutt's previous report of 51 patients in the *Lancet* of 1868,[143] but although "most of his observations were made upon patients in this asylum … as they occurred four years ago, I have not been able to find one patient alive who was then examined" (II:224–225). Aldridge's studies also involved some experimental work, to observe the effects of picrotoxine, a poison, for which he used cats (including kittens) and rats, indeed bemoaning the fact at one point that "some large

---

[139] For example, see Ogle (1860).

[140] Aldridge's findings in acute dementia were later referenced by William Gowers in his monograph on ophthalmoscopy (1879:163) but his citation to "West Riding Asylum Reports, vol. iii" was incorrect. It is possible that Gowers' references to "Arlidge" (1879:159, 226) should read "Aldridge" since the citations are to "West Riding Asylum Reports, vol. i" and "West Riding Asylum Reports, i, 1871, p.73", of which the latter is definitely by Aldridge. Gowers was presumably confusing Aldridge with John Thomas Arlidge (1822–1899) who spent some time at Hanwell and was resident medical officer at St. Luke's Hospital for Lunatics, and also published on lunacy (e.g. Arlidge 1870) despite pursuing a career as a physician (see John Thomas Arlidge | RCP Museum)

[141] Referencing Crichton Browne (1871e).

[142] Allbutt (1871a:278–280).

[143] Allbutt (1868c).

rats were the only animals I could obtain" (II:241). Aldridge's ophthalmo-scopic work was later mentioned by Crichton-Browne in the context of his own experimental work on picrotoxine.[144] Aldridge also observed the ophthalmological effects of laburnum poisoning (II:243).[145] Other authors mentioning Aldridge's ophthalmoscopic observations included Milner Fothergill (see Chap. 7) in his *WRLAMR* essay on "cerebral anaemia" (at IV:115), and Burman in a case where diagnosis rested largely on the examination by Dr. Aldridge "of the retina with the ophthalmoscope".[146]

In 1872, Aldridge was awarded the degrees MB CM by Aberdeen University, and MD in 1876.[147] Also in 1872, having "been connected with this Asylum as Clinical Clerk and Assistant Medical Officer for four years, and … rendered valuable service", he "entered upon the management of a private Asylum in the South of England".[148] This was located at Plympton in Devon, in which town Aldridge remained for the rest of his life, dying at the age of 71 in 1919.[149] He did not publish in the *Journal of Mental Science* but did make one brief contribution to the Abstracts of British and Foreign Journals section in the first volume of *Brain* (1878–1879).

J. Wilkie Burman (1846–1911)

Born in Southampton, James Wilkie Burman, whose father originated from Newtyle in Angus, was an Edinburgh graduate (MB 1868, MD 1871),[150] and was apparently a pupil there of William Turner, the Professor of Anatomy in the University (see Chap. 9).[151]

---

[144] Crichton Browne (1875a:443).

[145] The patient initials and age but not gender (EB, 30, female) differ from those of the patient with laburnum poisoning published previously by Crichton Browne (1871b) (CH, 28, female) in whom no ophthalmological findings were reported. The source of the poison in the latter case was a laburnum tree growing on the front lawn of the Asylum, but no source was specified in Aldridge's report.

[146] Burman (1873:62).

[147] *Lancet* 1872;2:245 (17th August; Medical News). Johnston (1906:8, 644).

[148] *Report* (1873:27). Aldridge himself noted that "During the last four years I have made ophthalmo-scopic examinations in almost every well-marked case [of acute dementia] that has occurred in the West Riding Asylum." (IV:292).

[149] Obituary: *Report and Transactions of the Devonshire Association for the Advancement of Science, Literature and Art* 1919;51:39–40. There may be a later link with another WRA alumnus, Patrick Nicol (*vide infra*).

[150] MB: *Edinb Med J* 1868;14(3):268 (Graduation in Medicine at the University of Edinburgh. Candidates who received the degree of Bachelor of Medicine). He received his degree at the same time as Churchill Fox (*vide infra*) and David Ferrier (Chap. 7). MD: *Lancet* 1871;2:245 (12th August; Medical News). *Alphabetical list of graduates of the University of Edinburgh …*, 1889:26, 129.

[151] Turner (1878:241).

Burman had two spells at WRA, initially as Clinical Clerk, prior to an AMO post at the Devon County Lunatic Asylum, Exminster, located just outside the city of Exeter.[152] He was then "appointed Assistant Medical Officer to the West Yorkshire Lunatic Asylum"[153] in 1871, when George Thompson moved to Bristol.[154] In his first publication in *WRLAMR* (of three in total), Burman was listed as "Assistant Medical Officer, West Riding Asylum; Late Assistant Medical Officer of the Devon County Asylum, and Clinical Assistant, West Riding Asylum" (I:129). According to Crichton-Browne, Burman took a position at WRA lower than he had previously held, thus displaying "his intelligent appreciation of the opportunities for study and observation which the West Riding Asylum affords, by sacrificing higher emoluments than are here offered in order to join our staff".[155] Burman had been elected to membership of the MPA in 1869, listed as Assistant Medical Officer, Devon Asylum.[156]

Burman had published case material whilst at the Devon Asylum,[157] and continued to publish material from Devon during his time at WRA,[158] including a response to a paper by Crichton-Browne on gangrene of the lung published in the *BMJ* in 1871.[159] In this response, Burman reported examining the records of all patients dying at the Devon Asylum from 1845 to 1869, a total of 1325 deaths from all causes,[160] an endeavour which might have been

---

[152] In the *Lancet* 1869;1:350 (6th March; Medical Appointments), *BMJ* 1869;1:227 (6th March; Medical Appointments), and *J Ment Sci* 1869–1870;15(April 1869):165 (Appointments), Burman was noted to be "late Resident Clinical Clerk" at West Riding Asylum. It is thus possible that he may have taken up the Clinical Clerk vacancy at "West Riding of Yorkshire Lunatic Asylum" advertised in *BMJ* 1868;2:628 (12th December; Medical Vacancies).

[153] *Lancet* 1871;2:246 (12th August; Medical Appointments). Also *Medical Times and Gazette* 1871;2:208 (12th August; Appointments); *Medical Press and Circular* 1871;12:152 (16th August; Appointments); *J Ment Sci* 1871–1872;17(October 1871):469 (Appointments). Also *Lancet* 1871;2:308 (26th August; Medical Appointments) noting the appointment of his successor in Devon: "J.W. Burman … resigned, and appointed to the West Riding of Yorkshire Lunatic Asylum".

[154] *Report* (1872:32).

[155] *Report* (1872:32). Quoting this passage in part, Finn (2012:179–180 and n574) cited "'Medical Director's Journal', 27th January 1875 (WYAS C85/1/13/3)". I have not been able to see this: in my reading of WYAS C85/1/13/3 (on 19/11/2024) I found the first two entries to be for 29th October 1874 and 29th April 1875. Moreover, Finn's dating seems odd, as it is more than six years after Burman's first arrival at WRA as an unpaid Clinical Clerk, and more than a year after his departure to a medical superintendency elsewhere. It does not tally with the date of Crichton's Browne's comments in his *Report* (1872). Benham (*vide infra*) may also have taken "a position at WRA lower than he had previously held".

[156] *J Ment Sci* 1869–1870;15(October 1869):464 (Psychological News. New members).

[157] For example, Burman (1870).

[158] Burman (1872a). Although published in March 1872, the paper is as from "West Riding Lunatic Asylum, Wakefield, Nov. 1871".

[159] Crichton Browne (1871a).

[160] Burman (1871).

attractive to Superintendent Crichton-Browne when he was, according to his letter to Charles Darwin (1st June 1869), seeking assistance to examine "the mass of interesting material which is as it were going to waste … in this huge hospital for want of accurate observation & which might be of immense value".[161]

Burman's first *WRLAMR* paper was "A contribution to the statistics of general paralysis; with remarks" (I:129–151), which was later noted by Crichton-Browne (VI:173) to be amongst the "valuable investigations into particular aspects of general paralysis" undertaken at WRA.

Burman also undertook experimental work at Wakefield. For his study "On conia, and its use in subcutaneous injection" (II:1–40) he used cats, dogs, rabbits, pigeons, frogs, and guinea-pigs. He reported "great difficulty in getting dogs" whereas "a good supply of [rabbits] one can always procure" (II:10). This work also involved self-experimentation, Burman injecting himself with conia as well as other medical officers at the asylum (Wood, Courtenay, Mitchell; II:16) and the chief attendant (Beaumont).[162] A paper by Burman on the potential value of conia in the treatment of acute mania appeared in *The Practitioner*, a "monthly journal of therapeutics", in the same year,[163] in which he acknowledged Crichton-Browne for permission to publish seven cases (identified by Register number and date of admission) and cited the Superintendent's earlier publication on conium in the treatment of acute mania published in the *Lancet* of 1872 (Crichton-Browne's paper did not mention Burman).[164] All the patients referred to by Crichton-Browne were admitted to WRA in 1871, all those by Burman in 1872, so no duplicate publication was involved.

In Burman's final *WRLAMR* paper, published in 1873, entitled "Heart disease and insanity" (III:216–257), he was listed as "Deputy Medical Director"

---

[161] Darwin Correspondence Project, "Letter no. 6769,"

https://www.darwinproject.ac.uk/letter/?docId=letters/DCP-LETT-6769.xml (accessed 10/04/2023). See also Pearn (2010).

[162] One reviewer opined that this paper was "the most valuable contribution to English therapeutics that this decade has yet seen" (*Birmingham Medical Review* 1872;1:265). A review of what I presume to be the same work appears as "Burman on conia" in *Br Foreign Med Chir Rev* 1873;51(102):444–445. However, this refers to a "pamphlet", but as the title of the work and its pagination ("Pp 40") are identical to II:1–40 I presume the anonymous author of the review may have seen an offprint or reprint of the *WRLAMR* paper. See Chap. 6 for discussion of reprints of *WRLAMR* articles.

[163] Burman (1872b). He refers to his *WRLAMR* publication on conia at 337n1.

[164] Crichton Browne (1872a). It has been suggested that this paper represented an early example of an attempt at controlled drug evaluation in mental illness, albeit with many methodological shortcomings from the perspective of current clinical trials (Adams 2010). As noted by McDowall (*J Ment Sci* 1873–1874;19(April 1873):142), Crichton-Browne's paper was also included in the *American Journal of Insanity* 1872;29(July):118–132.

of the West Riding Asylum.[165] Tabulating the results of 500 postmortem examinations, he found the incidence of heart disease in the insane to be scarcely more common than in the general population of the West Riding.[166]

During his time at WRA Burman also published in the *Journal of Mental Science*[167] and the *Medical Times and Gazette*[168] (a later paper also included cases seen at WRA[169]). He manned one of the stalls at the 1872 medical *conversazione*, displaying pathological specimens, and he also demonstrated some animal experiments.[170] He also manned the pathological specimens table at the *conversazione* in 1873, along with McDowall. He supplied some clinical notes on a patient he had seen to John Lowe (III:213).

Burman left Wakefield in 1873 to "fill the office of Medical Superintendent of the Wilts County Asylum",[171] so worked at WRA as AMO for only about two years. Between 1873 and 1878, as Medical Superintendent at the Wiltshire County Asylum for Insane in Devizes,[172] he continued to publish,[173] and also referred a "very remarkable human brain" reported on by William Turner in 1878.[174] By late 1879, as "Late Medical Superintendent of the Wilts County Lunatic Asylum", Burman was living in Richmond, London,[175] but in 1880 was appointed "Medical Officer and Public Vaccinator to the No, 3

---

[165] This was also the affiliation given in Burman (1872b). In a list of British Medical Association members in Yorkshire published in the *BMJ* at the end of 1871, "Burman, James W" was listed as "Medical Superintendent of the West Riding Asylum, Wakefield", evidently an error, since this appears just seven names beneath "Browne, J Crichton" who had the same (correct) designation. See *BMJ* 1871;2:778 (30th December).

[166] Burman's paper on heart disease (III:216–257) is also discussed by Wallis (2017a:70–71).

[167] Burman (1872–1873). Finn (2012:181) reported five publications by Burman in the *Journal of Mental Science*, but I find six in all, published between 1873 and 1880. The first of these, from WRA, was later cited by Maudsley (1875:694). Also noted in Cox and Marland (2022:190) and footnotes 190, 191.

[168] Burman (1873).

[169] Burman (1874–1875b:248–250) (Cases II and III).

[170] *Yorkshire Post and Leeds Intelligencer* 27th November 1873, p.3 (West Riding Asylum. Medical Conversazione); *Leeds Mercury* 27th November 1873, p.7 (Medical Conversazione at the West Riding Asylum).

[171] *Report* (1874:28).

[172] *Lancet* 1873;2:687 (8th November; Medical Appointments); *BMJ* 1873;2:563 (8th November; Medical Appointments); *J Ment Sci* 1873–1874;19(January 1874):645 (Appointments).

[173] For example, Burman, 1873–1874, 1874 (in which he is designated as "Resident Medical Officer and Superintendent of the Wiltshire County Asylum, Devizes"), 1874–1875a, b.

[174] Turner (1878). The review of this paper in the "Abstracts of British and foreign journals" section of *Brain* (1878–1879;1:133–134), possibly written by Crichton-Browne (137), stated that the patient "died in the Wilts County Asylum" (133) but did not mention Burman.

[175] Burman (1879a, b).

District of the Hungerford Union".[176] As late as 1885 he was still publishing on the subject of his WRA work on the use of conia in acute mania.[177]

Charles Henry Mayhew

The *Lancet* issue of 16th January 1869 carried the notice:

> MAYHEW, Mr. C., of King's College Hospital has been appointed Clinical Clerk at the West Riding of Yorkshire Lunatic Asylum, Wakefield, vice Aldrige, promoted.[178]

Mayhew first appeared in the *Medical Directory* in 1871 with an address in Ipswich, but this did not mention his prior appointment at WRA.

His single paper in *WRLAMR*, on "Acute delirious melancholia" (I:252–260), showed his affiliations to be "Associate of King's College, Assistant House-Surgeon to the Stockport Infirmary, formerly Clinical Assistant, West Riding Asylum". He did not publish in either the *Journal of Mental Science* or subsequently in *Brain*.

"Dr. Charles Mayhew", presumably the same man, cropped up many years later in one of Crichton-Browne's "notebooks" published in the last decade of his life, in which, *a propos* the question of handedness, he reported that "I got my friend Dr. Charles Mayhew to examine the prisoners in Pentonville Prison" with results from 975 prisoners, but no date for this study was vouchsafed.[179]

J. Bywater Ward (1844–1898)

John Bywater Ward was born in Leeds and was a graduate of Cambridge University as well as Leeds School of Medicine.[180] He was a Clinical Clerk at WRA in 1869, replaced by George Henry Pedler (*vide infra*). By the time of his solitary paper in *WRLAMR*, "On the treatment of insanity by the hypo-

---

[176] *Lancet* 1880;1:348 (28th February; Medical Appointments).

[177] Burman (1885).

[178] *Lancet* 1869;1:106 (16th January; Medical Appointments) [capitals in original]. Also *J Ment Sci* 1869–1870;15(April 1869):165 (Appointments) which also indicated that Aldridge was "promoted".

[179] Crichton-Browne (1937:51). Based on this information, I presume Mayhew worked as a doctor in the prison medical service.

[180] Obituary: *J Ment Sci* 1899;45(January 1899):220–221.

dermic injection of morphia" (I:152–163), his affiliation was listed as "Assistant Medical Officer Warwick County Asylum; Late Clinical Assistant, West Riding Asylum". He was elected member of the MPA in 1871.[181]

Ward's *WRLAMR* paper mostly recounted the effects of morphia in patients suffering from mania, one of them (at least) from Warwick, and one case reported to Ward by Aldridge at WRA (I:157). Ward's conclusion was that "In some of the cases of chronic mania the effect was indeed almost magical, and it is in these where I have seen most special benefit from its use" whereas in melancholia the results "have not been so good as might have been expected" (I:162).

From Warwick, Bywater Ward moved in 1872 to the superintendency of the Warneford Asylum in Oxford (and was replaced at Warwick by Oscar Woods, *vide infra*).[182] In 1897 he retired after 25 years as medical superintendent at the Warneford.[183] Despite his long superintendency, he never published in either the *Journal of Mental Science* or *Brain*, perhaps as a consequence of his "always imperfect" health, as reported in his obituary, as well as the administrative burdens of the post.

Bywater Ward's *WRLAMR* paper was later (1876) cited with approbation by Bodington: "For detailed information and cases treated by the hypodermic method, I refer you to a paper by Dr. Bywater Ward, in the first volume of the *West Riding Asylum Reports*, [*sic*], and would especially commend to you the passage with which he concludes. It is this: 'In the earlier stages of insanity, often seen in private practice, but rarely met with in asylums, I should expect that this mode of treatment would prove of great benefit.'".[184]

George Henry Pedler

George Henry Pedler was appointed Clinical Clerk at WRA in October 1869, *vice* JB Ward, appointed AMO Warwick County Lunatic Asylum.[185] In his Superintendent's Report for 1870 (published 1871), Crichton-Browne noted

---

[181] *J Ment Sci* 1871–1872;17(October 1871):443.

[182] *BMJ* 1872;2:483 (26th October; Medical Appointments); *J Ment Sci* 1872–1873;18(October 1872):474 (Appointments).

[183] *J Ment Sci* 1897;43(October 1897):889. He merited only one mention in the history of the Warneford Hospital by Parry-Jones (1976:21).

[184] Bodington (1876:143) (citing I:163).

[185] *Lancet* 1869;2:627 (30th October; Medical Appointments). Also *J Ment Sci* 1869–1870;15(January 1870):662 (Appointments).

that "Mr. PEDLER … resigned his position in May last on entering upon practice in London".[186]

Pedler published two papers in *WRLAMR*, on "Mollities ossium and allied diseases" (I:164–177) and on "Puerperal mania" (II:137–156), in both of which his affiliations were listed as "Fellow of the Obstetrical Society, and Late Clinical Assistant, West Riding Asylum". Of note with respect to the former paper, at the meeting of the Obstetrical Society of London held on 3rd May 1871, "Mr. PEDLER exhibited the Pelvis of a Woman, the subject of Mollities Ossium. She was an inmate of the West Riding Asylum for four years, and died there last January". This report noted the distortion and contraction of the bone, chemical analysis of which showed less than half to be true bone, less than a quarter of which was inorganic matter.[187] In Pedler's first *WRLAMR* paper he stated of the first patient, JM, "the particulars of which I have laid before the Obstetrical Society", that she was admitted in November 1866 and died on "January 2nd, 1871" and that her pelvis "has been shown at the Obstetrical Society" (I:165), confirming that this was the same patient. A more extensive chemical analysis of the bone was presented here, performed by "Mr. Alexander Pedler, F.C.S" (I:166). Eight cases were presented in all, four with postmortem examination.

In his second *WRLAMR* paper, Pedler reported on cases of puerperal mania seen at WRA over the 3½ years from 10th October 1869 to 10th May 1872. He identified 76 cases in 73 women of the 889 admitted to the female side during that period (II:151), four of whom died but "no deaths occurred from the disease uncomplicated by other serious visceral lesions" (II:156). A variety of medications was tried for the condition, including purgatives, emetics, diaphoretics and diuretics (II:148); chloral hydrate, conium, and bromide of potassium were noted to be valuable remedies.

Pedler did not subsequently publish in either the *Journal of Mental Science* or *Brain*. He was elected to the membership of the MPA in 1873.[188]

The *Medical Directory* recorded Pedler's address from 1871 as "6, Trevorterr. Knightsbridge, S.W. (Martyn and Pedler)" and that he was a graduate of King's College (London). A note in *The London Gazette* of 27th February 1874 informed readers that the partnership to carry on business as Surgeons between Pedler and one William Martyn at this address was dissolved by

---

[186] *Report* (1871:27) [capitals in original].

[187] *Medical Times and Gazette* 1871;1:586 (20th May; Obstetrical Society of London) [capitals in original]. Although one is hesitant to indulge in retrospective diagnosis, this was presumably a case of osteomalacia.

[188] *J Ment Sci* 1873–1874;19(October 1873):473.

mutual consent in September 1872 [*sic*].[189] As noted (*vide supra*), on 10th May 1876 a "meeting of the past medical officers and others associated with the West Riding Asylum" to honour Crichton-Browne on his departure from WRA was "held at 6, Trevor-terrace",[190] presumably Pedler's address in London.

Patrick Nicol (1847–1873)

Patrick Nicol, an Aberdeen graduate,[191] was a Clinical Assistant at WRA around 1869–1870. In his Superintendent's Report for 1870, Crichton-Browne stated that:

> Dr. NICOL who was a member of the clinique [*sic*] at the close of 1869, and who was afterwards appointed Assistant Medical Officer in the Sussex County Asylum, returned here in Autumn to fill Dr. MITCHELL'S place, during his absence for four months, on a visit to Continental Asylums.[192]

Indeed, in May 1870 it was announced that, as "late Clinical Clerk" at WRA, Nicol was appointed AMO to the Sussex County Lunatic Asylum, Hayward's-heath [*sic*].[193] Whilst there he made observations on skin conditions associated with insanity,[194] including a paper on othaematoma, or the asylum ear, which included observations made at WRA[195] (a subject later returned to at WRA by Lennox Browne; see Chap. 7).

Nicol published three papers in *WRLAMR*, in all of which he was described as "Physician to the Bradford Infirmary" as well as noting his previous associations with WRA and the Sussex County Asylum. These papers were "On progressive locomotor ataxy and some other forms of locomotor deficiency as found in the insane" (I:178–208); "Phthisis and insanity" (I:233–251; co-authored with W. Watson Dove); and "The mental symptoms of ordinary disease" (II:177–202).

From Bradford, in 1872, Nicol published some experimental work using the ophthalmoscope to observe vessels on the optic disc as a proxy for the

---

[189] *The London Gazette*, 27th February 1874, p.907.

[190] *Lancet* 1876;1:726 (13th May; Medical News).

[191] Johnston (1906:404, 614). MA 1866, MB CM 1869, MD 1871.

[192] *Report* (1871:27) [capitals in original].

[193] *Lancet* 1870;1:682 (7th May; Medical Appointments). Also *J Ment Sci* 1870–1871;16(July 1870):311 (Appointments), where "Haywards Heath" is given. A "Dr. Nicol" was elected to membership of the MPA in 1870 (*J Ment Sci* 1870–1871;16(October 1870):456).

[194] Nicol (1870a). This paper is described in Wallis (2017a:40).

[195] Nicol (1870b). The paper was noted by Yeats (1873) and Cobbold (1873).

cerebral circulation in rabbits during the administration of various drugs including chloral hydrate, potassium bromide, alcohol, quinine, ergot, and belladonna.[196] According to Aldridge (I:99), Nicol had made some ophthalmoscopic observations whilst at WRA in patients taking chloral hydrate, subsequently passing his notes to Aldridge.

Nicol never published in either the *Journal of Mental Science* or *Brain*. He was mentioned several times by Darwin in *The expression of the emotions in man and animals* (1872), the only WRA clinician aside from Crichton-Browne thus noted. He was subsequently one of those invited to the 1872 medical *conversazione* at WRA.[197] In 1873 he resigned from a position as Examiner in Medicine at the University of Aberdeen.[198] Lennox Browne, critiquing Nicol's 1870 othaematoma paper, referred to him as "the late Dr. Nicol" (V:153),[199] and indeed it appears that Nicol died at Plympton, Devon, in May 1873 and his remains were transported for burial in Aberdeen.[200] Had his health failed? Was he visiting Aldridge at Plympton (with whom he had overlapped at WRA)? Answers to these questions are currently not forthcoming.

William Lawrence (Alexander Lawrence, 1845–1926)

In his Superintendent's Report for 1870, Crichton-Browne stated that "Dr. LAWRENCE" succeeded Pedler, and "has since been elected Assistant Medical Officer in the Chester County Asylum".[201]

In the first volume of *WRLAMR*, "William Lawrence" appears as the author of "On the artificial feeding of the insane" (I:209–217), his affiliations listed as "Assistant Medical Officer Chester County Asylum; Late Clinical Assistant West Riding Asylum". It seems reasonable to presume that this is the same

---

[196] Nicol and Mossop (1872). Similar experiments were later described in *WRLAMR* (V:130–148) by John Hunter Arbuckle (*vide infra*). One wonders if these experimental studies may have been prompted by the previous clinical ophthalmoscopic observations at WRA by Allbutt (1868a, b, c) and by Aldridge (I:71–128 and II:223–253; his final paper, IV:291–304, is too late). Aldridge had observed the effects of chloral, ergot, and belladonna on retinal appearances.

[197] *Leeds Mercury* 17th October 1872, p.8 (Medical Conversazione at the West Riding Asylum).

[198] *BMJ* 1873;1:320 (22nd March).

[199] I have found no obituary for Nicol in either the *BMJ* or *J Ment Sci* in the period 1872–1876. Of note, his name does not appear amongst those former WRA staff who were listed as "Subscribers to the testimonial gift" for Crichton-Browne published in *Medical Times and Gazette* 1876;1:529–530 (13th May; Presentation to Dr. Crichton Browne).

[200] *Bath Chronicle and Weekly Gazette*, 15th May 1873, p.6.

[201] *Report* (1871:27) [capitals in original].

person as "LAWRENCE, A." [*sic*] whose appointment as Clinical Clerk at WRA, "vice P. Nicol," was noted in the *Lancet* of 11th June 1870.[202] The following week "Alex Lawrence" was noted to have been appointed at Wakefield, having previously been House-Surgeon and Superintendent of Chalmers's Hospital, Banff.[203] This presumption is further substantiated by the notification in the *Lancet* of 8th October 1870 that "LAWRENCE, A." was appointed AMO to the Cheshire Lunatic Asylum, Chester.[204] Patrick Nicol (I:184) noted that "I have been favoured by my friend Dr. Lawrence, second medical officer of the Cheshire Asylum, with brief notes of a … case"; their qualifications suggest that they were contemporaries at Aberdeen University.[205]

A "Dr. Lawrence" from Chester was one of those invited to the 1872 medical *conversazione* at WRA.[206] "Dr. A. Lawrence" was amongst those subscribing to Crichton-Browne's testimonial gift on his departure from WRA, presented on 10th May 1876.[207] Hence the *WRLAMR* paper is the only place, to my knowledge, in which the name "William Lawrence" is to be found.[208]

Alexander Lawrence eventually became the Superintendent at the Cheshire County Asylum.[209] He did not subsequently publish in either the *Journal of Mental Science* or in *Brain*. He died in November 1926, although this was not announced until July 1928 in the *Journal of Mental Science*.[210]

---

[202] *Lancet* 1870;1:861 (11th June; Medical Appointments) [capitals in original].

[203] *Lancet* 1870;1:893 (18th June; Medical Appointments [Anderson]).

[204] *Lancet* 1870;2:524 (8th October; Medical Appointments) [capitals in original]; also *Lancet* 1870;2:692 (12th November; Medical Appointments [Hay]). The *Medical Directory* of 1871 (453) lists Alexander Lawrence as AMO at Chester Asylum. In a further twist, "Dr. James Lawrence, Chester County Asylum" was reported as elected to the membership of the MPA in 1872 (*J Ment Sci* 1872–1873;(October 1872):460.). As this same notice is, to my reading, in error with the spelling of the names of three other WRA clinicians, *viz.* Courtenay, Benham, and Major, I thought it possible that it might in fact refer to Alexander Lawrence, but later lists of MPA members give Alexander Lawrence's date of joining as 1870, as does his obituary in *J Ment Sci* 1928;74(July 1928):569.

[205] Johnston (1906:279). MA 1866, MB CM 1869, MD 1872.

[206] *Leeds Mercury* 17th October 1872, p.8 (Medical Conversazione at the West Riding Asylum).

[207] *Medical Times and Gazette* 1876;1:529–530 (13th May; Presentation to Dr. Crichton Browne).

[208] Is it possible that Crichton-Browne had confused his Clinical Assistant's name with that of the surgeon (Sir) William Lawrence (1783–1867) who, amongst other appointments, was surgeon to Bethlem Hospital, and an Honorary MPA member from 1863? Crichton-Browne had met him in 1862, "a meeting vividly remembered by me even after seventy years" (Crichton-Browne 1932:133–137, quotation at 133–134).

[209] In his history of the Chester County Lunatic Asylum, Murphy (2004:16) noted that "In June 1910 Dr. Lawrence resigned as medical superintendent after a service of forty years at the asylum". In addition, "A.H. Lawrence" is noted as Resident Medical Superintendent 1896–1910 (Murphy 2004:40). His date of appointment as superintendent is given as 1895 by Lord (1928:363) and in *J Ment Sci* 1928;74(July 1928):569.

[210] Obituaries: Lord (1928); *J Ment Sci* 1928;74(July 1928):569.

J. Hay

> HAY, J., M.B., C.M., M.R.C.S.E., has been appointed Clinical Clerk at the West Riding Lunatic Asylum, Wakefield, vice A. Lawrence.[211]

Aside from this note, dated November 1870, I have not been able to find anything further about "J. Hay".[212] None of the "Hay" entries in the *Medical Directory* lists an appointment at WRA. No one of this name appears in the Superintendent's *Report* for 1870. Evidently, not all WRA Clinical Clerks left a "footprint" in terms of publications, perhaps in part because not all were aiming for a career in asylum medicine. Another possible explanation for a brief and unrecorded stay as WRA Clinical Clerk was "summary removal … on account of misconduct or neglect".

E. Churchill Fox

Edwin Churchill Pigott Fox was an Edinburgh graduate (MB, CM 1868).[213] In his Superintendent's *Report* for 1870, Crichton-Browne stated that Churchill Fox followed Dr. Lawrence as Clinical Assistant at WRA, a position he held at the same time as Watson Dove.[214] He left in early 1871 to become Assistant Medical Officer at the Stafford County Asylum.[215]

He published only a single, very brief, paper in *WRLAMR*, "Ergot of rye in the treatment of mental diseases" (I:261–265), perhaps no more than a filler for the last few available pages of the volume. The subject matter overlapped with a paper Crichton-Browne had published earlier in the year in *The Practitioner*.[216]

---

[211] *Lancet* 1870;2:692 (12th November; Medical Appointments). Also *J Ment Sci* 1870–1871;16(January 1871):644 (Appointments).

[212] Hay was not mentioned in the listing of WRA AMOs and Clinical Assistants/Clerks presented in Finn (2012:181–184).

[213] *Edinb Med J* 1868;14(3):267 (Graduation in Medicine at the University of Edinburgh. Candidates who received the degrees of Bachelor of Medicine and Master in Surgery). He received his degrees at the same time as Burman and David Ferrier. *Alphabetical list of graduates of the University of Edinburgh …*, 1889:38.

[214] *Report* (1871:27).

[215] *Report* (1872:32).

[216] Crichton Browne (1871e). A commentary on this paper appeared in *J Ment Sci* 1871–1872;17(July 1871):286–290 (Psychological Retrospect). Also *Medical Record* 1871–1872;6:394.

Fox was elected MPA in 1877 at which time he was listed as in Bristol.[217] He did not publish in either the *Journal of Mental Science* or *Brain*.

Henry Sutherland (1841–1901)[218]

Henry Sutherland was appointed Clinical Clerk in succession to Churchill Fox in February 1871 and acted as Assistant Medical Officer between the departure of George Thompson (to Bristol) and the arrival of Wilkie Burman (from Devon).[219] According to Crichton-Browne, Sutherland "acquitted himself in that capacity in a manner worthy of his name and antecedents",[220] these being his father, Alexander John Sutherland, and grandfather, Alexander Robert Sutherland, both of whom had been Physician to St. Luke's Hospital for the Insane in London (A.J. had been the first President of the Association of Medical Officers of Asylums and Hospitals for the Insane, forerunner of the MPA, in 1854; prior to 1854 there was no permanent Presidency, each meeting electing a Chairman). Henry Sutherland had been educated at both Cambridge (BA 1867) and Oxford (MB, MA 1869; MD 1872), and his clinical qualification was listed in the *Medical Directory* as from St George's and Bethlehem Royal Hospital. He was admitted Member of the Royal College of Physicians (MRCP) in 1870,[221] and also became a member of the MPA in the same year.[222] He was appointed lecturer on Psychological Medicine at the Westminster Hospital, London, in 1872.[223]

---

[217] *J Ment Sci* 1877–1878;23(October 1877):434. The reference to Bristol may raise the possibility that Churchill Fox was in some way related to the extensive family of Edward Long Fox (1761–1835) who established the private Brislington House Asylum in Bristol in 1806 (Smith 2008). Long Fox had 15 daughters and 8 sons, but currently I have no further information as to whether Churchill Fox featured amongst his many descendants.

[218] Biographical material on Sutherland may be found in Todd and Ashworth (1991:398). His "Estimated birth year" in the 1871 census is 1842, a native of St Margaret's, London, but his obituary (*Lancet* 1901;2:1544) stated he was born on 28th December 1841. Hence, as for Crichton-Browne, the year of birth estimated by the census was wrong.

[219] Sutherland is listed in the 1871 census as "Assistant Officer", aged 29, and a member of Crichton-Browne's household. Note that Thompson was also listed as part of Crichton-Browne's household in the April 1871 census.

[220] *Report* (1872:32).

[221] *Lancet* 1870;1:214 (5th February; Medical News).

[222] *J Ment Sci* 1870–1871;16(October 1870):456. The words of Dr. Batty Tuke as reported here are somewhat oblique: "I have to propose the following six gentlemen as ordinary members of the Association. The first name I am sure will be received with very great pleasure by this Association, as it is one very familiar to us; I refer to Dr. Alexander [*sic*] Sutherland. I cannot refrain from expressing the gratification I feel at seeing the son of my old friend with us to-day." However, Henry Sutherland appears in subsequent lists of MPA members with his joining year given as 1870. Alexander John Sutherland had died in 1867 at the age of 55 (*Medical Times and Gazette* 1867;1:149 (9th February; The late Dr. Sutherland)).

[223] *BMJ* 1872;2:286 (14th September; Changes in the Hospitals and Medical Schools).

Despite the brevity of his time at WRA, Sutherland achieved a longer chronological spread of papers in *WRLAMR* (4 in total, one each in volumes I, II, III, and VI) than anyone else other than Crichton-Browne. In the first of these papers, "Arachnoid cysts" (I:218–232), his affiliation was given as Physician to the St George's, Hanover Square, Dispensary, and Late Assistant Medical Officer, West Riding Asylum (Sutherland referenced this paper in another publication some years later[224]). In all his subsequent *WRLAMR* publications (II:53–72; III:299–314; VI:108–119) he was listed as Lecturer on Insanity to the Westminster Hospital School of Medicine, where he had been appointed in 1872.[225]

Sutherland continued to work in the field of asylum medicine after leaving WRA and to present[226] and publish work related to mental disorders.[227] Amongst these publications was one directly related to his work on arachnoid cysts undertaken at WRA: "The following paper is an abstract from researches made some years ago and published in the first volume of the West Riding Asylum Medical Reports, edited by Dr. (now Sir) James Crichton Browne, M.D., F.R.S. The sketches were made from the subjects, and are now published for the first time", all ten cases being alluded to.[228] A book published in 1890 listed Sutherland's affiliation on the title page as "Physician to and Proprietor of Newlands House and Otto House Private Lunatic Asylums".[229]

He was presumably the "Dr. Sutherland (Private Asylums)" who, when giving evidence published in the Report of the Committee of the London County Council on a Hospital for the Insane (1889–1890), echoed Crichton-Browne's views regarding the position of an asylum pathologist:

---

[224] Sutherland (1877a). As Crichton-Browne explained (II:116), "If a large quantity of blood is extravasated on the surface of the hemispheres, without causing death, a coagulum is formed, absorption of fluid takes place, a membrane of low organization is developed round the clot, and an arachnoid cyst is the result". Crichton-Browne himself later published on the subject and mentioned "The writings of … Dr. Henry Sutherland" (Crichton Browne 1875:171). Viets (1938:480) adjudged Sutherland's paper on arachnoid cysts to refer to subdural haematomas and hence to be "a pioneer effort of marked importance".

[225] *J Ment Sci* 1872–1873;18(July 1872):310.

[226] For example, he presented at the Royal Medical and Chirurgical Society, 22nd April 1873, "On the histology of the blood of the insane" (Sutherland 1873; also 1885–1886); and at the Section of Psychology, British Medical Association Annual Meeting, Cambridge, 11th August 1880, on "Cases of alcoholic insanity in private practice" (N = 200, F:M = 100:100; *J Ment Sci* 1880–1881;26(October 1880):460). Also *BMJ* 1880;2:375 (4th September). This presentation was an update of Sutherland (1874), which documented three cases. Also, to the Medico-Psychological Association meeting at Bethlem Hospital on 18th May 1883 on "Prognosis in cases of refusal of food" (*Medical Times and Gazette* 1883;1:590), later published (Sutherland 1883–1884). This list of presentations does not presume to be comprehensive.

[227] For example, Sutherland (1872, 1873, 1873–1874, 1874, 1875a, b, 1877a, b, 1877–1878, 1878, 1879a, b, 1883, 1883–1884, 1886, 1892). This list of publications does not presume to be comprehensive.

[228] Sutherland, 1889.

[229] Sutherland (1890).

His duties should chiefly consist of carefully superintending post mortem examinations and histological investigations; keeping a record of the etiology, duration, and termination of the cases; and of the effects of various drugs upon the patients. He should be assisted by two clinical assistants, who should keep up the case-books under his direction. This plan has been carried out efficiently in the West Riding Asylum.[230]

Sutherland seems to have had a recurrent interest in food refusal, its treatment and prognosis, in the insane.[231] Although the *WRLAMR* article on this subject was by Lawrence (I:209–217), Sutherland noted many years later, in his contribution to Hack Tuke's (1892) *Dictionary of psychological medicine*, that:

At the West Riding Asylum, where there were occasionally as many as six patients to be fed three times a day, the writer was in the habit of making the melancholiacs [*sic*] hold one another down to be fed in turn. After a few trials the effect became so ridiculous that the patients used to laugh at one another, and eventually saw the folly of refusing food, and took it properly.[232]

Sutherland may also have taken an interest in neurological matters. He wrote a review of one of the papers published by David Ferrier in *WRLAMR*, on "Labyrinthine vertigo. Menière's disease" (V:24–39), which appeared in the *London Medical Record* in 1876,[233] and from 1889 was a member of the Neurological Society of London (founded 1886).

He died at the age of 59.[234] He never published in *Brain* but had a number of publications in the *Journal of Mental Science*.[235]

---

[230] Burdett (1891:199).

[231] Sutherland (1872, 1875a, 1883–1884, 1892).

[232] Sutherland (1892:495) (compare with Sutherland, 1872; cited in Chap. 3). His father, A.J. Sutherland, had apparently used chloroform to lessen the difficulties of forcible feeding, see *J Ment Sci* 1857–1858;4(October 1857):40 and Sutherland (1892:500n).

[233] Sutherland (1876). He became a member of the Medical Society of London in the same year.

[234] Obituaries: *BMJ* 1901;2:1642–1643 ("W.J.M.") noted the fact that Sutherland had published in *WRLAMR*, and also stated that he was a member of the Neurological Society (at 1643); *Lancet* 1901;2:1544 noted that he studied "at the West Riding County Lunatic Asylum at Wakefield, where he was resident assistant medical officer under Dr. (now Sir) James Crichton Browne" and "published various papers in the West-Riding Asylum Medical Reports [*sic*]" as well as his membership of the Neurological Society.

[235] Finn (2012:183) reported five publications in the *Journal of Mental Science*, but I find only four. I presume Finn included the report on the Section of Psychology of the British Medical Association Annual Meeting, Cambridge, 1880, where Sutherland was one of the secretaries and Crichton-Browne was the President (*J Ment Sci* 1880–1881;26(October 1880):460–471).

W. Watson Dove (Born?1848)[236]

William Watson Dove, a graduate of St Bartholomew's Hospital, London, was a Clinical Clerk at WRA in 1871,[237] leaving in July, after which he moved to an AMO post at the Somersetshire County Asylum at Wells.[238] This was acknowledged in the affiliation of his solitary *WRLAMR* paper, "Phthisis and insanity" (I:233–251), co-authored with Patrick Nicol. He was elected member of the MPA in 1871.[239] He never published in either the *Journal of Mental Science* or *Brain*. The 1877 *Medical Register* listed him as a resident of Alexandria, Egypt.

John W. F. Watson

Crichton-Browne reported that "MR. JOHN W. F. WATSON, of University College Hospital was appointed in his [Watson Dove's] stead, and faithfully performed his duties until failing health necessitated his resignation."[240]

The *Medical Directory* of 1873 includes "WATSON, JNO. WILCOCKS" LSA 1871 (Univ. Coll) as late Clinical Assistant at WRA, and in 1874 "John Wilcocks Watson" appears, i.e. there is no "F" in these entries. However, "Dr. J. Ferra Watson" was amongst those subscribing to Crichton-Browne's testimonial gift presented on 10th May 1876.[241]

Other than these brief notes, no other definitive information about Watson has been found. Finn reported that he published in neither the *Journal of Mental Science* nor *Brain*.[242] The Index to the Australian Medical Association Archive includes an entry for a John Wilcocks Watson dated 1875.

---

[236] "Estimated birth year" in the 1871 census where he was listed as a native of Calcutta, Bengal.

[237] Watson Dove was listed in the 1871 census as "Assistant Officer", aged 23, and a member of Crichton-Browne's household.

[238] *Lancet* 1871;2:179 (29th July; Medical Appointments); *J Ment Sci* 1871–1872;17(October 1871):469 (Appointments). *Report* (1872:32).

[239] *J Ment Sci* 1871–1872;17(October 1871):443.

[240] *Report* (1872:32–33) [capitals in original].

[241] *Medical Times and Gazette* 1876;1:529–530 (13th May; Presentation to Dr. Crichton Browne). The John Ferra Watson (1816–1886) who founded a private lunatic asylum at Heigham Hall in Norfolk is a possibility, although unlikely as he would have been aged 56 in 1872. I have found no other connection with Crichton-Browne.

[242] Finn (2012:181).

Herbert C. Major[243] (1850–1921)[244]

Herbert Coddington Major was an Edinburgh graduate (MB CM 1871)[245] who was initially appointed as a Clinical Assistant at WRA in 1871. Crichton-Browne reported this as following the departure of Henry Sutherland in August 1871 (*sic*, although Sutherland's appointment at Westminster Hospital dates to 1872), noting that Major was "a distinguished graduate of the University of Edinburgh, and an approved student of PROFESSOR LAYCOCK'S class of Medical Psychology".[246] However, in the *Lancet* announcement of his post, this was stated to be "vice W.W. Dove" when Watson Dove went to Wells (*ca.* July 1871).[247] Thereafter, having been "an indefatigable Clinical Clerk for twelve months", in 1872 Major was "promoted to the position of Assistant Medical Officer, which he now occupies with credit".[248] Following Burman's departure in 1873 he became "chief of the Medical Staff".[249]

Major (Fig. 5.2) developed an interest in neuropathology, and evidently this work was already well underway by this time. At the Psychological Section of the Annual (40th) British Medical Association meeting held in Birmingham (6th to 9th August 1872), Crichton-Browne showed "some beautifully

---

[243] This section is based in part on Larner (2024c). Although one of the most significant figures in the history of WRA, the only other biographical work devoted to Major, to my knowledge, is Todd and Ashworth (n.d.:151–178). Sources which mention him in passing include Ashworth (1975:70,72) and Todd & Ashworth (1991:416–417). Further biographical material may be found, alongside assessment of some of his work in brain histology and cytoarchitectonics, in Larner and Triarhou (2024a, b).

[244] Reynolds and Broussolle (2022:293) gave Major's dates as (1850–1920) but these authors did not cite any primary source(s) to support their claim. Whilst the date of birth is correct (see St Helier baptisms 1842-1909 Martin to Mauger – Jerripedia (theislandwiki.org)), the date of death given by these authors is certainly wrong, for which see Major's obituary in *BMJ* 1921;2:542 (1st October; Obituary).

[245] *Alphabetical list of graduates of the University of Edinburgh ...*, 1889:60.

[246] *Report* (1872:32) [capitals in original].

[247] *Lancet* 1871;2:308 (26th August; Medical Appointments) gave his name as "Magor, H.C." [*sic*]. Ditto *Medical Press and Circular* 1871;12:196 (30th August; Appointments); also *J Ment Sci* 1871–1872;17(October 1871):470 (Appointments). His baptism record (St Helier baptisms 1842-1909 Martin to Mauger – Jerripedia (theislandwiki.org)) gives his surname as "Mauger" [*sic*], which has the same pronunciation as Major, and might possibly account for this variant spelling. Another possible error with the spelling of Major's name may occur in *J Ment Sci* 1872–1873;18(October 1872):460 where "Dr Herbert Mayo, West Riding Asylum" was amongst the names proposed and elected as new members of the MPA. Herbert Mayo was a noted clinician and physiologist who died in 1852 (Bradley 2017). Yet another nominal error occurs in Major's entry in the *Medical Directory* of 1872, wherein he was listed as "MAJOR, Herbert Codrington", corrected in the 1873 edition to "Coddington".

[248] *Report* (1873:27). This promotion was also reported in *Lancet* 1872;2:173 (3rd August; Medical Appointments); *Medical Times and Gazette* 1872;2:139 (3rd August; Appointments); *Medical Press and Circular* 1872;14:122 (7th August); *BMJ* 1872;2:179 (10th August; Medical Appointments); and *J Ment Sci* 1872–1873;18(October 1872):474 (Appointments).

[249] *Report* (1874:28).

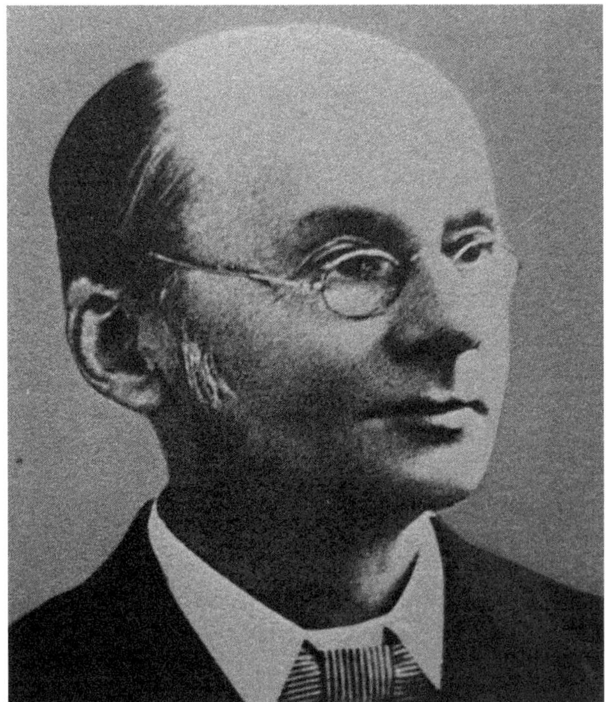

Fig. 5.2 Herbert Coddington Major

prepared sections of Brain-Structure [*sic*] in Health and Disease, the work of Dr. Herbert C. Major, of the West Riding Asylum".[250] As per the pre-meeting notification of scheduled papers,[251] where Crichton-Browne was listed to present a paper on "Instruments for Measuring the Depth of the Grey Matter of the Brain", the meeting report confirmed that, as well as Major's prepared sections, Crichton-Browne "also exhibited an ingenious glass instrument, *of his own device*, for measuring the depth of the grey matter of the brain"[252] (Major's name does not appear in the list of those attending the meeting[253]). I take this to be the tephrylometer,[254] described by Major in the second of his papers in *WRLAMR*, titled "A new method of determining the depth of the grey matter of the cerebral convolutions" (II:157–176), in which he reported that "I was led to devise an instrument which I have called the Tephrylometer"

---

[250] *BMJ* 1872;2:221 (24th August) [capitals in original].

[251] *BMJ* 1872;2:136 (3rd August).

[252] *BMJ* 1872;2:221 (24th August) [my italics].

[253] *BMJ* 1872;2:191–192 (17th August).

[254] Sloffer (2023:44) erred with "typhrylometer".

(II:160).[255] Perhaps the confusion as to who devised this instrument arose from the *BMJ* correspondent, but I am not aware that any correction was ever published.

Aside from neuropathology, Major also had clinical duties, some vignettes of which survive. He was called upon by Burman to attend him after one of his self-experiments with subcutaneous injection of conia (II:31). He collaborated with Clifford Allbutt (Chap. 7), to the extent of doing most of the work in a study later published in *WRLAMR* by Allbutt ("The electric treatment of the insane"; II:203–222). On 12th November 1874 Major saw a patient in status epilepticus, later reported by Wallis (V:267). He attended the medical *conversazione* and there is published evidence that he presided over one of the stalls at the meetings held in 1872, 1873, 1874, and 1875.[256] Clinical notes by Major and Charles Frederick Newcombe (*vide infra*) were used by Crichton-Browne to prepare a report of a patient with puerperal mania, pelvic haematocele, and sudden death, which appeared in the *Lancet* in 1874.[257]

Major was soon publishing in the *Lancet* himself, on the subject of brain histology,[258] as well as in *WRLAMR* to which he was the most frequent contributor aside from Crichton-Browne, publishing six papers in all between 1872 and 1876. His other *WRLAMR* publications were "On the minute structure of the cortical substance of the brain, in a case of chronic brain wasting" (II:41–52)[259]; "Observations on the histology of the brain in the insane" (III:97–112); "Observations on the histology of the morbid brain" (IV:223–239); "On the morbid histology of the brain in the lower animals" (V:160–170); and "The histology of the island of Reil" (VI:1–10).[260] He also provided a microscopic section for one of Milner Fothergill's publications (III:124).

---

[255] Major's priority was evident to reviewers, e.g. *Br Foreign Med Chir Rev* 1873;51:377. "Dr. Major's tephrylometer" was used in a pathological study by Batty Tuke (1873:451).

[256] For 1872: *BMJ* 1872;2:474–475 (26th October; Medical Conversazione at the West Riding Asylum); *Medical Press and Circular* 1872;14:360 (23rd October; Conversazione and lecture by Professor Turner). For 1873: *Yorkshire Post and Leeds Intelligencer* 27th November 1873, p.3 (West Riding Asylum. Medical Conversazione); *Leeds Mercury* 27th November 1873, p.7 (Medical Conversazione at the West Riding Asylum). For 1874: *Medical Times and Gazette* 1874;2:609 (28th November; Annual Conversazione at the West Riding Asylum). For 1875: *BMJ* 1875;2:680 (27th November; The West Riding Asylum); *Leeds Mercury* 20th November 1875, p.3 (Medical Conversazione at Wakefield Asylum).

[257] *Lancet* 1874;1:54 (10th January; West Riding Asylum). Clinical observations by Major are also mentioned in Crichton Browne (1874b:180).

[258] Major (1874). On the same topic, Major (1875–1876a).

[259] The condition of "brain wasting" was also addressed in Crichton Browne (1871d).

[260] Viets (1938:480–481) adjudged that "The work of Major at West Riding alone would serve to give the hospital neurological immortality" although he acknowledged that Ferrier "was to make the greater contribution".

Major also had time to complete his thesis, *Histology of the brain in apes*, for the MD degree of Edinburgh University in 1875,[261] which received the gold medal.[262] In this work he illustrated the lamination of the cerebral cortex as having six layers, a finding repeated elsewhere.[263] He also published opportunistic studies on the brain of a baboon and of a "white whale" (beluga),[264] obtained respectively from the Zoological Gardens, London, and from the Westminster Aquarium, reflecting an interest in comparative neurology.[265] Arbuckle (*vide infra*) later described Major as "the first authority on the minute structure of the cerebral cortex of man and monkeys".[266]

Lest it be thought that Major was "dry as dust", devoted only to his microscopical studies, it may be noted that he also joined in the amateur theatricals at the Asylum. For example, in the "Dramatic Performance" of the comedy "Faint heart never won fair lady", staged at WRA on 12th February 1875, he appeared as "GUZMAN (a Gentleman, who by becoming a Page turns over a new leaf, as he usually uses his *High Powers* on more distinguished parts)".[267]

On Crichton-Browne's departure from WRA, Major was appointed Medical Director in his place in January 1876.[268] He co-edited the sixth (and final) volume of *WRLAMR* (his affiliation in VI:1–10 was given as "Medical Director") but he never published in *Brain*. Part of his "inheritance" was the probability that further asylum accommodation would be needed in the West Riding due to the (apparent) increase in the numbers of patients suffering from insanity, as reported at the meeting of the Leeds Board of Guardians in April 1876.[269] This may have stimulated his interest in statistical tables of the causes of insanity, a scheme which spread to asylums nationally in the

---

[261] *BMJ* 1875;2:251 (21st August; Medical News), which notes his Jersey origin.

[262] *Alphabetical list of graduates of the University of Edinburgh* …, 1889:60, 128. Some material from this thesis was later published in Major (1877a). Larner (2024c:2144) noted the handwritten thesis to be 67 pages in length; in fact, there are 65 numbered pages, with two unnumbered pages with drawings (Figures 11–14) intercalated between pages 53 and 54 (Major 1875).

[263] Major (1875–1876b, 1877a), and VI:1–10. Discussed in Larner and Triarhou (2024b).

[264] Major (1875–1876b, 1879), respectively.

[265] On the collaboration between those engaged in animal experimentation and marine laboratories and metropolitan zoos, see Stahnisch (2010:142).

[266] Arbuckle (1876b:209).

[267] WYAS C85/1382, programme for "West Riding Asylum, Wakefield" [capitals and italics in original]. Lawson, Wallis, and (possibly) Davy also appeared in this production. Major also performed in the farce "The Day after the Wedding" on 17th November 1874 in the role of "Colonel Freelove"!

[268] *BMJ* 1876;1:142 (29th January; The West Riding Asylum); *Lancet* 1876;1:229 (5th February; Medical Appointments); *Medical Press and Circular* 1876;21:149 (16th February; Appointments); *J Ment Sci* 1876–1877;21(April 1876):168 (Appointments).

[269] *Lancet* 1876;1:581 (15th April).

following decade.[270] Major was also appointed Lecturer on Mental Diseases at the Leeds School of Medicine in place of Crichton-Browne.[271]

Unlike his predecessor, Major is said to have opposed the provision of beer as an item of the Asylum dietary, apparently on the grounds of its addictive potential.[272] He had previously written to the *Lancet* to question a report of possible adulteration of beer with "coeculus indicus".[273] Accordingly, beer was discontinued at WRA in 1882,[274] an action not calculated to court popularity with the patients (as a cost-cutting measure it may have been approved of by the Committee of Visitors).

Aside from occasional case reports,[275] Major's output of publications slowed in the late 1870s and early 1880s. In his final *WRLAMR* paper, on the histology of the Island of Reil, he expressed the intention "in this and subsequent papers" (VI:3) to address specific questions, but to my knowledge there was no subsequent publication on the subject. He spoke at the Section of Psychology of the British Medical Association Annual Meeting in Cork in 1879, a "Discussion on the prevention of insanity", where he read a paper on behalf of "Dr Rabagliati" (for whom, see Chap. 7).[276]

Major resigned the WRA superintendency in 1884 on grounds of ill-health, to be succeeded by Bevan-Lewis. As the *Journal of Mental Science* noted:

Dr. Major has … by his individual efforts in varied histological research advanced science *pari passu* with the fulfilment of the routine duties of administration, although unfortunately at the sacrifice of his health.[277]

He later resurfaced in Bradford, working at Bradford Infirmary as an Honorary Physician (1885), later becoming a Consulting Physician (1898).[278]

---

[270] Major (1877b, 1884–1885).

[271] *BMJ* 1876;2:356 (9th September); *Medical Times and Gazette* 1876;2:341 (16th September); *J Ment Sci* 1876–1877;22(October 1876):506 (Appointments).

[272] *J Ment Sci* 1883–1884;29(July 1883):251. Ashworth (1975:71). Perhaps, in addition, Major's neuropathological studies had acquainted him with the deleterious morphological effects of alcohol on the brain, or possibly he was aware of the publication by Lawson (*vide infra*) "On the symptomatology of alcoholic brain disorders" which appeared in the inaugural volume of *Brain* (1878;1(2):182–194).

[273] Major (1877c).

[274] Wallis (2017a:194 and n64), citing "WYAS C85/1/12/4 Annual reports [*sic*] of Medical Superintendent (1880–1886). *Report of the Committee of Visitors and of the Medical Superintendent of the West Riding Pauper Lunatic Asylum, for the year 1882.* (Wakefield: W.H. Milnes, 1883). Report of the Medical Superintendent, 12." (not seen by me).

[275] For example, Major (1879–1880, 1882–1883).

[276] *J Ment Sci* 1879–1880;25(October 1879):447–449.

[277] *J Ment Sci* 1885;30(January 1885):654 (Retirement of Dr. Major from the West Riding Asylum).

[278] Finn (2012:177) stated that Major remained in Bradford until 1897.

There were existing connections between WRA and Bradford—former WRA Clinical Assistant Patrick Nicol (*vide supra*) had been a Physician at the Infirmary, and *WRLAMR* contributor and *conversazione* attendee Andrea Rabagliati was surgeon to the Infirmary—but whether these contacts were relevant to Major's move to Bradford is unknown (Nicol had died more than ten years earlier). Major remained a member of the MPA, with a Bradford address.

Thereafter Major moved to Bedford in 1900 as Honorary Pathologist to the Bedford County Hospital. He retired to Jersey in 1907, having married Mary Ann Balleine there in 1906. Major died in 1921, in relative obscurity, having moved in 1920 to Oxford. Some 10 years later, the Medical Charitable Society for the West Riding of the County of York received a legacy of £500 under the terms of the will of the late Mrs. M.A. Major "in memory of her husband, Dr. Herbert Coddington Major, formerly of the West Riding Asylum".[279]

John Lowe

John Lowe, an Edinburgh graduate,[280] was a Clinical Assistant at WRA in 1871, taking the place of Watson.[281] In early 1872 he was replaced by Courtenay, having been appointed AMO at the Durham County Lunatic Asylum, Sedgefield,[282] whence he gained a publication in the *Lancet*.[283] "Dr. Lowe" from Sedgefield was one of those invited to the 1872 medical *conversazione* at WRA.[284] Later in 1872 he was appointed AMO to the South Yorkshire Asylum, Wadsley, Sheffield,[285] assisting Dr. Samuel Mitchell, the first Medical Superintendent there.[286] Subsequently Lowe returned to WRA,

---

[279] *BMJ* 1931;2:270–271.

[280] *Alphabetical list of graduates of the University of Edinburgh* …, 1889:54.

[281] *Report* (1872:33). His selection as a Clinical Clerk is also mentioned in *Report* (1873:27).

[282] *Medical Times and Gazette* 1871;2:786 (23rd December; Appointments); *Lancet* 1872;1:98 (20th January; Medical Appointments); *J Ment Sci* 1871–1872;17(January 1872):628 (Appointments).

[283] Lowe (1872).

[284] *Leeds Mercury* 17th October 1872, p.8 (Medical Conversazione at the West Riding Asylum).

[285] *Lancet* 1872;2:693 (9th November; Medical Appointments). Also noted in *Medical Press and Circular*, 1872;14:428 as "South Yorkshire Asylum" (13th November) and 1872;14:493 as "Sheffield Lunatic Asylum" (4th December). Also *J Ment Sci* 1872–1873;18(January 1873):632 (Appointments).

[286] Of Mitchell and Lowe, Thorpe (1972:12) stated "both of Edinburgh and transferred from Wakefield Asylum".

as "Pathologist and Assistant Medical Officer",[287] and attended the 1873 *conversazione* presiding over a stall displaying scientific and surgical instruments.[288]

His various career moves were reflected in his single publication in *WRLAMR*, "On electro-excitability in mental and nervous diseases" (III:196–215), where his affiliations were listed as "Assistant Medical Officer, South Yorkshire Asylum; Late Assistant Medical Officer, Durham County Asylum; and Clinical Assistant, West Riding Asylum". He was elected a member of the MPA in July 1872 at the same time as Herbert Major.[289] He never published in either the *Journal of Mental Science* or *Brain*. In the *Medical Directory* of 1876 (861) his address was in Galashiels and in 1877 (887) in Edinburgh as "Paroch. Med. Off. Cramond".

E. Maziere Courtenay (1845–1912)

Edward Mazière Courtenay (the accent was not used in his *WRLAMR* paper) studied medicine at Trinity College Dublin and determined early on a career in asylum medicine. He was appointed Clinical Assistant at WRA in January 1872, replacing John Lowe.[290] During his time in Wakefield, he acted as a subject for Burman's experiments with injections of conia (II:16). He later moved to an AMO post at the Derby County Asylum,[291] as noted in the affiliation given in his solitary paper in *WRLAMR*, "The use of opium in the treatment of melancholia" (II:254–277).[292] He was elected a member of the MPA in 1872[293] (and again as an Honorary Member in 1891). "Dr. Courtenay" of Derby was one of those invited to the 1872 medical *conversazione* at WRA.[294]

Courtenay was later, in June 1873, appointed Medical Superintendent of the District Asylum, Limerick,[295] whence he published a case report in the

---

[287] *Lancet* 1873;2:895 (20th December; Medical Appointments). Also *Medical Press and Circular*, 1873;16:582 (24th December; Appointments); *BMJ* 1873;2:771 (27th December; Medical Appointments).

[288] *Yorkshire Post and Leeds Intelligencer* 27th November 1873, p.3 (West Riding Asylum. Medical Conversazione); *Leeds Mercury* 27th November 1873, p.7 (Medical Conversazione at the West Riding Asylum).

[289] *J Ment Sci* 1872–1873;18(October 1872):460.

[290] *Lancet* 1872;1:98 (20th January; Medical Appointments). Also *J Ment Sci* 1872–1873;18(April 1872):152 (Appointments); *Report* (1872:33).

[291] *Report* (1873:27). Also *J Ment Sci* 1872–1873;18(July 1872):310 (Appointments) where his name is given as "Courtenay, E. Maguire [*sic*]".

[292] This paper did not mention Bywater Ward's previous work at WRA investigating morphia (I:152–163).

[293] *J Ment Sci* 1872–1873;18(October 1872):460 where his name is given as "E. Maguire Courtney [*sic*]".

[294] *Leeds Mercury* 17th October 1872, p.8 (Medical Conversazione at the West Riding Asylum).

[295] *Medical Press and Circular* 1873;15:564 (25th June; Appointments).

Journal of Mental Science[296] but he never appeared in the pages of *Brain*. He held the post in Limerick until 1890 when he became an Inspector of Lunatics and Member of the Board of Control of Asylums in Ireland,[297] in which role he was instrumental in the reform of Irish asylums.[298]

T. W. McDowall (Died 1936)[299]

Thomas William McDowall was a graduate of the University of Edinburgh (MD 1866)[300] where he apparently came under the influence of Thomas Laycock.[301] His arrival at WRA was heralded in the Superintendent's *Report* for 1872 thus:

> On the resignation of DR. MITCHELL it was felt that, notwithstanding the diminution in the number of patients, which contemporaneously took place, no reduction of the Medical Staff could be recommended; so that a third permanent Assistant Medical Officer and Pathologist was appointed in the person of Dr. T.W. McDOWALL, who adduced high testimonials of efficiency from the Inverness and Perth District Asylums, in which he had served for several years, and who has entered upon his duties here with ardour.[302]

Evidently, then, McDowall was a man with some asylum experience, and he had already had publications in the *Journal of Mental Science*[303] and been elected to the MPA (in 1870). In 1873, described as "a zealous member of his profession", he "assumed the duties of Departmental Assistant on the male side" at WRA.[304] He manned one of the stalls at the 1873 *conversazione*, along with Burman, displaying pathological specimens.[305]

---

[296] Courtenay (1889).

[297] *J Ment Sci* 1890;36(April 1890):309–310 (The new inspectors of lunatic asylums).

[298] Obituaries: *BMJ* 1913;1:52 (4th January); *J Ment Sci* 1913;59(January 1913):179–181.

[299] Biographical material on McDowall may be found in Todd and Ashworth (1991:399).

[300] *Alphabetical list of graduates of the University of Edinburgh …*, 1889:56.

[301] James (1996:374–375).

[302] *Report* (1873:27) [capitals in original].

[303] For example, McDowall (1872–1873), in which his opening remarks referred to the clinical lectures of Mr. Syme, the Edinburgh surgeon and the father-in-law of Joseph Lister. He also published a case series of patients with insanity and intercurrent scarlatina from Inverness District Asylum (McDowall 1871–1872).

[304] *Report* (1874:28).

[305] *Yorkshire Post and Leeds Intelligencer* 27th November 1873, p.3 (West Riding Asylum. Medical Conversazione); *Leeds Mercury* 27th November 1873, p.7 (Medical Conversazione at the West Riding Asylum). The latter gives his name as "T.W. McDavall" [*sic*].

He published only a single paper in *WRLAMR*, "On the power of perceiving colours possessed by the insane" (III:129–152), hence unrelated to pathology. McDowall indicated that "the present paper is only a preliminary one, containing chiefly a brief abstract of the opinions and cases recorded by previous observers, with some of the results obtained by myself" and that "I shall be able to give next year an absolutely accurate account of all the cases examined" (III:130) although, to my knowledge, no later paper on this subject ever appeared. His assessment technique required the patient to pick out a skein or two of coloured worsted, from about 120 skeins spread on a white tablecloth, to match the colour of the one he held in his hand (III:148–149). His finding was that 9 out of 324 women tested and 13 of 302 men were "more or less colour-blind". Many years later (>50!) Crichton-Browne recalled that "My colleague, Dr. T.W. McDowell [*sic*], at my suggestion carried out an inquiry as to the power of perceiving colours possessed by the insane" and he reiterated McDowall's results, noting that the percentages (under 3 percent in women, and about 6 percent in men) indicated a higher prevalence than reported in the community at large at that time (2 percent).[306]

McDowall continued to publish in the *Journal of Mental Science* whilst at WRA, also in *The Practitioner* on the subject of guarana for sick headache.[307] He was amongst those who received Ferrier's thanks at the end of his seminal *WRLAMR* paper on cortical localisation (III:96). He appears also to have had an interest in the history of insanity.[308]

In 1874 McDowall was appointed Medical Superintendent of the Northumberland Lunatic Asylum at Morpeth.[309] During his tenure there he became Professor of Psychological Medicine at the University of Durham College of Medicine, Newcastle-upon-Tyne. He had multiple publications in the *Journal of Mental Science*, around 40 in all, many of them retrospects, mostly of American and French literature, and also translated from the German a paper by Rabow entitled "On the composition of the urine of the insane".[310] He also contributed to Hack Tuke's (1892) *Dictionary of psychological medicine* (Bearded women, I:128–129; Erysipelas in asylums, I:460–461),

---

[306] Crichton-Browne (1926:49). He stated that the patients were "subjected to the Helmholtz test".

[307] McDowall (1873).

[308] McDowall (1873–1874). This paper ends "(*To be continued.*)" (398) but I have found no later paper on this subject by McDowall. Perhaps he had insufficient time once appointed as a Medical Superintendent to pursue studies which had previously "employed my leisure" (386).

[309] Medical Director's Journal 29th April 1874 (WYAS C85/1/13/2). *Lancet* 1874;1:284 (21st February; Medical Appointments); *J Ment Sci* 1874–1875;20(April 1874):166 (Appointments); *Medical Press and Circular* 1874;17:171 (25th February; Appointments).

[310] *J Ment Sci* 1877–1878;23(July 1877):222–242. This paper did not cite similar work by Merson published in *WRLAMR* (IV:63–93; *vide infra*).

but he never published in *Brain*. He was the first of the WRA "old boys" after Crichton-Browne to be appointed President of MPA, in 1897.[311]

At a dinner held in honour of Crichton-Browne in 1931, the former Medical Director acknowledged that McDowall was still surviving.[312] McDowall's name appeared in the Obituary column of Honorary Members of the MPA in the *Journal of Mental Science* issue of January 1937.[313]

Oscar T. Woods (ca.1848–1906)

According to the *Medical Press and Circular* of 23rd October 1872, Oscar Thomas Woods "M.B. Dub., L.R.C.S.I.", late Clinical Clerk at WRA, was appointed AMO to the Warwick County Asylum,[314] replacing there J.B. Ward, a former WRA Clinical Clerk (*vide supra*). Woods was recorded as being present at the WRA *conversazione* of 15th October 1872, presiding over "Stall C" upon which were arranged a "large number of scientific and surgical instruments belonging to the Asylum, together with others" loaned from elsewhere.[315] He was elected to the membership of the MPA in 1873.[316]

Although he did not publish in *WRLAMR* or *Brain*, Woods did later publish in the *Journal of Mental Science* from his post in Warwick.[317] In a listing of MPA members published in 1877 he appeared as "Medical Superintendent, Asylum, Killarney".[318] in County Kerry, having moved there after three years at Warwick. After fourteen years, he became superintendent at Cork District Asylum, and he was President of the MPA in 1901, delivering the presidential address at the meeting held in Queen's College, Cork. He died at the age of 58, one of his obituaries recording that his written contributions were "less

---

[311] It was Crichton-Browne who moved the vote of thanks following McDowall's Presidential Address to the MPA, in response to which McDowall dwelt "at some length on his association with Sir C. Browne [*sic*] at Wakefield" (*J Ment Sci* 1897;43(October 1897):702–703).

[312] *J Ment Sci* 1931;77(July 1931):658.

[313] *J Ment Sci* 1937;83(January 1937):xl. Obituary: *BMJ* 1936;2:446 (29th August).

[314] *Medical Press and Circular* 1872;14:361 (23rd October; Appointments). Also *BMJ* 1872;2:483 (26th October; Medical Appointments); *Medical Times and Gazette* 1872;2:476 (26th October; Appointments); *J Ment Sci* 1872–1873;18(January 1873):632 (Appointments); *Report* (1873:27).

[315] *Medical Press and Circular* 1872;14:360 (23rd October; Conversazione and lecture by Professor Turner).

[316] *J Ment Sci* 1873–1874;19(October 1873):473.

[317] Woods (1874–1875); also Woods (1874); an example of duplicate publication. Finn (2012:184) recorded seven publications in all by Woods in the *Journal of Mental Science*, most dating from the late 1880s and beyond.

[318] *J Ment Sci* 1877–1878;23:x. Of note (*vide infra*), Thomas Outterson Wood appeared in the same list, as "Medical Superintendent General Lunatic Asylum, Isle of Man".

numerous than they would have been could he have commanded more leisure and more detachment of mind".[319]

W. Crochley S. Clapham (ca.1848–1923)

William Crochley Sampson Clapham was a native of Wakefield. He trained at Cambridge and Guy's Hospital and served as a surgeon in the Franco-Prussian War of 1870. He was selected as a Clinical Clerk at WRA in 1872, working alongside John Lowe and W. Bryan Wood.[320] He was appointed Resident Clinical Assistant in late 1872, *vice* "T.O. Woods [*sic*]",[321] presumably meaning Oscar T. Woods who had recently been appointed AMO to the Warwick County Asylum.[322] Clapham continued in the Clinical Assistant role into 1873,[323] and was subsequently appointed AMO to the Hoxton House Asylum, London, in February 1873.[324] Hence it would appear that he was a Clinical Assistant at WRA for only 3–4 months.

Despite this, Clapham published three papers in *WRLAMR*, the first in 1873 as "Fellow of the London Anthropological Society; Late Clinical Assistant West Riding Asylum" and the latter two both in 1876, when his affiliation was designated simply as "West Riding Asylum". The anthropological connection may perhaps explain his particular interests as manifested in these *WRLAMR* papers. The first two papers had the same title, "The weight of the brain in the insane" (III: 285–298; VI:11–26), whilst the third, a joint effort with Henry Clarke (for whom, see Chap. 7), was on "The cranial outline of the insane and criminal" (VI:150–169). Clapham later published in

---

[319] Obituary: *J Ment Sci* 1906;52(October 1906):841, which also noted that "He began his studies in insanity, like so many men of his time, at the West Riding Asylum, Wakefield"; *cf. BMJ* 1906;2:455 (25th August), which did not mention WRA, saying that "He began his career in asylum work … as medical officer to the Warwickshire Asylum".

[320] *Report* (1873:27). Crichton-Browne referred to him here as "Crochley Clapham" but Finn (2012:125) referred to him as "William Clapham".

[321] *Lancet* 1872;2:693 (9th November; Medical Appointments); also *J Ment Sci* 1872–1873;18(January 1873):631 (Appointments) with the same error in Woods' initials. Clapham's appointment was also noted in *Medical Press and Circular* 1872;14:428 (13th November; Appointments).

[322] *J Ment Sci* 1874–1875;20(April 1874):166 (Appointments) recorded a "Wood, Thomas O.", presumably Thomas Outterson Wood, with whom Oscar T. Woods might potentially have been confused. Outterson Wood was appointed Medical Superintendent of the Isle of Man Lunatic Asylum, Douglas, in 1876 (*Medical Press and Circular* 1876;21:84) and later wrote on the history of the Medico-Psychological Association (Outterson Wood 1896).

[323] *Report* (1874:28).

[324] *Lancet* 1873;1:291 (22nd February; Medical Appointments); *Medical Press and Circular* 1873;15:197 (26th February; Appointments).

Brain on related topics, "On skull mapping" (1878)[325] and "Head measurements" (1880), and elsewhere.[326]

In an August 1875 paper Clapham reported experience gained on a trip around the world of nearly two years duration. In Hong Kong, at the postmortem of a patient who died after a fall whilst sea-sick, the pathological changes were reported to be similar to those he had previously seen in a patient examined during his time at WRA "who died in the 'status'". Accordingly, Clapham subsequently tried amyl of nitrite, a remedy which Crichton-Browne had found helpful for epileptic status at WRA (III:153–174), in individuals with sea-sickness, finding it "eminently satisfactory" in 121 of 124 trials.[327]

Clapham eventually returned to the North of England, to work at The Grange at Rotherham and also as Physician to the Sheffield Royal Hospital. "Mr. C. Clapham" of York was one of those accepting invitations to the 1875 medical *conversazione* at WRA.[328]

He was elected a member of the MPA in 1878,[329] and over the next 20 years continued to publish and present on occasion on topics related to head shape and insanity,[330] including two contributions to Hack Tuke's (1892) *Dictionary of psychological medicine.* One such was a paper presented to the MPA meeting at Sheffield in February 1898 on the comparative intellectual value of the anterior and posterior cerebral lobes, wherein Clapham discussed the newer, "lobar phrenology" of David Ferrier (see Chap. 7), as against the older, "lobular phrenology" of Gall and Spurzheim, and presented data from measurements he had made in 4000 heads.[331]

Clapham was elected as an Ordinary Member of the Neurological Society of London in 1887. He was appointed Honorary Physician to the Sheffield Public Hospital and Dispensary in 1891 and ten years later as Consulting Physician to the Royal Hospital, Sheffield.[332] He published a sympathetic

---

[325] A subsequent editor of *Brain* was, more than 100 years later, to label this work on skull mapping as "verging on phrenology" (Kullmann 2019).

[326] Clapham (1878). Clapham's findings in Pelew Islanders were later commented on by Crichton-Browne (1931:36–37).

[327] Clapham (1875). He was listed here as having a doctorate, "Ph.D.". The paper was also mentioned in *Medical Record* 1875;10:728.

[328] *Leeds Mercury* 20th November 1875, p.3 (Medical Conversazione at Wakefield Asylum).

[329] *J Ment Sci* 1878–1879;24(October 1878):498.

[330] For example, Anon. (1881–1882) and Clapham (1892a, b, 1898a).

[331] Clapham (1898b).

[332] *Medical Press and Circular* 1891;52:696 (30th December; Appointments) which credited him as "M.D. Brux.". *Medical Press and Circular* 1901;71:186 (13th February; Appointments). The latter appointment was noted by Neve and Turner (1995:407n48).

obituary for John Charles Bucknill (see Chap. 9).[333] He died at the age of 75 in 1923.[334]

W. Bryan Wood

W. Bryan Wood was selected as a Clinical Clerk in 1872, along with John Lowe and Crochley Clapham.[335] During his time in Wakefield, he acted as a subject for Burman's experiments with injection of conia (II:16). He served on one of the stalls at the 1872 medical *conversazione*,[336] but resigned in early 1873 to be replaced by John Galton.

William Dyson Wood (1844–1900)

A possible source of confusion with "W. Bryan Wood" is a similarly named clinician, William Dyson Wood, who trained under James Syme (1799–1870) in Edinburgh and then worked as Assistant Surgeon at the West Riding House of Correction in Wakefield from around 1868 to 1879,[337] where his father, William Wood, also an Edinburgh graduate, was the Surgeon. He helped to manage an outbreak of enteric fever at the prison in 1875,[338] for which the Visiting Justices of the West Riding Prison made him a grant of £100. At the same time, his father was recommended the grant of a superannuation allowance of £200 a year on his resignation "in consequence of injury received in the performance of his duty".[339] In addition to his prison work, Dyson Wood did have some contacts with WRA: for example, he attended the medical *conversazione* in 1875.[340] Crichton-Browne reported many years later that, when "Assistant Medical Officer of the West Riding Prison", Dyson Wood "made some observations for me on the then routine punishment of three days in a dark cell with bread and water and found that the loss of weight was always considerable and in some cases amounted to 3 lb. … I requested Mr. Dyson Wood to have a number of prisoners undergoing that punishment

---

[333] Clapham (1897).

[334] Obituary: *J Ment Sci* 1923;69(October 1923):592–593. He was here listed as "M.D., F.R.C.P.Edin.".

[335] *Report* (1873:27). I have not found his name in the *Medical Directory*.

[336] *BMJ* 1872;2:474–475 (26th October; Medical Conversazione at the West Riding Asylum).

[337] *Lancet* 1868;2:529 (17th October; Medical Appointments).

[338] *Lancet* 1875;1:317 (27th February) and *Lancet* 1875;1:556 (17th April); the latter report stated that 17 persons died including two members of officers' families.

[339] *Medical Times and Gazette* 1875;2:511 (30th October).

[340] *BMJ* 1875;2:680 (27th November; The West Riding Asylum).

supplied with the ordinary prison diet while sojourning in the dark cell, but such was the rigidity of prison government in those days that the experiment was not allowed".[341]

G.W. Baroll

In the Superintendent's *Report* for 1873, "MR. G.W. BAROLL" was listed as one of the clinical assistants in that year, following Clapham and preceding Galton.[342] From 1874 through 1878 the *Medical Directory* lists a George William Barroll [*sic*] with qualifications in 1867 but with "*Address uncommunicated*"; he disappeared thereafter.

John C. Galton (ca.1840–1903)[343]

John Charles Galton was appointed Clinical Assistant in early 1873,[344] "vice Wood, resigned",[345] this referring presumably to W. Bryan Wood, rather than Oscar T. Woods.

Born in Exeter, Galton was educated at Oxford before qualifying M.R.C.S. in 1866 from St Bartholomew's Hospital. His obituary in the *BMJ*[346] stated that he then continued his studies in Vienna, and there was certainly a publication from Vienna dated 1872,[347] but prior to this there were publications from Oxford in 1869. He specialised in comparative anatomy, under the instruction of Professor Rolleston, publishing works on the six-banded armadillo and the aardvark in the *Transactions of the Linnean Society of*

---

[341] Crichton-Browne (1926:97–98). Had he confused Dyson Wood with Henry Clarke (see Chap. 7) who reported such a study (*Brain* 1878–1879;1(2):210–4) undertaken at Crichton-Browne's suggestion? It may also be mentioned here that Dyson Wood published on Hamlet, as did many nineteenth-century psychiatrists, specifically a pamphlet entitled *Hamlet from a psychological point of view*. This was reviewed in *J Ment Sci* 1871–1872;17(April 1871):133–134 and also *Br Foreign Med Chir Rev* 1871;48:140–142. This work was not considered by Bynum and Neve (1985) but its drift seems to run counter to their view that nineteenth-century clinical opinion generally accepted that Hamlet was insane.

[342] *Report* (1874:28) [capitals in original].

[343] Biographical material on Galton may be found in Lazar (2013:101–103).

[344] *Report* (1874:28).

[345] *Lancet* 1873;1:292 (22nd February; Medical Appointments); *Medical Press and Circular* 1873;15:197 (26th February; Appointments); *J Ment Sci* 1873–1874;19(April 1873):168.

[346] Obituary: *BMJ* 1903;2:173–174. (I thank Elizabeth Larner for drawing my attention to this reference, 16/11/2023.) Also Willett 1904a:cxxii-cxxiii; 1904b:16–17; Willett made no mention of Galton's time at WRA but noted that he "translated some German medical works into English".

[347] Galton (1872). Possibly also Galton (1874), where no affiliation was given.

London,[348] of which society he became a Fellow (FLS). His obituary stated that on return from Vienna he was lecturer in comparative anatomy at Charing Cross Hospital Medical School, but at the outbreak of the Franco-Prussian War (i.e. 1870) volunteered for foreign military service and "for the next seven or eight years" spent most of his time abroad as a military surgeon. Clearly this chronology is confusing, as seemingly contradictory to his known attendance at WRA in 1873 (which is not mentioned in his *BMJ* obituary).

He contributed a single paper to *WRLAMR*, "Notes on the condition of the tympanic membrane in the insane – Part I" (III:258–272). Despite the title, no "Part II" ever appeared. He also published a letter in the *BMJ* based on the findings at a post-mortem performed "this evening" (15th July 1873) at WRA.[349]

He made other contributions whilst at WRA which, with the benefit of hindsight, proved to be of greater importance. Firstly, he translated *Die Hirnwindungen des Menschen* (as *On the convolutions of the human brain*) from the original German text by the anatomist Alexander Ecker (1816–1887).[350] This work was later used by David Ferrier for the nomenclature of the human convolutions and in transposing his animal cortical localisations onto human brains.[351] Evidently a fine draughtsman, Galton also produced illustrations for Ferrier's 1873 *WRLAMR* paper on cortical localisation (III:30–96)[352] accompanied by his characteristic monogram, and was amongst those who received Ferrier's thanks at the end of this contribution. He also provided an illustrated microscopic section to Milner Fothergill (III:124 and n1).

He later published a single review and some abstracts of British and foreign journals in *Brain*. He was a Fellow of both the Linnaean and Zoological Societies and was elected a Fellow of the Royal Medical and Chirurgical Society of London in 1883. He was living in Upper Cheyne Row, Chelsea, when he died at the age of 63.

---

[348] Galton (1869a, b).

[349] Galton (1873).

[350] Reviews of Galton's translation of Ecker appeared in *Lancet* 1873;2:524 (11th October; Reviews and Notices of Books); *Nature* 1873;8:526–527 (23rd October; Ecker's "Convolutions of the Brain"); *BMJ* 1873;2:486 (25th October; Reviews and Notices); *Br Foreign Med Chir Rev* 1874;53(105):118–119 (Ecker on [*sic*] cerebral convolutions). Elsewhere it was described as a "capital translation" (*Lancet* 1873;2:908). For Alexander Ecker, see Lazar (2013:98–100) and Larner (2025g).

[351] Ferrier (1876:297, 298 (Fig. 59), 302 (Fig. 61)).

[352] This work was described by Lazar (2013).

Edward G. Levinge (1852–1929)

Edward George Levinge qualified in Ireland.[353] He was listed in the Superintendent's *Report* for 1873, "MR. E. LEVINGE", as one of the Clinical Assistants, following the name of Galton and preceding that of Tyler Smith.[354] It was recorded in the *Lancet* appointments section in September 1873 that he was appointed Assistant Medical Officer to the Borough Lunatic Asylum, Newcastle-upon-Tyne,[355] and subsequently that "Levinge" was replaced as Clinical Assistant at WRA by F. Wright (*vide infra*).[356] Levinge was noted as an unpublished correspondent to the *Lancet* from Wakefield in September 1873.[357] He was elected to membership of the MPA in 1874.[358] He did not publish in *WRLAMR* and does not appear to have published in the *Journal of Mental Science* or *Brain*. However, the authors of a case from the Hants County Asylum were "indebted to Edward G. Levinge, M.B., late Assistant Medical Officer, Hants County Asylum" published in 1877,[359] and Levinge himself had a publication in the *BMJ* in 1878 when he was Assistant Medical Officer at the Bristol Lunatic Asylum, a case in which the pathological details were provided by "My friend, Dr. Bevan Lewis, of the West Riding Asylum".[360]

Some years later, in 1887, Levinge was appointed Medical Superintendent to the Sunnyside Mental Hospital, Christchurch, New Zealand,[361] the first mental asylum to be opened in that city, in 1863. He appears to have remained in New Zealand until his death in 1929.

---

[353] *Lancet* 1871;1:558 (22nd April; Medical News. College of Physicians, Ireland).

[354] *Report* (1874:28) [capitals in original].

[355] *Lancet* 1873;2:473 (27th September; Medical Appointments). Also *J Ment Sci* 1873–1874;19(January 1874):645 (Appointments).

[356] *Lancet* 1873;2:508 (4th October; Medical Appointments [Wright]). Also *J Ment Sci* 1873–1874;19(January 1874):646 (Appointments).

[357] *Lancet* 1873;2:476 (27th September; Communications, Letters, &c.)

[358] *J Ment Sci* 1874–1875;20(October 1874):476

[359] *BMJ* 1877;1:164–165 (10th February; Hants County Asylum; Congenital hydrocephalic imbecility: post mortem examination: abnormally heavy brain: remarks. (Under the care of Dr. Hanley.)). The case was later cited by Clapham (1892a:164) as "recorded by Dr. Levinge", although the two do not appear to have overlapped at WRA.

[360] Levinge (1878:53). Levinge and Bevan-Lewis do not appear to have overlapped at WRA.

[361] *J Ment Sci* 1887–1888;33(October 1887):482.

E. Tyler Smith (1848–1901)

Ernest Louis Tyler Smith appeared in the Superintendent's *Report* for 1873 as one of the Clinical Assistants at WRA in 1873.[362] He assisted Herbert Major at the 1873 *conversazione* at the stall displaying microscopical preparations.[363] He was the son of William Tyler Smith (1815–1873),[364] a noted London obstetric physician from the late 1840s and President of the Obstetrical Society in 1861–1863. Crichton-Browne mentions "a very able paper, communicated to the Obstetrical Society by Dr. [William] Tyler Smith in 1861" (I:11).

Ernest Louis Tyler Smith appeared in the *Medical Directory* from 1876 (M.B. Camb. 1875; L.R.C.P. Edin. 1874) with an address in Hounslow, Middlesex, and from 1877 as "late Clin. Asst. York W. Riding Lunat. Asyl." as well as Fellow of the Obstetrical Society.[365] As of 1879 he appears as Ernest Louis Tyler-Smith [*sic*, with hyphen].[366]

F. Wright

"F. Wright" was appointed Clinical Assistant around October 1873,[367] in place of Levinge.[368] He was in turn replaced by Newcombe (*vide infra*) in early 1874.[369] Based on the entry in the *Medical Directory* of 1874 for Frederick Wade Wright, a Leeds graduate whose details included Clinical Assistant at WRA, this was in all likelihood the "Wright, F.W." whose appointment as Assistant Medical Officer to the Royal Lunatic Asylum at Aberdeen was

---

[362] *Report* (1874:28).

[363] *Yorkshire Post and Leeds Intelligencer* 27th November 1873, p.3 (West Riding Asylum. Medical Conversazione); *Leeds Mercury* 27th November 1873, p.7 (Medical Conversazione at the West Riding Asylum).

[364] Shepherd (1980:24).

[365] Finn (2012:183) listed Tyler Smith as "Author of 'Influence of Alcoholism in the Causation & Aggravation of Disease'" (not dated) but at time of writing I have not been able to identify this work.

[366] Another "saga of the inconsistent hyphen," perhaps? (See Crichton-Browne and Bevan-Lewis in this Chapter, and Hughlings Jackson in Chap. 7.) Another of William Tyler Smith's sons, Giulio Cowley Tyler Smith (1849–1909) reportedly changed his name to "Tyler-Smith" in later life (see Wikipedia entry for Giulio Cowley Smith, accessed 13/09/2024).

[367] *Lancet* 1873;2:508 (4th October; Medical Appointments); *Medical Press and Circular* 1873;16:337 (8th October; Appointments); *J Ment Sci* 1873–1874;19(January 1874):646 (Appointments).

[368] Unlike Levinge, Wright did not appear in Finn's listing (2012:181–184) of junior clinicians at WRA in the Crichton-Browne years.

[369] *Lancet* 1874;1:285 (21st February; Medical Appointments).

announced at the same time as Newcombe's move to WRA.[370] "Dr. F.W. Wright" was amongst those subscribing to Crichton-Browne's testimonial gift presented on 10th May 1876.[371] He does not appear in the Superintendent's *Report* for 1873, nor in the *Journal of Mental Science.*

C.E. Watson

In the Superintendent's Report for 1873, "MR. C.E. WATSON" was reported "at the present time" as Clinical Assistant along with Newcombe.[372] He was recorded at the 1874 *conversazione*: one of the tables was "superintended by Mr. C. E. Watson, of King's College, assisted by Mr. Bracey, the Apothecary of the Asylum, … fitted with numerous specimens of new drugs, and many magnificent samples of crystallised alkaloids, etc., lent by Messrs. Smith, of Edinburgh".[373] It may be that he was also at the 1873 *conversazione*, as it is recorded that a "Mr Watson" manned the table displaying drugs and medicinal preparations.[374]

Charles F. Newcombe (1851–1924)[375]

Charles Frederick Newcombe was noted to be Clinical Assistant "at the present time" in the Superintendent's *Report* for 1873 (dated 29th January 1874),[376] but his appointment as Clinical Assistant, *vice* Wright, was noted in the medical journals in early 1874.[377] Later that year he was appointed AMO at the Lancashire Lunatic Asylum, Rainhill,[378] to be replaced at WRA by

---

[370] *J Ment Sci* 1874–1875;20(April 1874):166 (Appointments); *Medical Press and Circular* 1874;17:40 (14th January; Appointments).

[371] *Medical Times and Gazette* 1876;1:529–530 (13th May; Presentation to Dr. Crichton Browne).

[372] *Report* (1874:28) [capitals in original]. I have not found his name in the *Medical Directory.*

[373] *Medical Times and Gazette* 1874;2:609 (28th November; Annual Conversazione at the West Riding Asylum).

[374] *Yorkshire Post and Leeds Intelligencer* 27th November 1873, p.3 (West Riding Asylum. Medical Conversazione); *Leeds Mercury* 27th November 1873, p.7 (Medical Conversazione at the West Riding Asylum). The other Watson, John W.F., would seem to have left WRA by this time (*vide supra*).

[375] Biographical material on Newcombe may be found in Low (1982) and Todd and Ashworth (1991:400).

[376] *Report* (1874:28).

[377] *Lancet* 1874;1:285 (21st February; Medical Appointments); *J Ment Sci* 1874–1875;20(April 1874):166 (Appointments); *Medical Press and Circular* 1874;17:171 (25th February; Appointments).

[378] Medical Director's Journal 29th April 1874 (WYAS C85/1/13/2). *BMJ* 1874;1:761 (6th June; Medical Appointments). See also *J Ment Sci* 1874–1875;20(July 1874):326 (Appointments); *Medical Press and Circular* 1874;17:482 (3rd June; Appointments).

Robert Lawson. Rainhill was Newcombe's primary affiliation when his only paper in *WRLAMR* was published, in the fifth volume, on "Epileptiform seizures in general paralysis" (V:198–226). Therein, Newcombe thanked Herbert Major "who kindly supplied me with notes of several … cases, taken from the records of the West Riding Asylum" (V:219). Prior to this, clinical notes by Newcombe and Major had been used by Crichton-Browne to report a patient with puerperal mania, pelvic haematocele, and sudden death, published in the *Lancet* in 1874.[379] Newcombe was later elected to membership of the MPA (1876),[380] and published a single article in *Brain* (which referenced the paper by "Nichol" [*sic*] in the first volume of *WRLAMR*), but nothing in the *Journal of Mental Science.*

He emigrated to the USA in 1884, later moving to Victoria, British Columbia, Canada, where he became an authority on local natural history and ethnology.[381]

Robert Lawson (?1846–1896)[382]

Robert Lawson was an Edinburgh graduate (1871),[383] apparently with links to Thomas Laycock since he later recorded himself in the *Medical Directory* (1879) as "Asst. to Prof. of Pract. of Med. and Med. Psychol. Univ. Edin. 1871-72" (also in *WRLAMR*, IV:240). According to an obituary, Lawson was selected by Laycock as his "class assistant for 1871-2 and imbued him with the shrewd and original thinking for which the chair of medicine was then celebrated".[384] These connections and attributes were likely to have impressed Crichton-Browne. Lawson was appointed Clinical Assistant at WRA in 1874,

---

[379] *Lancet* 1874;1:54 (10th January; West Riding Asylum)

[380] *J Ment Sci* 1876–1877;22(October 1876):489. Crichton-Browne was elected an Honorary Member at the same meeting.

[381] Obituary: *Nature* 1924;114(2877):903–904, which made no mention of Newcombe's medical work in the United Kingdom. See also Low (1982). Crichton-Browne (1937:93) later wrote of "a brilliant young physician, once a pupil of mine, who had to give up a successful practice in England and emigrate to Canada because of his wife's insane jealousy of every lady patient he attended". Might this pupil have been Newcombe?

[382] Biographical material on Robert Lawson may be found in Larner and Gardner-Thorpe (2012) (reprinted in adapted form as "Robert Lawson (ca. 1846–1896): alcoholic amnesia before Korsakoff" in Larner 2019b:142–144).

[383] *Alphabetical list of graduates of the University of Edinburgh …*, 1889:52. MB CM, 1871; MD 1881.

[384] *J Ment Sci* 1896;42(October 1896):474 (Dr Robert Lawson).

vice Newcombe.[385] At some point in 1874 or 1875 he was promoted to "Pathologist and Assistant Medical Officer" (V:40).[386]

Based on his publication record, Lawson was evidently one of the most industrious juniors to work at WRA. He was author on four papers in *WRLAMR*: "On the hourly distribution of mortality in relation to recurrent changes in the activity of vital functions" (IV:240–264); "On the physiological action of hyoscyamine" (V:40–84); "Hyoscyamine in the treatment of some diseases of the insane" (VI:65–84); and "Clinical notes on conditions incidental to insanity" (VI:120–149), the latter co-authored with Bevan-Lewis. In addition to these four papers, he also published extensively elsewhere in the medical literature during his years at WRA, manifesting his involvement in both clinical and experimental work.[387] As regards the former, other clinical cases appearing in the medical press were "reported by" or "indebted to" him.[388] As regards the latter, Crichton-Browne noted his "valuable assistance" with his own experimental programme.[389] Lawson attended the WRA medical *conversazione* in 1874 and 1875, on both occasions presiding over a display of selected specimens from the pathological museum.[390]

One of Lawson's principal interests was therapeutics[391] and in particular the physiological and therapeutic actions of hyoscyamine (V:40–84 and VI:65–84 respectively),[392] an alkaloid obtained from henbane (*Hyoscyamus niger*), and injected hypodermically. Lawson investigated both the experimental and

---

[385] *Lancet* 1874;1:822 (6th June, Medical Appointments); *Medical Press and Circular* 1874;17:503 (10th June; Appointments); *J Ment Sci* 1874–1875;20(July 1874):326 (Appointments).

[386] This was also his affiliation in Lawson (1875a). He was denoted simply as "Pathologist to the West Riding Lunatic Asylum" in Lawson (1875b).

[387] Lawson (1874, 1875a, b, c, 1876a, b).

[388] For example: *BMJ* 1875;1:774 (12th June; West Riding Asylum. Case of apoplexy of the cerebellum); *Lancet* 1876;2:50–51 (8th July; West Riding Asylum. Case of epilepsy of traumatic origin; Haemorrhage from vessels at the base of the brain. (Under the care of Dr. Major.)); *BMJ* 1876;2:430–431 (30th September; West Riding Lunatic Asylum. Cases of disease and extravasation into the cerebellum. (Under the care of Dr. Major.)). This listing does not claim to be comprehensive.

[389] Crichton Browne (1875a:542).

[390] For 1874: *Leeds Mercury* 21st November 1874, p.7 (Medical Conversazione at Wakefield Asylum). For 1875: *Medical Times and Gazette* 1875;2:603 (27th November; Conversazione at the West Riding Asylum); *Leeds Mercury* 20th November 1875, p.3 (Medical Conversazione at Wakefield Asylum).

[391] Lawson (1874, 1875a). Is it possible that Lawson was influenced in these interests by Lauder Brunton, a physician noted for his work in therapeutics (see Chap. 7)? Lauder Brunton visited WRA at some point in 1874, so may possibly have overlapped with Lawson's time there.

[392] Also Lawson (1876b). The article in *J Ment Sci* 1876–1877;22(October 1876):434–439 (Clinical notes and cases) entitled "The therapeutic action of hyoscyamine" is based on Lawson (1876b); and that in *J Ment Sci* 1877–1878;23(October 1877):368–372 (Occasional notes of the Quarter) entitled "Dr Lawson on the treatment of certain cases of insanity by hyoscyamine" (which concludes "*West Riding Reports for 1877* [*sic*]") is based on *WRLAMR* VI:65–84. The WRA alumnus Geroge Thompson later (1888) advocated use of hyoscine, also derived from henbane, for the treatment of mania, but did not reference Lawson's work on hyoscyamine.

clinical use of hyoscyamine, in the latter reporting good results in recurrent, acute and subacute mania, monomania of suspicion and the excitement of senile dementia, and even reporting cures of patients with chronic mania and often with chronic alcoholism, finding that hyoscyamine worked where bromide of potassium and tincture of cannabis had failed.[393]

Lawson left WRA in 1877, appointed AMO to the Middlesex Lunatic Asylum, Banstead.[394] At the meeting of the Physiological Society in London on 15th February 1877 when David Ferrier was in the chair he introduced as a guest "Mr. Robert Lawson"[395]; although their respective sojourns at WRA do not appear to have overlapped, they may possibly have encountered one another, or, as I think more likely, Lawson had an introduction to Ferrier from Crichton-Browne.[396] Lawson was also subsequently a contributor to *Brain*, including one of the earliest descriptions of amnesia in alcoholics, long predating the description which gained eponymous fame for Sergei Korsakoff (1854–1900), published in 1887.[397] At the time of this paper, Lawson was working as the Medical Superintendent of the Wonford House Lunatic Asylum in Exeter. He also published in the *Journal of Mental Science*, on the (alleged) epilepsy of Shakespeare's Othello,[398] by which time he was Deputy Commissioner in Lunacy in Scotland, appointed 1878,[399] a post in which he died after 18 years of service in 1896. According to his obituary, Crichton-Browne "valued him as one of the ablest and most agreeable assistants he ever had".[400] He sent congratulations to Crichton-Browne on his knighthood in 1886.[401]

---

[393] Crichton-Browne (1865) had published on bromide of potassium during his time in Newcastle.

[394] *BMJ* 1877;1:409 (31st March; Medical Appointments). Also *Medical Press and Circular* 1877;23:300 (11th April; Appointments); *Lancet* 1877;1:669 (5th May; Medical Appointments [Plaxton]).

[395] Sharpey-Schafer (1927:43–44).

[396] Another possibility, which I think less likely, is an introduction through Bevan-Lewis, if he was already in touch with Ferrier regarding his cortical lamination paper (Lewis and Clarke 1878) which Ferrier presented to the Royal Society. More likely, I think, Bevan-Lewis was introduced to Ferrier by Crichton-Browne.

[397] Lawson (1878–1879). Draaisma (2009:163–164) described Lawson's paper as the "most promising account" of alcoholic amnesia reported in the medical literature before Korsakoff.

[398] Lawson, 1880 (cf. Larner 2007 for a different opinion on Othello's loss of consciousness; reprinted in Larner 2019b:176). One may perhaps suspect the influence of Bucknill here, as both a former superintendent of the Devon County Lunatic Asylum in Exeter and a commentator on the works of Shakespeare, viz. *The Psychology of Shakespeare* (1859) and *The Medical Knowledge of Shakespeare* (1860). The asylum doctors with an interest in the works of Shakespeare also included John Conolly who published *A Study of Hamlet* (1863) (Renvoize 1991:44; Scull et al. 1996:80). In this context, see also Bynum and Neve (1985).

[399] *Medical Press and Circular* 1878;26:324 (16th October; Appointments); *J Ment Sci* 1878–1879;24(January 1879):698 (Appointments).

[400] Obituary: *J Ment Sci* 1896;42(October 1896):474.

[401] Crichton-Browne (1926:191–192).

Robert Lawson Tait (1845–1899)

A possible, if unlikely, source of confusion with Robert Lawson is a similarly named clinician, Robert Lawson Tait, unlikely since he was generally known as Lawson Tait.[402] An Edinburgh graduate, he worked as house surgeon at Wakefield Infirmary between 1867 and 1870 before moving to Birmingham.[403] Hence, he arrived in Wakefield shortly after Crichton-Browne. Both were acknowledged in Netten Radcliffe's 1870 report on the sanitation of Wakefield, and both were correspondents with Darwin, so the comment by one of Lawson Tait's biographers that he "developed a close friendship with Dr Crichton Browne" is neither impossible nor implausible. Indeed, in a letter to the *BMJ* published in September 1870 Tait referred to Crichton-Browne as "my distinguished friend" and reported, following a visit to the Asylum farm where he found the milk to have a "peculiarly disagreeable smoky taste", that Crichton-Browne "had sometimes occasion to send away milk and cream from his table, which was unfit to use on account of this smoky taste", comments bespeaking a certain close familiarity.[404] Many decades later Crichton-Browne wrote that "I was always on very friendly terms with Lawson Tait".[405] However, the suggestion that Tait "may well have collaborated in his [Crichton-Browne's] research into mental conditions" is highly unlikely as Tait was a surgeon and, at least eventually, against animal experimentation as a means of understanding human physiology.[406] However, according to his 1871 paper "On the myoidema [*sic*] of phthisis" Tait did see patients at WRA:

> In order further to extend my experience of the value of the myoidema, and to avoid any possible source of error, I examined a number of the inmates of the West Riding Lunatic Asylum, having been permitted to do so by the courtesy of my friend, Dr. Crichton Browne. A table of these observations I append, and it

---

[402] Biographical material on Lawson Tait may be found in: Leyland (1888:II:144–155), who mentioned only "a brief sojourn at Wakefield" (144); Shepherd (1980) and Marland (1987:415–416); D'Arcy Power, revised Sewell, https://doi.org/10.1093/ref:odnb/26919

[403] In his biography, Shepherd (1980:16–29) gave these dates for Tait's time in Wakefield, as did Reader (1971:692), although Marland (1987:415) said 1867 to 1871. Tait's appointment in Birmingham dates to 1870, although he was certainly in Wakefield in 1871 for his marriage to Sybil Stewart, daughter of a Wakefield solicitor, at the Parish church (now Cathedral) on 28th June.

[404] Tait (1870). Of note, this letter, dated 17th September, is addressed as from "Waterloo Street, Birmingham".

[405] Crichton-Browne (1930:122).

[406] Shepherd (1980:28–29). The reference Shepherd gave here was "Viets, H.R. (1938) 'Crichton Browne 1840–1938'. Bull. Of Inst. Of Hist. Med. 6, 472" which I cannot find. Viets's paper, on *WRLAMR*, begins on page 477 of this volume, and there is a picture of Crichton-Browne on the facing page. The preceding paper, on an entirely different topic, covers pages 467–476. Tait was never a visiting surgeon to the Asylum, a position more usually awarded to more senior local practitioners (see Chap. 2).

will be seen they fully bear out my former conclusions. Amongst the insane phthisis is well known to be extremely prevalent, so that it is not surprising to find fascicular irritability in a large percentage of the insane, and the nodule in many of those who, at the time of examination, were losing weight.[407]

The table referred to included 90 patients.[408] Lawson Tait's name later appeared on the "List of the gentlemen invited" to the 1872 medical *conversazione* at WRA.[409]

John Merson (1846-?1936)[410]

John Merson, who had his medical training at the University of Aberdeen, came to WRA in 1873, succeeding McDowall as Pathologist, having already spent three years as Assistant Medical Officer in the Northumberland County Asylum. According to Crichton-Browne, his "solid attainments have already been brought into requisition, during his residence here as a Supernumerary".[411] He was promoted to the degree of MD at the University of Aberdeen in 1874.[412]

He attended the WRA *conversazione* of 1873, at a stall displaying photographs and stereoscopes,[413] and again in 1875, at a stall showing a "magnificent collection of photographs of insane patients now or formerly resident in the Asylum".[414] He published three papers in *WRLAMR*, "The urinology of general paralysis" (IV:63–93); "On the influence of diet in epilepsy" (V:1–23); and "The climacteric period in relation to insanity" (VI:85–107), all as Assistant Medical Officer.[415]

---

[407] Tait (1871:324).

[408] Ibid., 325–326.

[409] *Leeds Mercury* 17th October 1872, p.8 (Medical Conversazione at the West Riding Asylum.). I have found no information to indicate whether or not he attended.

[410] Biographical material on John Merson may be found in Bickford (1981:51–52, 1983:28–29) and Bickford and Bickford (1983:87–88), although their suggested date of death ("c1933") does not tally with my findings.

[411] *Report* (1874:28).

[412] *Medical Times and Gazette* 1874;2:197 (15th August; Medical News). Johnston (1906:365). MA 1866, MB CM 1870, MD 1874.

[413] *Yorkshire Post and Leeds Intelligencer* 27th November 1873, p.3 (West Riding Asylum. Medical Conversazione); *Leeds Mercury* 27th November 1873, p.7 (Medical Conversazione at the West Riding Asylum). The latter gave his name as "John Moxon" [*sic*].

[414] *Medical Times and Gazette* 1875;2:603 (27th November; Conversazione at the West Riding Asylum); *Leeds Mercury* 20th November 1875, p.3 (Medical Conversazione at Wakefield Asylum).

[415] Merson's work on epilepsy (V:1–23) was recalled many years later by Crichton-Browne (1895:75, 1927:41) in a lecture on dreamy states.

At the time of Crichton-Browne's departure from WRA, Merson was reportedly the "Deputy Medical Director", and it was he who presented the illuminated vellum memorial to Crichton-Browne on behalf of the staff of WRA in March 1876.[416] However, when elected to the membership of the MPA, as noted in October 1877, he was listed as "Senior Assistant Medical Officer".[417]

Merson was later appointed Medical Superintendent of Hull Borough Asylum, in succession to John Wallis (*vide infra*).[418] Bickford reported that in this role Merson was "competent" and that he "reduced the provisions supplied to patients ... and stopped the issue of beer. ... He came to Hull as a bachelor but soon announced his forthcoming marriage to a widow with children who had been Matron at Wakefield".[419] Merson superintended the move from the Old Asylum in Hull's Argyle Street to the new purpose-built asylum at De La Pole Farm in 1883. Comments from his Asylum Report appeared in the *Journal of Mental Science* in 1890,[420] but otherwise he published neither in this journal nor in *Brain*.

Reporting on the Hull Borough Asylum in 1889, by this time "situated six miles from Hull, at Cottingham", Hack Tuke stated that it was "Dr. Merson ... to whom the satisfactory state of the existing asylum is really due".[421] Merson made medical news in 1897 when it was reported that he was "rendered unconscious by a violent blow to the back of the head with a cricket bat, by one of the inmates. His condition for some time caused much anxiety, but he is now making slow but steady progress.".[422] Indeed it seems to have had no impact on his longevity: he was to remain in office at Hull for nearly fifty years.[423] At a dinner in honour of Crichton-Browne held in 1931, the former WRA Medical Director acknowledged that Merson, along with McDowall,

---

[416] *Medical Times and Gazette* 1876;1:365–366 (1st April; Dr. Crichton Browne).

[417] *J Ment Sci* 1877–1878;23(October 1877):434.

[418] *Medical Press and Circular* 1878;26:466 (4th December; Appointments); *J Ment Sci* 1878–1879;24(January 1879):698 (Appointments).

[419] Her name was Harriet Castledine. See Bickford (1981:51 and, especially, 1983:31–32).

[420] *J Ment Sci* 1890;36(July 1890):424.

[421] Hack Tuke (1889a:369, 1889b:15). Hack Tuke (1889b:24, 31) also referred to Merson.

[422] *BMJ* 1897;2:320 (31st July; Medical News). Cited by Macmillan (2011–2012:35). Also *J Ment Sci* 1897;43(October 1897):885. No update on his health is to be found in the *BMJ*, but he certainly wrote to the Journal early in the following year, *BMJ* 1898;1:196 (15th January; Letters, Communications, Etc.). Based on the timing, I suspect this unpublished correspondence may have related to the untimely death of John Wallis, his predecessor as superintendent at the Hull Asylum (*vide infra*). Bickford (1983:71) dated the cricket bat incident to 1898, stating that "Dr. Merson was umpiring ... when a patient he had given out attacked him so violently that he was concussed, and on sick leave for months".

[423] Bickford (1981:52). Bickford and Bickford (1983:88), said that he retired from Hull in March 1924, to live in Selby. Their conclusion was that "he was an administrator rather than a doctor".

was still surviving.[424] Merson's name appeared in the Obituary column of the *Journal of Mental Science* issue of January 1937.[425]

William T. Benham (Born 1847)

In the *Lancet* issue of 18th April 1874 the following announcement appeared:

> BENHAM, W.T., M.D. (Assistant Medical Officer at the Bristol City and County Asylum), has been appointed Pathologist and Assistant Medical Officer to the West Riding Asylum, Wakefield.[426]

In the Medical Director's Journal for 29th April 1874, Crichton-Browne wrote that:

> Dr. W.T. Benham who had served for two years as Assistant Medical Officer in the Bristol Asylum and who had come here gratuitously as a Clinical Assistant was with the approval of the Chairman temporarily appointed in his [McDowall's] stead. He has discharged his duties most efficiently and I now beg to submit his testimonials and recommend his appointment.[427]

William Thomas Benham received his medical training in both Aberdeen and Bristol. His appointment in Bristol dated from 1872,[428] so he would presumably have known and been known to George Thompson, an erstwhile WRA AMO who had moved to Bristol Asylum as Superintendent in 1871 (if so, one might speculate as to whether Thompson may have provided Benham with one of the testimonials spoken of by Crichton-Browne). Benham was elected member of the MPA in 1872.[429] He published a paper from Bristol in

---

[424] *J Ment Sci* 1931;77(July 1931):658.

[425] *J Ment Sci* 1937;83(January 1937):xl.

[426] *Lancet* 1874;1:571 (18th April; Medical Appointments) [capitals in original]. Also *BMJ* 1874;1:565 (25th April, Medical Appointments) which gave his first name. Also *Medical Press and Circular* 1874;17:372 (29th April; Appointments).

[427] Medical Director's Journal 29th April 1874 (WYAS C85/1/13/2).

[428] Benham's appointment as "Assistant Resident Medical Superintendent of the Bristol Lunatic Asylum" was listed in *Medical Press and Circular* 1872;13:266 (20th March), ditto *J Ment Sci* 1872–1873;18:152 (April 1872; Appointments). Both the *Lancet* and *BMJ* gave his Bristol post as Assistant Medical Officer.

[429] *J Ment Sci* 1872–1873;18(October 1872):460 where his name was given as "W.S. Benham [*sic*]" but the affiliation, Bristol Asylum, was correct.

1873,[430] the same year he received his MD degree from the University of Aberdeen.[431]

Benham undertook experimental work at WRA as shown in his two *WRLAMR* publications, "On the therapeutic value of cold to the head" (IV:152–178) and "The actions of nicotine" (IV:305–317). "Dr. T. W. Benham" presided over one of the tables at the 1874 medical *conversazione*, "A stall for scientific and surgical instruments", and later in the evening "demonstrated Ludwig's Strom-uhr as a method of determining the amount of blood passing through any vessel in a given time".[432]

Benham also published a single paper in the *Journal of Mental Science*,[433] although the patient reported had been seen in Bristol rather than in Wakefield. He never published in *Brain*. According to the *Medical Press and Circular* of 9th December 1874, Benham was appointed "Physician-in-Chief to the Chilian [*sic*] Government Lunatic Asylum at Santiago".[434]

A possible source of confusion here is the similarly named clinician, Harry Arthur Benham, younger brother of William Thomas, born 1856, who became Medical Superintendent in Bristol in succession to George Thompson in 1890.[435]

J. Davy

DAVY, Dr. J., Clinical Assistant at the West Riding Lunatic Asylum, Wakefield.[436]

---

[430] Benham (1873).

[431] *BMJ* 1873;2:245 (23rd August; University of Aberdeen). Johnston (1906:38). MB CM 1871, MD 1873.

[432] *Medical Times and Gazette* 1874;2:609 (28th November; Annual Conversazione at the West Riding Asylum).

[433] Benham (1874–1875).

[434] *Medical Press and Circular* 1874;18:517 (9th December; Appointments). Also *Medical Times and Gazette* 1874;2:649 (5th December; Appointments); *BMJ* 1874;2:758 (12th December; Medical Appointments); *J Ment Sci* 1874–1875;20(January 1875):663 (Appointments).

[435] Tobia (2017:56) stated that "Dr Thompson retired and was replaced by Dr. Harry Bentham [*sic*], whose older brother William had been an assistant to Dr. Thompson." Is it likely that both a William Benham and a William Bentham could have worked in close succession for Thompson at Bristol? Dr. H.A. Benham appears as a member of the MPA from 1872, and as Medical Superintendent of City and County Asylum, Stapleton, near Bristol. I suggest that Tobia, *passim*, was thus in error with "Bentham", rather than "Benham". For Harry Benham's qualifications, see Johnston (1906:38). MB CM 1880, MD 1883.

[436] *Medical Press and Circular* 1875;19:21 (6th January; Appointments). Also *J Psychol Med Ment Pathol* 1875;1:x [after 154].

This notification appeared in the appointments section of the *Medical Press and Circular* in January 1875. However, this appointment may have finished very quickly, possibly even before it had begun, since just over a month later we read in the same journal's appointments section:

> DAVY, Mr. J., Assistant Resident Medical Officer to the Chorlton Union Workhouse.[437]

However, in the "Dramatic Performance" staged at WRA on 12th February 1875, the comedy "Faint heart never won fair lady", a "Dr. Davy" played the role of "PEDRO. His first appearance".[438] If this was, in fact, his first and last appearance at WRA, there was consequently a vacancy, shortly to be filled by one of the most notable figures in the history of the Asylum.

In the *Medical Directory* (408) for 1876, a "John Davy" was listed, with details "W. Riding Co. Asyl. Wakefield", ditto 1877, but in 1878 he was recorded as "*Address uncommunicated*" and the WRA affiliation disappeared thereafter.[439]

William Bevan-Lewis[440] (1847–1929)[441]

Like John Galton, William Bevan-Lewis had already made several career moves before arriving at WRA, such that he was older than some of his predecessors, such as Herbert Major. Born in Cardigan in the west of Wales, he trained at Guy's Hospital in London, qualifying in 1868. He gained initial

---

[437] *Medical Press and Circular* 1875;19:132 (10th February; Appointments).

[438] WYAS C85/1382. Other roles were taken in this production by Drs Lawson, Wallis, and Major.

[439] Davy was not mentioned in the listing of WRA AMOs and Clinical Assistants/Clerks presented by Finn (2012:181–184).

[440] As for both Crichton-Browne (*vide supra*) and Hughlings Jackson (Chap. 7), Bevan-Lewis is a subject for a "saga of the inconsistent hyphen" (using the terminology of Critchley and Critchley 1998:177–179, 181) since, as is the case for Hughlings Jackson and Crichton-Browne, there is inconsistency in the hyphenation of his name. As for Hughlings Jackson and Crichton-Browne, I have used the ultimate form, hence Bevan-Lewis (as per Larner and Triarhou 2023), which he adopted around 1906, with the exception of citations in the Bibliography where the specific usage in each paper is followed (as for Crichton Browne and Crichton-Browne), hence some of his publications appear as "Lewis B." or "Bevan Lewis W." or "Bevan-Lewis W." The hyphen was absent in his publications in *WRLAMR* and *Brain*, likewise in the three editions of his two textbooks, but it was present by the time of his address "On the Formation of Character" to the nursing staff at the York Retreat (November 1906) and in his presidential address to the Medico-Psychological Association (Bevan-Lewis 1909) and in his obituaries.

[441] There is no full-length (i.e. book-length) biography of Bevan-Lewis to my knowledge, but some shorter biographical pieces are available, for example Todd and Ashworth (n.d.:179–233), Hoole (2013), Triarhou (2021:59–63), and Larner and Triarhou (2023). The latter forms the basis for the account presented here.

experience as an Assistant Medical Officer at Buckingham County Asylum at Aylesbury[442] and at Norwich Borough Asylum but, having married young, was obliged to pursue private practice in Cardigan which he reportedly found uncongenial. He first appeared in the *Medical Directory* in 1871 at a post in Rotherham. He was appointed as Clinical Assistant at WRA in early 1875 "vice Watson, resigned",[443] to be replaced by "L. Jones" as "Medical Officer to the Pembrey Copper and Colliery Works, the Bury [*sic*] Port Smelting Company, the Pembrey White Lead Works, and the Bury [*sic*] Port and Gwendraeth Valley Railway Company".[444]

Like Major, Bevan-Lewis (Fig. 5.3) started to publish early in his WRA career, not only in *WRLAMR* but elsewhere.[445] He had an evident interest in neuropathology, as shown by his first paper in *WRLAMR*, "On the histology of the great sciatic nerve in general paralysis of the insane" (V:85–104), which confirmed the opinion of Major concerning morbid changes in the peripheral nerves of patients with GPI (V:86), and in this type of work Lewis noted that he was encouraged by Major.[446] He also did some experimental work, "Calorimetric observations upon the influence of various alkaloids on the generation of animal heat" (VI:43–64), and a collaborative paper with Robert Lawson, "Clinical notes on conditions incidental to insanity" (VI:120–149). He attended the medical *conversazione* in 1875, manning a table with Major displaying microscopical preparations.[447]

Also like Major, Bevan-Lewis joined in the amateur dramatic performances at the Asylum, for example on 12th November 1875 he appeared as "Mr. Euclid Facile" in the farce "Twice Killed" and also in the following "grand fairy extravaganza" of "The Invisible Prince".[448]

---

[442] *J Ment Sci* 1869–1870;15:165 (April 1869; Appointments).

[443] *Lancet* 1875;1:390 (13th March; Medical Appointments). Also noted in *Medical Press and Circular* 1875;19:242 (17th March; Appointments) and *BMJ* 1875;1:828 (19th June; Medical Appointments). I have no explanation for the disparity of 3 months between these announcements. Also *J Psychol Med Ment Pathol* 1875;1:x [after 154], concurrent with Davy. Shorvon and Compston (2019:381) erred in stating that Crichton-Browne "appointed Bevin [*sic*] Lewis in 1871 [*sic*] as pathologist at the West Riding Lunatic Asylum".

[444] *Lancet* 1875;1:810 (5th June; Medical Appointments). The Carmarthenshire town is in fact "Burry Port" or Porth Tywyn.

[445] For example, Lewis (1876a, b, 1877) and Bevan Lewis (1877–1878). Arbuckle (1876b:212) misdated Lewis (1876a) as appearing in the *Medical Times and Gazette* issue of 3rd March, rather than 4th March.

[446] Lewis (1876a:248).

[447] *BMJ* 1875;2:680 (27th November; The West Riding Asylum); *Medical Times and Gazette* 1875;2:603 (27th November; Conversazione at the West Riding Asylum); *Leeds Mercury* 20th November 1875, p.3 (Medical Conversazione at Wakefield Asylum).

[448] WYAS C85/1382, programme for "Theatre Royal, Stanley-cum-Wrenthorpe". Mrs. Lewis also appeared in "Twice Killed"; Drs Lawson and Arbuckle and Mr. Bracey appeared in both productions.

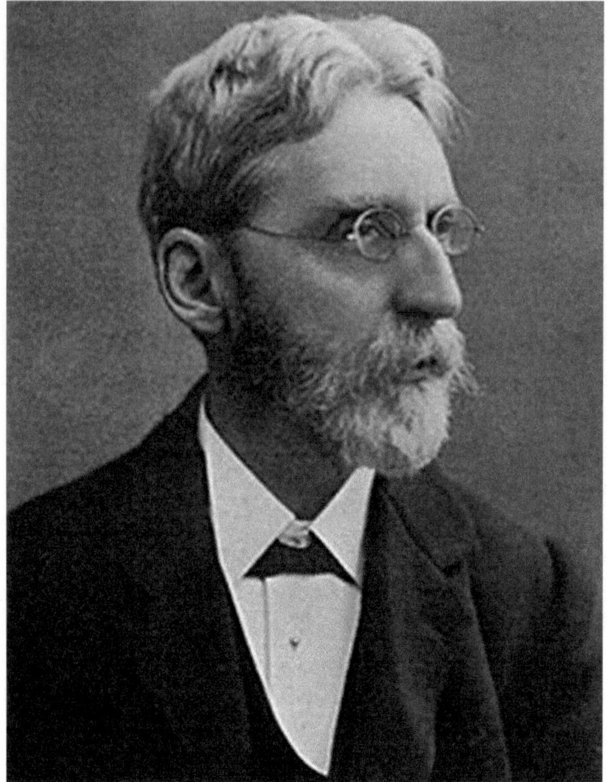

Fig. 5.3 William Bevan-Lewis

Bevan-Lewis's career after Crichton-Browne's departure was the most distinguished of any of the WRA staff of the era. He was prolific contributor to both *Brain* and the *Journal of Mental Science*. In addition, he was co-author with Henry Clarke (for whom, see Chap. 7) of a seminal paper on cerebral cytoarchitectonics which was communicated to the Royal Society by David Ferrier (see Chap. 7) on 24th January 1878. Building on the work of Meynert, Bevan-Lewis and Clarke illustrated for the first time the large pyramidal ("ganglionic") cells previously described by Betz ("Betz cells") and showed their distribution, thus localising the motor area anterior to the fissure of Rolando. As for cortical lamination, a subject on which Major had previously published, Bevan-Lewis and Clarke made only a single mention of Major, to the effect that he "follows Baillarger in regarding the cortex of the vault and that of the central lobe as consisting of six layers".[449] In contrast, Bevan-Lewis and Clarke favoured a five-layered model of the motor area, following the scheme of Meynert. Their only reference to Major's papers on the subject was to his 1876 *WRLAMR* publication (VI:1–10) but not to his other studies which had described cortical lamination in the brains of non-human primates and man.[450] Bevan-Lewis's subsequent paper in the inaugural issue of *Brain* (April 1878), "On the comparative structure of the cortex cerebri", was an extension of this work and repeated his views about pentalaminar and hexalaminar cortices: "There is a five and a six-laminated cortex, each typical of a certain definite area: but, whilst the six-layered formation is found extensively spread over the convolutions of the parietal and other regions, the *five-laminated* type is pre-eminently characteristic of the motor area of the brain".[451] This work included comparative studies in various animals (rat, rabbit, pig, sheep, cat, ocelot, Barbary macaque) and was supported by a government grant.

A series of six papers on "Methods of preparing, demonstrating, and examining cerebral structure in health and disease" by Bevan-Lewis appeared in *Brain* between 1880 and 1882, subsequently forming the subject matter of his first book, *The Human Brain. Histological and Coarse Methods of Research. A Manual for Students and Asylum Officers*, which was published in 1882.[452] These various studies not only demonstrated his facility with microscopic techniques but also the use of the freezing microtome to cut thin sections of brain tissue. His familiarity with various staining techniques was instrumental in his description of "spider cells" (what would now be termed astrocytes) in the cortex of brains from patients with general paralysis of the insane. He also made use of the photographic facilities established at WRA by Crichton-Browne to illustrate his works. He was acknowledged in the preface to the second edition of David Ferrier's *The functions of the brain* (1886), the first

---

[449] Lewis and Clarke (1878:42). For further discussion of this paper, see Triarhou (2021:59–63) and Larner and Triarhou (2024b:1659–1661). The latter authors questioned whether Bevan-Lewis's omission of references to Major's works was mere oversight or wilful exclusion; certainly, a general pattern of minimal or non-citation of his colleague appears to emerge. He certainly knew of Major's work since it was displayed at the table which he shared with Major at the 1875 *conversazione* (*BMJ* 1875;2:680; see Chap. 8). Finn (2012:155–157, 171) noted the pioneering contributions of both Major and Bevan-Lewis to cortical cytoarchitectonics.

[450] Major (1875, 1875–1876a, b, 1877a).

[451] Lewis, 1878–1879:80 [italics in original] (this paper is listed, along with others, in Table 6.4).

[452] Bevan Lewis (1882). In his Preface, he stated that "Prompted by the editors of *Brain*, ... the author contributed to the pages of that journal a series of articles on 'Methods of Preparing, Demonstrating, and Examining Cerebral Structure in Health and Disease.'" (1882:v). Does this mean he was in contact with all four of them, or that they spoke collectively when inviting contributions to *Brain*? I think it would seem likely that Crichton-Browne was the main mover in this instance, with his interest in brain pathology and his personal promotion of Bevan-Lewis.

edition of which Bevan-Lewis cited in a case report of epileptiform convulsions in general paralysis of the insane, with localisation of discharging lesions.[453] He also assisted at least two WRA alumni, Levinge and Plaxton, by contributing pathological reports in their publications.[454]

Bevan-Lewis became Superintendent of WRA in 1884 following Major's resignation and remained in the post for 26 years. During this time, he inaugurated an outpatient department (1889), reconstructed the pathology department to include a complete outfit of laboratories by 1895, and oversaw the planning and building of a new acute hospital on the site (opened in 1900). He also witnessed the founding of further branches of WRA, the third and fourth respectively, at Menston (1888) and Storthes Hall outside Huddersfield (1904).

Bevan-Lewis's magnum opus, *A Text-book of Mental Diseases*, first appeared in 1889 (second edition 1899) and was dedicated to Sir James Crichton-Browne "In admiration of the vigorous intellect, commanding eloquence, and untiring energy brought to bear on the scientific aspects of psychological medicine during his directorate of the West Riding Asylum". The book summarised Bevan-Lewis's wealth of neuropathological and clinical experience, including observations on the deleterious effects of alcohol on the brain.[455] It was acknowledged to be "without doubt, the best English book of its kind" by the reviewer in the *Journal of Mental Science*.[456] Bevan-Lewis also contributed to Hack Tuke's (1892) *Dictionary of psychological medicine* (Psycho-physical methods, II:1022–1024; Reaction-time in certain forms of insanity, II:1063–1067) and the chapter on the pathology of the nervous system in the first edition (1899) of the multi-volume *A System of Medicine* edited by Clifford Allbutt (for whom, see Chap. 7).[457] Throughout his years at Wakefield, Bevan-Lewis was also Lecturer and Examiner in Mental Diseases to the Yorkshire College, later the University of Leeds; this post became a professorship when the Leeds school of medicine became a University Faculty. He was elected to the membership of the MPA in 1879[458] and became President in 1909. He finally retired from the superintendency of WRA in 1910.[459]

---

[453] Lewis (1877:530).

[454] Levinge (1878) and Plaxton (1878–1879).

[455] Bevan Lewis (1889).

[456] Anonymous review in *J Ment Sci* 1890;36:242–248, quote at 242.

[457] Bevan Lewis (1899). He did not appear in the second edition, published in 1911.

[458] *J Ment Sci* 1879–1880;25(October 1879):435.

[459] Obituaries: *Lancet* 1929;2:954–955; *BMJ* 1929;2:833–834; *J Ment Sci* 1930:76:383–388 [by JS Bolton].

John Hunter Arbuckle (ca.1845–1918)

As Clinical Assistant, John Hunter Arbuckle, a Glasgow graduate, presided over the drug-stall at the 1875 WRA *conversazione* which was "rich in new medicinal agents".[460] In the same year he had his only publication in *WRLAMR*, "On the appearance of the retina and choroid during the administration of certain drugs" (V:130–148). His experimental work was mentioned by Lawson (V:51n1).

He later published, in the capacity of "Clinical Assistant to the West Riding Asylum", some ophthalmological cases but as none had any documented mental health issues it is not clear if these patients were seen at WRA or elsewhere; the dating of the first case, 26th April 1873, predates Arbuckle's time at WRA.[461] He also published details on histological methods which referenced publications in *WRLAMR* by Sankey (see Chap. 7) and Major, as well as Bevan-Lewis;[462]; and a patient from WRA in whom "Dr Major believed she had an intra-cranial tumour … At his request I made a minute examination of her eyes with the ophthalmoscope on 6th October 1875".[463]

Arbuckle took the Diploma in Public Health, possibly in 1875, and later became Medical Officer of Health in Kilmarnock, date uncertain.[464] He did not publish in either the *Journal of Mental Science* or *Brain*.[465]

John Wallis (?1844 or?1846–1897)[466]

John Michael Augustus Wallis, or John Augustus Michael Wallis (sources differ), was, according to some sources, born in Waterford, Ireland, to others in Cornwall, his family only later removing to the south of Ireland. He studied medicine in Dublin and subsequently gained his medical qualification and

---

[460] *Medical Times and Gazette* 1875;2:603 (27th November; Conversazione at the West Riding Asylum). *BMJ* 1875;2:680 stated that Arbuckle was "with Mr. Bracey" on this stall which, as Bracey was the Asylum dispenser, would be appropriate. Likewise, *Leeds Mercury* 20th November 1875, p.3 (Medical Conversazione at Wakefield Asylum).

[461] Arbuckle (1876a).

[462] Arbuckle (1876b).

[463] Arbuckle (1876c).

[464] He was appointed house surgeon to the Stanley Hospital, Liverpool, according to *Medical Press and Circular* 1877;23:362 (2nd May; Appointments).

[465] Obituary: *Glasgow Med J* 1918:89(3):155. This does not mention his time at WRA.

[466] As an illustration of the uncertainty about Wallis's date of birth, Bickford and Bickford (1983:136) headline his entry in their biographical dictionary as "(1846–97)" but then report "B at Waterford, Sept 1844"! Johnston (1906:572) has "Sep. 1844".

later his MD from Aberdeen.[467] He was AMO at the Durham County Asylum from 1867. After seven years there, he travelled on the Continent and in the United States before his appointment at WRA.

Wallis contributed a single paper to *WRLAMR*, "On the therapeutic value of chloral hydrate in epileptic convulsions" (V:257–270). In the same year, experimental work on chloral hydrate (CCl_3CHO), a compound related to chloroform, was published in the *BMJ* by Crichton-Browne.[468] Wallis "superintended" one of the tables at the 1874 *conversazione*, "An excellent table of photographs, illustrative of cases at present or formerly in the Asylum".[469] He was elected to membership of the MPA in 1876.[470]

Wallis's affiliation in his *WRLAMR* paper was given as "Medical Superintendent, Hull Borough Asylum. Late Assistant Medical Officer, West Riding Asylum". Bickford reported of Wallis's time at Hull that he "was rather detached. … he described physical conditions in detail and he was interested in the shape of patients' skulls. He was a good superintendent but not personally concerned about the patients. He asked for an increase in salary when he married; it was refused".[471] This may explain why he was only briefly superintendent at Hull, leaving in 1878, to be succeeded by another WRA alumnus, John Merson (*vide supra*). Wallis was then superintendent at the Lancashire County Lunatic Asylum at Whittingham (the fourth Lancashire county asylum),[472] a post he held for 15 years before becoming a Commissioner in Lunacy,[473] replacing Cleaton, a former WRA superintendent (see Chap. 2). Wallis suffered from heart disease and died suddenly at the end of 1897.[474] His obituary in the *Journal of Mental Science* described him as "not a

---

[467] Johnston (1906:572). MB 1875, MD CM 1883.

[468] Crichton Browne (1875a). He had also published notes on the drug's "inconveniences and dangers" (Crichton Browne 1871c).

[469] *Medical Times and Gazette* 1874;2:609 (28th November; Annual Conversazione at the West Riding Asylum).

[470] *J Ment Sci* 1876–1877;22(October 1876):490. Crichton-Browne was elected an Honorary Member at the same meeting.

[471] Bickford (1981:51).

[472] *J Ment Sci* 1878–1879;24(January 1879):698 (Appointments), where his name is given as "WALLIS, J.M.A." [capitals in original].

[473] Mellett (1981, esp. 250). *Biographies of Medical Lunacy Commissioners* 1828–1912. http://studymore. org.uk/6biom.htm (accessed 09/12/2023) gave a different date of birth, "about 1846".

[474] Obituaries: *BMJ* 1898;1:120 (8th January); *J Ment Sci* 1898;44(April 1898):452–453. These are very similar, verbatim in parts. The *BMJ* obituary reported he was aged 52; if correct this is difficult to square with a birth date in either 1844 or 1846 since he died on 30th December 1897. Bickford (1981:51) said he died from a "ruptured aneurism" but gives no anatomical location; Bickford and Bickford (1983:136) stated "D of heart disease".

voluminous writer", noting his *WRLAMR* paper and also a paper in the *Journal of Mental Science* from his time at Whittingham.[475] He never published in *Brain*.

Joseph W. Plaxton

Joseph William Plaxton was a graduate of Hull. He is included in Finn's list of those working as either medical officers or clinical clerks at WRA during the Crichton-Browne era between 1866 and 1876,[476] but his appointment as AMO at WRA (in place of Lawson) clearly postdates Crichton-Browne's departure from WRA,[477] although it is just possible that he might have overlapped with his superintendency if he had previously been a Clinical Assistant (hence his inclusion here). His AMO appointment occurred in the same year in which he was elected to the MPA, at the same time as Churchill Fox and Merson.[478]

Plaxton did not publish in *WRLAMR* (unsurprisingly, as it may have become defunct by the time he arrived at WRA) nor in *Brain* but did have one publication in the *Journal of Mental Science* from WRA, which included a pathological report by Bevan-Lewis.[479] He was appointed medical superintendent of the Lunatic Asylum in Ceylon (as it then was) in 1878,[480] whence he had further publications in the *Journal of Mental Science*, but it appears he was not happy there ("In the happier times before the folly of exchanging England for Ceylon had overtaken me"[481]) and later moved to the Jamaica Lunatic Asylum, Kingston, Jamaica.[482]

---

[475] Wallis (1894).

[476] Finn (2012:183).

[477] *Lancet* 1877;1:669 (5th May; Medical Appointments); *Medical Press and Circular* 1877;23:382 (9th May; Appointments); *J Ment Sci* 1877–1878;23(July 1877):307 (Appointments). Scrimgeour (2015:310) recorded Plaxton's forthright opinion of one Asylum patient as "A sweet sample of the knave and fool", dated 1st August 1878.

[478] *J Ment Sci* 1877–1878;23(October 1877):434.

[479] Plaxton (1878–1879).

[480] *J Ment Sci* 1878–1879;24(January 1879):698 (Appointments).

[481] Plaxton (1880–1881:559). This paper listed him as "MRCP", which I presume was a typographical error for "MRCS". The latter is found in Plaxton (1881–1882).

[482] For example, Plaxton, 1888–1889. This paper listed him as "MRCS".

Discussion

WRA was atypical in the period 1866 to 1876 in that, unlike other county asylums of the era which were staffed by a Medical Superintendent and one or possibly two Assistant Medical Officers, several clinicians were often working at WRA at any one time. For example, the 1871 national census documented four clinicians at WRA in addition to Crichton-Browne (Thompson, Aldridge, Watson Dove, Sutherland). Furthermore, a listing of the Resident Staff which appeared in *WRLAMR* in 1872 (II:308) included Deputy Medical Director (Mitchell), Assistant Medical Officers (Aldridge, Burman, and Major) and Clinical Assistants (W.B. Wood and Oscar T. Woods). Moreover, in addition to the resident staff documented in this Chapter there were also visiting clinicians (to be discussed in Chap. 7). These staffing numbers evidently reduced the social isolation which was a typical aspect of asylum medicine as a specialty "with only superficial ties with the rest of the medical enterprise",[483] and may also have fostered education and promoted esprit de corps.

Accepting certain assumptions concerning the correct identification of particular individuals (i.e. "W.P. Ledgard" = William Edward Ledgard; "William Lawrence" = Alexander Lawrence; "J.W.F. Watson" = John Wilcocks Watson; "Baroll" = Barroll; "F. Wright" = Frederick Wade Wright), and noting missing data for certain individuals (Hay, Wood, Barroll, C.E. Watson, Davy), some observations and generalisations may be made regarding the WRA resident staff between 1866 and 1876. The data presented here indicate heterogeneity amongst the junior staff in terms of their origins, training, seniority, and career intentions, as might be anticipated in any medical institution. There is also a range from those who made significant intellectual contributions (Major, Bevan-Lewis) and/or became leaders in the field (McDowall, Woods, Bevan-Lewis) to those otherwise not biobibliographically identifiable (Hay, Barroll, Davy).

As for their origins, a few were locals: several came from and/or trained in nearby Leeds (Thompson, Aldridge, Bywater Ward, Wright) although to my knowledge Clapham was the only one to originate from Wakefield itself. The preponderance of those training and/or gaining qualifications in Scotland is perhaps not unexpected, considering Crichton-Browne's early career pathway in Edinburgh, and the widely held perception that Scottish medical training was superior to that obtainable in England in this period. Perhaps of note, however, is that although many had Edinburgh connections and/or qualifications (Oxley, Ledgard, Mitchell, Burman, Fox, Watson Dove, Major, Lowe,

---

[483] Scull (1979:176).

McDowall, Tyler Smith, Lawson) several others had connections with Aberdeen (Aldridge, Nicol, Lawrence, Wright, Newcombe, Merson, Benham, Davy, Wallis) but with only one graduating from Glasgow (Arbuckle). With respect to Edinburgh, it has been suggested[484] that Crichton-Browne, much influenced himself by Thomas Laycock, recruited from his course. How many of the Edinburgh trainees coming to WRA had passed through or were exposed to Laycock's teaching has not been examined here,[485] but it was a recorded factor in the training of at least three (Major, McDowall, and Lawson).[486] Irish connections are also evident in the resident WRA staff (Courtenay, Woods, Levinge, Wallis).[487]

As for their qualifications, many of those appointed to the WRA resident staff had some combination of the standard London "College and Hall" qualifications of MRCS Eng, LRCP Lond, and LSA (Ledgard, Thompson, Aldridge, Mayhew, Bywater Ward, Pedler, Hay, Watson Dove, J.W.F. Watson, Clapham, Galton, Wright, Benham, Bevan-Lewis, Plaxton). However, the suggestion that Crichton-Browne recruited from the course in mental diseases taught by W.H.O. Sankey at University College London[488] does not seem tenable, the evidence gathered here suggesting that only one member of WRA resident staff had been through that course (J.W.F. Watson). Of note, few WRA resident staff had Oxbridge connections (Cambridge: Bywater Ward, Sutherland, Clapham, Tyler Smith; Oxford: Sutherland, Galton). Two of those appointed to WRA were Fellows of the Linnean Society (Fryer, Galton).

This latter point also bears on the question of experience gained prior to appointment at WRA. Appointment as "FLS" indicated or implied some research experience in the study of natural history. Generally, however, whatever energy or enthusiasm the resident staff brought to their work at WRA,

---

[484] Finn (2012:73n249).

[485] In 1868, Laycock observed of his course that "the attendance is … very small compared with the number of students" (Laycock 1867–1868:587). Crichton-Browne's father, William Browne (see Chap. 7), recorded in a lecture read before Professor Laycock's class of Medical Psychology that "for two consecutive years I offered, with the cordial concurrence of Professor Laycock, a prize to his class for an essay on 'Psychical Aspects of Disease,' for which no competitor appeared. The signal failure of the proposal confirmed me in my opinion that the profession disregarded such an element in observation and diagnosis, that the subject was foreign to such studies as are at present encouraged, and that new efforts were required to direct attention to states of the system having a powerful but unestimated influence upon disease" (Browne 1865–1866:336). Is it possible that David Ferrier (see Chap. 7), who began his Edinburgh medical studies in 1865, was in one of these classes? Or did Browne refer to an earlier period?

[486] Ditto David Ferrier and Milner Fothergill (see Chap. 7). Hollander (1921:405) listed among Laycock's students "James Crichton Browne, Hughlings Jackson, David Ferrier, Lauder Brunton, MacKendrick, William Rutherford, Stirling, and Thomas Clouston".

[487] More detail on the Irish contingent who received some of their training at WRA along with their subsequent career trajectories may be found in Larner (2025h).

[488] Finn (2012:73n249).

few appointees had any training in a research background, many being at too junior a stage in their careers. This was perhaps an active choice by Crichton-Browne, seeking men he could mould for a future career in a scientifically-oriented asylum medicine, although mature graduates were also appointed (e.g. McDowall, Galton, Bevan-Lewis). A record of publication before arrival at WRA was the exception.[489]

Whilst some of the junior men appointed to posts at WRA may well have been "birds of passage",[490] with little or no intention of remaining within the specialty of asylum medicine, this was unlikely to be the case at WRA in this period, most especially for the clinical clerks and assistants who were unpaid for their services, merely receiving board and lodging for the opportunity to gain clinical experience. Many followed the standard route of training in asylum medicine, both during and following their time at WRA: appointment as an Assistant Medical Officer; membership of MPA (e.g. see Table 5.1); publications, ideally in the *BMJ*, *Lancet*, or the *Journal of Mental Science*; and eventual appointment as an asylum superintendent, in either the public or private sector. Whether the changes instituted by Crichton-Browne at WRA[491] made any difference to the prospects of his AMOs, clinical clerks and assistants, is difficult to say but certainly several went on to become Medical Superintendents at other asylums (Table 5.2) and three eventually became President of the MPA (McDowall, Woods, Bevan-Lewis) in indirect succession to Crichton-Browne.

Was it possible to bridge the divide between asylum medicine and the career of a physician, or were the two mutually incompatible? In this context, a consideration of Crichton-Browne will be deferred until later (see Chap. 10), but of the other resident WRA clinicians documented in this chapter, it is my contention that only two came even close to achieving this combination: Henry Sutherland and Crochley Clapham (again, both considered in Chap. 10). Both eventually held an appointment as "Physician" and both had membership of one of the Royal Colleges of Physicians. Only one other WRA resident clinician later gained an appointment as a physician: Patrick Nicol, at

---

[489] The only examples I am aware of are: McDowall (1871–1872, 1872–1873) and Galton (1869a, b, 1872).

[490] This terminology is taken from Dodds et al. (1890:44).

[491] Crichton Browne (1868–1869).

Table 5.2 WRA Assistant Medical Officers/Clinical Clerks/Clinical Assistants 1866–1876 subsequently appointed to public asylum Medical Superintendent and other significant positions

Name	Superintendency	Appointment
THOMPSON, George	Bristol	1871–1890
MITCHELL, Samuel	Sheffield (South Yorkshire, second West Riding Asylum)	1872–1888
BURMAN, J. Wilkie	Wiltshire County Lunatic Asylum, Devizes	1873–1878
WARD, J. Bywater	Warneford Asylum, Oxford	1872–1897
LAWRENCE, Alexander	County Asylum, Chester	?1895/6–1910
MAJOR, Herbert C.	West Riding Asylum, Wakefield	1876–1884
COURTENAY, E. Mazière	District Asylum, Limerick	1873–1890 Inspectors of Lunatics, Ireland 1890–1910
McDOWALL, T.W.	Northumberland, Morpeth	1874–? MPA President 1897
WOODS, Oscar T.	District Asylum, Killarney, County Kerry	1875–1889 or 1890
	Cork District Asylum Cork	1890–1906 MPA President 1901
LEVINGE, Edward G.	Sunnyside Mental Hospital, Christchurch, New Zealand	1887–?
LAWSON, Robert	Wonford House Asylum, Exeter	1877–?1878 Deputy Commissioner in Lunacy in Scotland 1878–1896
MERSON, John	Borough Asylum, Hull	1878–1924
BEVAN-LEWIS, William	West Riding Asylum, Wakefield	1884–1910 MPA President 1909
WALLIS, John A.M.	Borough Asylum, Hull	1875–1878
	Lancaster County Asylum, Whittingham	1878–1893 Lunacy Commissioner 1894–1897

Superintendencies of private asylums: Aldridge (Plympton, Devon); Sutherland (Newlands House and Otto House, London); Clapham (The Grange, Rotherham)
Superintendence of overseas asylums: Benham (Santiago, Chile); Plaxton (Ceylon; Kingston, Jamaica)

Bradford Infirmary.[492] He did not, however, have the Membership[493] and his post-WRA publications quickly petered out, possibly as a consequence of the demands of his clinical role and certainly because of his early death. Other WRA alumni sometimes styled themselves as physician (Mitchell as "Physician to the Sheffield Hospital and Dispensary", I:27; Aldridge as "Physician to the Plympton House Asylum", IV:291) but they were clearly asylum doctors, entirely unlike the physicians (Allbutt, Ferrier, Hughlings Jackson, Lauder Brunton, Milner Fothergill) to be discussed later (Chap. 7).

As for research and publications, it is doubtful that any of the resident staff were able to maintain these pursuits after leaving WRA, again with the possible exception of Sutherland and Clapham (see Bibliography). A few later published in the early volumes of *Brain* (Aldridge, Clapham, Galton, Lawson, Bevan-Lewis, Newcombe; see Table 6.4) but more appeared in the *Journal of Mental Science* (Table 6.5). Even for the most productive during their time at WRA (e.g. Burman, Lawson, Benham), publication became at best occasional and at worst non-existent once confronted with the realities of senior roles within asylum medicine. One might argue that Lawson in particular had demonstrated the potential to develop a research programme encompassing both clinical and experimental work but once departed from WRA, and particularly once appointed a Lunacy Commissioner in Scotland, such possibilities were at an end. At WRA itself, Major and, particularly, Bevan-Lewis tried to maintain the ethos of a research school alongside the clinical and administrative demands of the Asylum, with some success,[494] albeit not with the renown achieved in the Crichton-Browne era.

It may therefore be redundant to ask whether any of the resident WRA staff during the years of the Crichton-Browne research school made any contributions specifically to the origins and development of neurology. Here we might distinguish between neurology as professional discipline and neurology as a body of specialised knowledge referring to the physiology and clinical phenomenology of the nervous system. Accepting that any such judgment must

---

[492] I exclude Herbert Major here, for although he was eventually appointed as a both an Honorary and then Consulting Physician in Bradford, this was after the self-determined cessation of his career in asylum medicine at WRA.

[493] Other than Sutherland and Clapham, I do not find convincing evidence that any other resident WRA clinician ever gained either membership or fellowship at any of the Royal Colleges. Plaxton is denoted "MRCP" on one of his papers (Plaxton 1880–1881) but I think this was a typographical error for "MRCS". Even Crichton-Browne was neither FCRPEd nor FRCP, despite being both FRSE and FRS (further discussed in Chap. 10).

[494] For research in the Bevan-Lewis era, see Wallis (2017a). Bolton (1928:612) suggested that in the later years of Bevan-Lewis's superintendency "the administration of the hospital had become beyond his powers. … He was essentially a recluse and an enthusiast, and a hard worker with few interests beyond his scientific investigations".

rest on the benefit of hindsight (or, dependent upon one's point of view, the condescension of posterity), I would argue that the resident staff made no contribution to the origins of neurology as a discipline. For example, Thompson's advocacy for the sphygmograph is now no more than a historical footnote, and Aldridge's exploration of the uses of the ophthalmoscope was derivative from the works of other clinicians, such as Allbutt, his teacher, and Hughlings Jackson (both discussed in Chap. 7). Clapham and Sutherland were both later elected to the Neurological Society of London (see Chap. 10) but made no specific contribution. Major's work in cortical cytoarchitectonics was largely overlooked, Bevan-Lewis's less so, but their findings had no impact on clinical practice.

Since most resident WRA staff were determined on a career in asylum medicine, and hence followed the prescribed pathways for such a career, this conclusion is unsurprising. This trajectory, with the inevitability of administrative burden, may explain why few maintained any output of publications. As regards neurology as a body of specialised knowledge, I would argue that the publications in *WRLAMR* by the resident staff contributed no significant or enduring advance, no citation classic. Crichton-Browne aside, none of the resident staff was elected FRS, and none appears in the *Oxford Dictionary of National Biography* to my knowledge. The pharmacological and physical therapies explored in the various forms of insanity and in epilepsy as documented in *WRLAMR* (discussed in Chap. 6) have not survived into the modern therapeutic armamentarium. The most important clinical observation by one of the WRA alumni, Lawson's description of alcoholic amnesia,[495] postdated his time at WRA, and was largely neglected by posterity, eponymous fame devolving on another clinician (Korsakoff).

The calibre and contributions of these resident WRA clinicians may be compared with those non-resident clinicians who either contributed to the house journal, the *WRLAMR*, and/or who visited WRA to undertake clinical or experimental investigations. These individuals will be discussed in a subsequent chapter.

---

[495] Lawson (1878–1879).

Part III

Journal

In the end the asylum, where man could be systematically observed and studied, was one of the birthplaces of the idea of the "human sciences".[1]

There are difficulties for the historian making the attempt to map or quantify the influence of any periodical.[2]

[1] Khalfa J. Introduction. In: Foucault, 2006:xix.
[2] Richardson (1992:96).

6

The *West Riding Lunatic Asylum Medical Reports (WRLAMR)*

The foundation of specialist journals is instrumental not only for the wide dissemination of research findings but also for focusing and binding a nascent profession. Whilst there was a profusion of new journals in Great Britain in the early nineteenth century, including the *Lancet* and the *British Medical Journal*, their clinical focus was general rather than specialised. The inception of a dedicated journal at the West Riding Asylum, the *West Riding Lunatic Asylum Medical Reports*, provided a vehicle for the communication of the research findings of the local faculty. It later attracted contributions from other clinicians, either working at the Asylum by invitation or who became associated with the Asylum through a shared interest in diseases of the brain. After the sixth and final issue of the journal, many of the personnel involved with the *West Riding Lunatic Asylum Medical Reports* were subsequently instrumental in the foundation of another journal with overlapping interests and which contributed significantly to the development of British neurology: *Brain: a journal of neurology*.

The *West Riding Lunatic Asylum Medical Reports* (henceforward *WRLAMR*), the house journal of the West Riding Asylum at Wakefield (WRA), first appeared in 1871,[1] edited by "J Crichton Browne" (*sic*, without hyphen). The journal was published in London by J. & A. Churchill, retailing at seven

---

[1] Bolton (1928:608) stated that "In 1870 the first volume of the *West Riding Reports* was published", certainly an error, although preparations for its publication may have been in progress in 1870. Other examples of misdating of *WRLAMR* may be found in Crammer (1996:219) who gave "(1870–1876)" and O'Connor (1991:485) who stated that "important work in neurology was published in the *Reports* in 1868–75".

© The Author(s), under exclusive license to Springer Nature Switzerland AG 2026
A. J. Larner, *The West Riding Asylum and the Origins of British Neurology 1866-1876*,
https://doi.org/10.1007/978-3-032-12591-0_6

shillings and sixpence.[2] In all, six volumes of *WRLAMR* were published,[3] appearing on an annual basis, the last four iterations from the publisher Smith, Elder & Co. These volumes have been recognised to contain a number of seminal papers in both the clinical and experimental domains of neurology. Although mentioned in passing in historical scholarship relating to WRA,[4] to Crichton-Browne,[5] and to medical journals as a nineteenth-century cultural phenomenon,[6] they have attracted little dedicated attention.[7] An emerging discipline needs a dedicated journal, and the interface between asylum medicine and neurology as practiced at WRA was no exception.

Origins and Aims of *WRLAMR*

The aims of *WRLAMR* were stated explicitly in the preface to the first volume by Crichton-Browne (I:iii–v) in what might now be considered, to use modern parlance, a "mission statement". He observed that:

> In the harmless, but vindictive, attacks which have been recently directed against the public lunatic asylums of this country, it has been a frequent charge that no scientific work is accomplished in them.

Accordingly, he noted that "a belief is entertained that there has perhaps been some remissness on the part of those engaged in the superintendence of our hospitals for the insane in publishing the results of their observations," perhaps in part due to the "absence of any immediate stimulus to the arrangement and elaboration of the materials collected, and to the want of any ready

---

[2] This was the price noted on the cover of volume I, and also according to an advertisement for the journal ("Now ready") appearing on the back cover of issues of the *Journal of Mental Science*, volume 17 (January 1872) and volume 18 (April 1872). No price appeared on the cover of volume II. As detailed on their covers, volumes III, IV, and V retailed at 8 shillings and sixpence, volume VI at 9 shillings and sixpence. Sloffer (2023:32n47) reported the cost was five shillings to subscribers based on a "note from the publisher between pages iv and v in the copy [of Volume I] at the Bodleian Library, Oxford". I have found no list of subscribers printed in any of the other volumes of *WRLAMR* that I have seen and indeed wonder whether it would in fact have been odd for an annual publication to have subscribers (other than, say, one emanating from a medical school with a large number of alumni).

[3] For reason(s) unknown, Star (1989:49,268) referred to only four volumes ("1871–74").

[4] Ashworth (1975:69), Gatehouse (1981), Todd and Ashworth (1991:400–401), Finn (2012:78–83), Sloffer (2023).

[5] Neve and Turner (1995:409–411).

[6] Shepherd (1992:201).

[7] To my knowledge, the only publications dedicated to *WRLAMR* are Viets (1938) and Larner (2023b). Neve and Turner (1995:409n64) judged the former to be "a detailed analysis". This chapter is based in part on, but much extended from, Larner (2023b).

channel of exposition". Hence "It is with a view to supplying this deficiency …
that the present volume has been projected".

What were the stimuli to the inception of this new journal? The question is
pertinent since many journals were already in existence at this time, not only
addressed to the general medical audience (e.g. *Lancet, British Medical Journal*
[henceforward *BMJ*], *Medical Times and Gazette, Medical Press and Circular*)
but also specifically to the subject matter of asylum medicine. In this latter
category, the *Journal of Psychological Medicine and Mental Pathology*, edited by
Forbes Benignus Winslow (1810–1874), had first appeared in 1848,[8] appearing quarterly until it ceased publication in October 1860. It was followed by
the *Medical Critic and Psychological Journal* which appeared in quarterly instalments between January 1861 and October 1863.[9] The *Journal of Psychological
Medicine and Mental Pathology* then reappeared between April 1875 and
January 1883, generally two issues per year, under the editorship of Lyttleton
Winslow, the son of the founding editor. The *Asylum Journal*, published under
the auspices of the Association of Medical Officers of Asylums and Hospitals
for the Insane (AMOAHI) and edited by John Charles Bucknill (1817–1897),
appeared from November 1853 and was later to become the *Asylum Journal of
Mental Science* (1855) and later still the *Journal of Mental Science* (1858). This
journal was to survive under this name for over 100 years.[10]

Crichton-Browne's initial preface to *WRLAMR* might be contrasted with
the prospectus of the *Asylum Journal* written by Bucknill in 1853:

> The aims and objects of the *Asylum Journal* will be, to afford a medium of inter-
> communication between men engaged in the construction and management of
> asylums, in the treatment of the insane, and in all subsidiary occupations; it will,
> therefore, embrace topics, not only interesting to medical men, but to visiting
> justices, asylum architects, and chaplains; nothing will be excluded which is not
> foreign to the modern system of the care and treatment of the insane. It will be
> a record of improvements and experiments in psycho-therapeutics; whether in
> medicine, hygiene, diet, employment and recreation; or, in the construction,
> fittings, organization, and management of asylums. It will notice new opinions
> in the physiology of the nervous system, and the neurological observations and
> discoveries of every kind.[11]

---

[8] In Winslow's obituary (*J Ment Sci* 1874–1875:20(April 1874):165–166) it was described as the
"Psychological Journal" (at 166).

[9] Crichton-Browne published a paper in the January 1863 issue of this journal (Crichton Browne 1863).

[10] Later still, in 1963, it became the *British Journal of Psychiatry*. For the history of the journal, see Walk
(1953), Tyrer and Craddock (2012).

[11] [Bucknill] (1853:6) (cited in *Lancet* 1854;1:367).

Whilst some overlap with Crichton-Browne's purposes might be detected here (e.g. experiments in psycho-therapeutics; new opinions in the physiology of the nervous system), much was not concordant with his plans (e.g. construction and management of asylums; interesting to … visiting justices, asylum architects, and chaplains). Moreover, by 1871, now under the editorship of Charles Lockhart Robinson and Henry Maudsley, the *Journal of Mental Science* was perceived to have shed its initial focus of practical asylum management in favour of more philosophical and speculative issues. Hence, Crichton-Browne may have sensed a niche in the market, with scope to appeal not only to asylum doctors but also to those pursuing "neurological observations and discoveries of every kind". The opportunity to advertise his own asylum and its work may also have been a factor.

Why a journal? The idea was not, in all likelihood, inherent. Crichton-Browne's father, William Browne, had given a lecture in 1837 regarding "What asylums ought to be",[12] but this contained no mention of, nor advocacy for, a programme of brain research as an ideal for the future asylum, let alone the need for a dedicated journal. Hence one must look elsewhere for possible triggers.

As previously noted (Chap. 5), it has been suggested that Crichton-Browne's "choice of Paris influenced the rest of his career, for clinical observation in hospital or asylum wards and the performance of autopsies, on the French model, became Crichton-Browne's basic approach to psychological medicine".[13] The inauguration of new medical journals was one of the methods used extensively by Jean-Martin Charcot (1825–1893) to communicate the findings of research undertaken by himself and his colleagues at the Salpêtrière Hospital, beginning with the *Archives de Physiologie Normale et Pathologique* in 1868, although the first journal devoted to neurology in which he was an "advisor", the *Iconographie photographique de la Salpêtrière*, did not appear until 1876, and the first of which he was the founder, *Archives de Neurologie*, not until 1880.[14]

Why now? Changes in both the institutional infrastructure (Chap. 3) and the faculty of resident clinicians (Chap. 4) at WRA may have meant that Crichton-Browne was now in a favourable position to inaugurate a journal. With access to a pathological laboratory and a photographic studio, and with an increased number of young clinical clerks or assistants hopeful for a career in asylum medicine, an adequate supply of material and authors to fill the

---

[12] Browne (1837:176–231).

[13] Oppenheim (1991:61–62).

[14] Goetz et al. (1995:95) (their Table 3.1).

pages of a journal may have seemed assured. Equally, provision of an adequate source of funding (*vide infra*) may have been key.

A dedicated house journal was not necessarily the limit of Crichton-Browne's ambitions with respect to publications. In February 1874, an item appeared in the *BMJ* informing readers that:

THERE will this year, we understand, be issued from the West Riding Asylum, in addition to the volume of medical reports, the first of what promises to be an important and valuable series of monographs upon mental diseases. Dr. Crichton Browne, who will edit these monographs, has conceived the project of combining the efforts of a number of independent investigators in the elucidation of one malady, so that, by their convergent labours, the pith of it may perchance be reached. Selecting general paralysis, an obscure and very fatal disease, with well marked and tolerably parallel psychical and physical symptoms, as the subject of the first essay, he has secured the co-operation of several able associates, who will explore it from various points and in various ways. Besides the members of the medical staff of the West Riding Asylum, Dr. Clifford Allbutt, Dr. Lauder Brunton, Dr. Batty Tuke, Dr. Ferrier, Dr. Milner Fothergill, and Dr. Rabagliati are to take part in the work, and Mr. Charles Darwin has promised to supply a contribution on the physiognomy of the disease.[15]

Crichton-Browne's correspondence with Darwin in December 1873 suggests, however, that, far from "promising", Darwin was not entirely willing to contribute ("I really think it will be impossible for me to write even a short essay on the subject"), believing that Crichton-Browne could do a better job than he could.[16] In the event, no such monograph came to pass. Although not perhaps one of medical literature's great "Might have beens", nevertheless one anticipates that such a volume would have been of interest. Its non-appearance may have been due to a number of factors including, but not limited to, Crichton-Browne being too busy, the task of coordinating multiple authors proving too difficult, the absence of a willing publisher, or the market being already supplied with adequate material on this subject.[17]

---

[15] *BMJ* 1874;1:210 (14th February; Monographs on mental diseases). It may be that Crichton-Browne had communicated this plan to the Editor of the *BMJ*, Ernest Hart (for whom, see Chap. 9).

[16] Darwin Correspondence Project, "Letter no. 9190," https://www.darwinproject.ac.uk/letter/?docId=letters/DCP-LETT-9190.xml, and "Letter no. 9193," https://www.darwinproject.ac.uk/letter/?docId=letters/DCP-LETT-9193.xml (both accessed 11/12/2024). Finn (2012:109n356) misdated the latter as 1870 rather than 1873. Finn (2012:127) also mentioned the proposed volume, noting that "Darwin turned down the invitation".

[17] Perhaps Buzzard (1874), had trumped Crichton-Browne's plans? Buzzard's book was reviewed in *Medical Times and Gazette* 1874;1:542–543 (16th May); *J Ment Sci* 1874–1875;20(July 1874):288–289.

Funding

Being made of paper, journals may, ultimately, grow from trees, but not on them, so sources of funding are required for their production and distribution, and possibly also for honoraria paid to the editor and/or authors, advertising, etc. Factors which influence cost include the extent of the print run, perhaps based on the estimated circulation, the cost of paper, etc. So how was *WRLAMR* financed? To my knowledge, there is no explicit statement which answers this question. Based on analysis of new medical journals published in the nineteenth century,[18] two possibilities may be suggested: that the journal was either the private property of the publisher, or the editor.[19]

Both J. & A. Churchill and Smith, Elder & Co. were well-established publishers who may have been prepared to take a risk on a new medical journal, perhaps at the suggestion of a persuasive would-be editor, such as Crichton-Browne. For these publishers, "editorial payments were certainly common if not universal"[20] so Crichton-Browne may have benefitted financially, as well as scientifically, from his work on the journal. Perhaps the change of publisher was because Smith, Elder & Co. offered better terms, or J. & A. Churchill no longer thought the financial risk viable.

If not the property of the publisher, *WRLAMR* may have been owned solely by Crichton-Browne,[21] or jointly with the Committee of Visitors who were persuaded to use some of the Asylum's budget, derived ultimately from the payments of local ratepayers whose interests were represented by the Committee, in order to help underwrite the costs. Perhaps some of the savings Crichton-Browne purportedly made elsewhere at WRA, as documented in his annual *Reports* to the Asylum's Committee of Visitors, were put towards the journal, as for the pathological laboratory. Certainly, he was used to handling large sums of money, if a later comment is true:

> When I was at the head of the West Riding Asylum, I had to sign cheques for £40,000 a year; I had a staff of 200 nurses and attendants under my control, a large farm, a butcher's shop, a bakery and a brewery, weaving sheds, for we wove

---

[18] Bynum and Wilson (1992).

[19] As was apparently the case with Bucknill and the *Asylum Journal* when first published (according to Russell 1988:299). It was certainly the case with Forbes Winslow and the *Journal of Psychological Medicine and Mental Pathology*, as an editorial in that journal in 1853 (most probably by Winslow; see Bewley 2008:130–131), responding to the plan for the new journal edited by Bucknill, stated "Having embarked a capital of some thousand pounds in establishing this journal" (Anon 1853:454).

[20] Bynum and Wilson (1992:43).

[21] In Chap. 8, the possibility that Crichton-Browne alone funded the annual medical *conversazione* held at WRA is discussed.

all our own clothes and made our own clothing, and all that I was responsible for. The magistrates looked to me to insure the efficient management of all these departments, and it was with the utmost difficulty I succeeded in getting any time for strictly medical and scientific work.[22]

However, little definitive information pertinent to the journal appears to be available, apart from "a note by the asylum's committee in 1875 that a grant of £40 be made towards the cost of their printing".[23] Each annual *Report* of WRA contained a "Balance Sheet for the Year" drawn up by the Asylum's Clerk and Steward. Of the recurrent items, three might potentially have included moneys which were put towards the funding of *WRLAMR*, namely "Stationery, Printing, and Advertising", "Books, Periodicals, and Music", and "Incidentals".[24]

What total cost might have been involved? Perhaps some clues might be found in the annual balance sheets of the Medico-Psychological Association (MPA), publishers of the *Journal of Mental Science*. The costs of printing, publishing, and advertising the *Journal of Mental Science* recorded in the Balance Sheet to July 1869 came to £192 15s 3d; to July 1870 came to £245 19s 11d; and to July 1871 came to £225 10s 0d.[25] These were substantial sums of money, representing by far largest recorded expenditure of the MPA in each of these years.[26] As for *WRLAMR*, the extent of the *Journal's* print run is unknown, but the MPA membership at this time was around 300.

Other potential sources of funding for *WRLAMR* merit consideration. Inclusion of advertisements may potentially defray journal production costs, but *WRLAMR* initially carried no advertisements. However, after the change of publisher from J. & A. Churchill to Smith, Elder & Co. in 1873 this policy changed. In the copies of *WRLAMR* digitised by Yale University (see Table 6.1 for links), two pages of advertisements for "Smith, Elder, & Co.'s Medical

---

[22] Burdett (1891:183). Cited by Shorvon and Compston (2019:343).

[23] Finn (2012:79), citing "Minutes of the Committee of Visitors", 29th April 1875 (WYAS C85/1/1/3).

[24] See Appendix 1 for a tabulation of these numbers, along with an analysis of serial costs using a cumulative sum (cusum) method.

[25] Numbers taken from *J Ment Sci* 1869–1870;15(October 1869):unpaginated, between 468–469; *J Ment Sci* 1870–1871;16(October 1870):unpaginated, between 458–459; *J Ment Sci* 1871–1872;17(October 1870):unpaginated, between 444–445. These years have been selected as those most likely to coincide with Hughlings Jackson's tenure as one of the two auditors of the MPA (1869–1871; see Chap. 7) although his signature did not appear on any of these balance sheets. If Jackson was, as some authors have claimed, a lifelong friend of Crichton-Browne, he may have been able to advise him on the costs of publishing this journal, but it is my impression that this is unlikely.

[26] Costs of the *Journal of Mental Science* appear to have been a recurrent problem for successive MPA treasurers: see Bewley (2008:85–88) (presenting data prepared by Fiona Subotsky).

Table 6.1 *West Riding Lunatic Asylum Medical Reports* contents by volume

Reference	Title	Author(s) and qualifications	Affiliation(s)
Volume I (1871)			
Available online at:			
https://wellcomecollection.org/works/v3kfekjk/items			
http://dbooks.bodleian.ox.ac.uk/books/PDFs/502369335.pdf			
https://archive.org/details/39002086346260.med.yale.edu			
https://darwin-online.org.uk/converted/pdf/1871_WestRiding_CUL-DAR.LIB.79.pdf			
I: i	[Title page]		
I: ii	[Epigraph]	Berkeley	
I: iii–v	Preface	[JCB]	
I: vi	[blank]		
I: vii–viii	Contents		
I: 1–26 [1]	Cranial injuries and mental diseases	James Crichton Browne [*sic*, without hyphen] MD FRSE	Medical Director West Riding Asylum, and Lecturer on Mental Diseases to the Leeds School of Medicine
I: 27–57 [2]	Observations on the physiological action of nitrous oxide	Samuel Mitchell MD	Deputy Medical Director West Riding Asylum, and Physician to the Sheffield Hospital and Dispensary
I: 58–70 [3]	The sphygmograph in lunatic asylum practice	George Thompson LRCP Lond	Medical Superintendent of the Bristol City and County Lunatic-Asylum; late Assistant Medical Officer, and formerly Clinical Assistant, at the West Riding Asylum, Wakefield
I: 71–128 [4]	The opthalmoscope [*sic*; cf. "Contents"] in mental and cerebral diseases	Charles Aldridge LRCP Lond	Assistant Medical Officer, Late Clinical Assistant, West Riding Asylum, Wakefield
I: 129–151 [5]	A contribution to the statistics of general paralysis; with remarks	J Wilkie Burman MB (Edin)	Assistant Medical Officer, West Riding Asylum; Late Assistant Medical Officer of the Devon County Asylum, and Clinical Assistant, West Riding Asylum
I: 152–163 [6]	On the treatment of insanity by the hypodermic injection of morphia	J Bywater Ward BA MB Cantab	Assistant Medical Officer Warwick County Asylum; Late Clinical Assistant, West Riding Asylum

(*continued*)

Table 6.1 (continued)

Reference	Title	Author(s) and qualifications	Affiliation(s)
I: 164–177 [7]	Mollities ossium and allied diseases	George Henry Pedler LRCP Lond, MRCS	Fellow of the Obstetrical Society, and Late Clinical Assistant, West Riding Asylum
I: 178–208 [8]	On progressive locomotor ataxy and some other forms of locomotor deficiency as found in the insane	Patrick Nicol MA MB	Physician to the Bradford Infirmary, Late Assistant Medical Officer, Sussex County Asylum, and Clinical Assistant, West Riding Asylum
I: 209–217 [9]	On the artificial feeding of the insane	William Lawrence MB	Assistant Medical Officer Chester County Asylum; Late Clinical Assistant West Riding Asylum
I: 218–232 [10]	Arachnoid cysts	Henry Sutherland MA MB Oxon MRCP Lond	Physician to the St George's, Hanover Square, Dispensary, and Late Assistant Medical Officer, West Riding Asylum
I: 233–251 [11]	Phthisis and insanity	Patrick Nicol MA MB	Physician to the Bradford Infirmary; Late Assistant Medical Officer, Sussex County Asylum; and Clinical Assistant West Riding Asylum
		W Watson Dove LRCPE MRCS	Assistant Medical Officer, Somerset County Asylum; Late Clinical Assistant, West Riding Asylum
I: 252–260 [12]	Acute delirious melancholia	Charles Henry Mayhew LRCP Lond MRCS	Associate of King's College, Assistant House-Surgeon to the Stockport Infirmary, formerly Clinical Assistant, West Riding Asylum
I: 261–265 [13]	Ergot of rye in the treatment of mental diseases	E Churchill Fox MB CM	Late Clinical Assistant, West Riding Asylum

(*continued*)

Table 6.1 (continued)

Reference	Title	Author(s) and qualifications	Affiliation(s)
Volume II (1872)			
Available online at:			
http://dbooks.bodleian.ox.ac.uk/books/PDFs/555022684.pdf			
https://archive.org/details/39002086346278.med.yale.edu			
II: i	[Title page with editor and publisher]		
II: ii	[Epigraph]	Emerson; Shakespeare	
II: iii	Preface	[JCB]	
II: iv	[blank]		
II: v–vi	Contents		
II: 1–40 [1]	On conia, and its use in subcutaneous injection	J Wilkie Burman MD (Edin)	Assistant Medical Officer, Male Division, West Riding Asylum; Late Assistant Medical Officer, Devon County Asylum; and Clinical Assistant, West Riding Asylum
II: 41–52 [2]	On the minute structure of the cortical substance of the brain, in a case of chronic brain wasting	Herbert C Major MB CM (Edin)	Assistant Medical Officer, Late Clinical Assistant, West Riding Asylum
II: 53–72 [3]	Menstrual irregularities and insanity	Henry Sutherland MA MB Oxon MRCP Lond	Lecturer on Insanity to the Westminster Hospital School of Medicine; Late Assistant Medical Officer, West Riding Asylum
II: 73–96 [4]	Experiments to ascertain the effects of ether and nitrous oxide combined, to which are added some general observations on stimulants	Samuel Mitchell MD	Medical Superintendent, South Yorkshire Asylum, Late Assistant Medical Officer, West Riding Asylum
II: 97–136 [5]	Cranial injuries and mental diseases	James Crichton Browne [*sic*, without hyphen] MD FRSE	Medical Director, West Riding Asylum, and Lecturer on Mental Diseases to the Leeds School of Medicine
II: 137–156 [6]	Puerperal mania	George Henry Pedler LRCP Lond, MRCS	Fellow of the Obstetrical Society, and Late Clinical Assistant, West Riding Asylum

(continued)

Table 6.1 (continued)

Reference	Title	Author(s) and qualifications	Affiliation(s)
II: 157–176 [7]	A new method of determining the depth of the grey matter of the cerebral convolutions	Herbert C Major MB	Assistant Medical Officer, Late Clinical Assistant, West Riding Asylum
II: 177–202 [8]	The mental symptoms of ordinary disease	Patrick Nicol MA MB	Physician to the Bradford Infirmary, Formerly Clinical Assistant, West Riding Asylum
II: 203–222 [9]	The electric treatment of the insane	T Clifford Allbutt MA MD (Cantab) FLS	Physician to the Leeds General Infirmary, &c.
II: 223–253 [10]	Ophthalmoscopic observations in general paralysis, and after the administration of certain toxic agents	Charles Aldridge LRCP Lond	Assistant Medical Officer, Late Clinical Assistant, West Riding Asylum
II: 254–277 [11]	The use of opium in the treatment of melancholia	E Maziere Courtenay MB AB TCD	Assistant Medical Officer, Derby County Asylum, Late Clinical Assistant, West Riding Asylum
II: 278–301 [12]	Impairment of language, the result of cerebral disease	W A F Browne MD FRCSE FRSE	Psychological Consultant, Crichton Royal Institution, Late Commissioner in Lunacy for Scotland
II: 302–306 [13]	The sphygmograph in epilepsy	George Thompson LRCP Lond	Medical Superintendent, Bristol County and City Lunatic-Asylum; Late Assistant Medical Officer and Clinical Clerk, West Riding Asylum

Volume III (1873)
Available online at:
https://archive.org/details/39002086346286.med.yale.edu

III: i	[Title page with editor and publisher]		
III: ii	[Epigraph]	Carlyle	
III: iii–iv	Preface	[JCB]	
III: v–vi	Contents		
III: 1–29 [1]	The convolutions of the human brain considered in relation to the intelligence	William Turner MB Lond	Professor of Anatomy in the University of Edinburgh

(*continued*)

Table 6.1 (continued)

Reference	Title	Author(s) and qualifications	Affiliation(s)
III: 30–96 [2]	Experimental researches in cerebral physiology and pathology	David Ferrier MA MD (Edin) MRCP	Professor of Forensic Medicine, King's College London; Assistant Physician to the West London Hospital
III: 97–112 [3]	Observations on the histology of the brain in the insane	Herbert C Major MB CM	Assistant Medical Officer, Late Clinical Assistant, West Riding Asylum
III: 113–128 [4]	The heart sounds in general paralysis of the insane	J Milner Fothergill MD MRCP	[No affiliation given]
III: 129–152 [5]	On the power of perceiving colours possessed by the insane	T W McDowall MD	Pathologist, and Assistant Medical Officer, West Riding Asylum
III: 153–174 [6]	Nitrite of amyl in epilepsy	James Crichton Browne [sic, without hyphen] MD (Edin) FRSE	Medical Director, West Riding Asylum, and Lecturer of Mental Diseases to the Leeds School of Medicine
III: 175–195 [7]	Observations on localisation of movements in the cerebral hemispheres, as revealed by cases of convulsion, chorea and "aphasia"	J Hughlings Jackson MD FRCP	Physician to the London Hospital and to the Hospital for the Epileptic and Paralysed[a]
III: 196–215 [8]	On electro-excitability in mental and nervous diseases	John Lowe MB CM (Edin)	Assistant Medical Officer, South Yorkshire Asylum; Late Assistant Medical Officer, Durham County Asylum; and Clinical Assistant, West Riding Asylum
III: 216–257 [9]	Heart disease and insanity	J Wilkie Burman MD (Edin)	Deputy Medical Director, West Riding Asylum, Wakefield
III: 258–272 [10]	Notes on the condition of the tympanic membrane in the insane—Part I	John C Galton MA (Oxon) MRCS FLS	Clinical Assistant, West Riding Asylum
III: 273–284 [11]	On the obscurer neuroses of syphilis	T Clifford Allbutt MA MD (Cantab) FLS	Physician to the Leeds General Infirmary
III: 285–298 [12]	The weight of the brain in the insane	W Crochley S Clapham Esq. LRCP (Lond)	Fellow of the London Anthropological Society; Late Clinical Assistant West Riding Asylum

(continued)

Table 6.1 (continued)

Reference	Title	Author(s) and qualifications	Affiliation(s)
III: 299–314 [13]	The change of life, and insanity	Henry Sutherland MD MA (Oxon) MRCP (Lond)	Lecturer on Insanity to the Westminster Hospital; Late Assistant Medical Officer West Riding Asylum; Physician to the St. George's Hanover Square Dispensary; Etc.
III: 315–349 [14]	On the anatomical, physiological, and pathological investigation of epilepsies	J Hughlings Jackson MD FRCP	Physician to the London Hospital, and to the Hospital for the Epileptic and Paralysed
Volume IV (1874) Available online at: https://archive.org/details/39002086346294.med.yale.edu			
IV: i	[Title page]		
IV: ii	[blank]		
IV: iii	[Title page with editor and publisher]		
IV: iv	[Epigraph]	Swedenborg	
IV: v	Preface	[JCB]	
IV: vi	[blank]		
IV: vii–viii	Contents		
IV: 1–23 [1]	On the physiological import of Dr Ferrier's experimental investigations into the functions of the brain	William B Carpenter MD LLD FRS	Corresponding Member of the Institute of France
IV: 24–29 [2]	On a case of recovery from double optic neuritis	J Hughlings Jackson MD FRCP	Physician to the London Hospital, and to the Hospital for the Epileptic and Paralysed
IV: 30–62 [3]	Pathological illustrations of brain function	David Ferrier MD MRCP	Professor of Forensic Medicine, King's College, London; Assistant-Physician to King's College, London.
IV: 63–93 [4]	The urinology of general paralysis	John Merson MA MD	Assistant Medical Officer, West Riding Lunatic Asylum
IV: 94–151 [5]	Cerebral anaemia	J Milner Fothergill MD Edin MRCP Lond	[No affiliation given]
IV: 152–178 [6]	On the therapeutic value of cold to the head	William T Benham MD Abdn	Pathologist and Assistant Medical Officer, West Riding Asylum

(continued)

Table 6.1 (continued)

Reference	Title	Author(s) and qualifications	Affiliation(s)
IV: 179–222 [7]	On inhibition, peripheral and central	T Lauder Brunton MD DSc Edin FRS MRCP	Casualty Physician and Lecturer on Materia Medica and Therapeutics at St Bartholomew's Hospital
IV: 223–239 [8]	Observations on the histology of the morbid brain	Herbert C Major MB Edin	Deputy Medical Director, West Riding Asylum
IV: 240–264 [9]	On the hourly distribution of mortality in relation to recurrent changes in the activity of vital functions	Robert Lawson MB CM Edin	Clinical Assistant, West Riding Asylum; Formerly Assistant to the Professor of Practice of Medicine and Medical Psychology at Edinburgh University
IV: 265–290 [10]	Acute dementia [cf. Contents: On acute dementia]	James Crichton Browne MD FRSE	Medical Director, West Riding Asylum; and Lecturer on Mental Diseases to the Leeds School of Medicine
IV: 291–304 [11]	Ophthalmoscopic observations in acute dementia	Charles Aldridge MB	Physician to the Plympton House Asylum; late Senior Assistant Medical Officer; formerly Clinical Assistant, West Riding Asylum, Wakefield
IV: 305–317 [12]	The actions of nicotine [cf. Contents: On the actions of nicotine]	William T Benham MD Abdn	Pathologist and Assistant Medical Officer, West Riding Asylum

Volume V (1875)
Available online at:
https://archive.org/details/39002086346302.med.yale.edu

V: i	[Title page]		
V: ii	[blank]		
V: iii	[Title page with editor and publisher]		
V: iv	[Epigraph]	[GH] Lewes	
V: v	Preface	[JCB]	
V: vi	[blank]		
V: vii–viii	Contents		
V: 1–23 [1]	On the influence of diet in epilepsy	John Merson MA MD	Assistant Medical Officer, West Riding Asylum, Wakefield
V: 24–39 [2]	Labyrinthine vertigo. Menière's disease	David Ferrier MD	Assistant Physician to King's College Hospital. Professor of Forensic Medicine, King's College, London

(*continued*)

Table 6.1 (continued)

Reference	Title	Author(s) and qualifications	Affiliation(s)
V: 40–84 [3]	On the physiological action of hyoscyamine	Robert Lawson MB Edin	Pathologist and Assistant Medical Officer, West Riding Asylum
V: 85–104 [4]	On the histology of the great sciatic nerve in general paralysis of the insane	W Bevan Lewis LRCP Lond, MRCS, FRMS	Clinical Assistant, West Riding Asylum; Formerly Assistant Medical Officer, Bucks County Asylum
V: 105–129 [5]	On temporary mental disorders after epileptic paroxysms	J Hughlings Jackson MD FRCP	Physician to the London Hospital and to the Hospital for the Epileptic and Paralysed
V: 130–148 [6]	On the appearance of the retina and choroid during the administration of certain drugs	John Hunter Arbuckle MD and CM Glas	Clinical Assistant, West Riding Asylum
V: 149–159 [7]	Othaematoma, or the insane ear	Lennox Browne FRCS Edin	Senior Surgeon to the Central London Throat and Ear Hospital, Surgeon, and Aural Surgeon to the Royal Society of Musicians, etc
V: 160–170 [8]	On the morbid histology of the brain in the lower animals	Herbert C Major MD Edin	Deputy Medical Director, West Riding Asylum, Wakefield
V: 171–187 [9]	Cerebral hyperaemia	J Milner Fothergill MD Edin MRCP Lond	Junior Physician to the West London Hospital
V: 188–197 [10]	A new process for examining the structure of the brain. With a review of some points in the histology of the cerebellum	H R Octavius Sankey	Undergraduate in Medicine of the University of London
V: 198–226 [11]	Epileptiform seizures in general paralysis	Charles F Newcombe MB	Assistant Medical Officer, Lancaster County Asylum, Rainhill. Late Clinical Assistant, West Riding Asylum
V: 227–256 [12]	The functions of the thalami optici	James Crichton Browne MD FRSE	Medical Director, West Riding Asylum

(*continued*)

Table 6.1 (continued)

Reference	Title	Author(s) and qualifications	Affiliation(s)
V: 257–270 [13]	On the therapeutic value of chloral hydrate in epileptic convulsions	J A M Wallis [cf. Contents: "A M Wallis"] MD	Medical Superintendent, Hull Borough Asylum. Late Assistant Medical Officer, West Riding Asylum
V: 271–283 [14]	Laryngoscopic observations in general paralysis	Lennox Browne FRCS Edin	Senior Surgeon to the Central London Throat and Ear Hospital, Surgeon to the Royal Society of Musicians, to Her Majesty's Italian Opera, etc
V: 284–292 [15]	Note on chronic mania	James Crichton Browne MD FRSE	Medical Director, West Riding Asylum

Volume VI (1876)
Available online at:
https://archive.org/details/39002086346310.med.yale.edu

VI: i	[Title page]		
VI: ii	[blank]		
VI: iii	[Title page with editor and publisher]		
VI: iv	[Epigraph]	Fiske	
VI: v	Preface	[HCM?]	
VI: vi	[blank]		
VI: vii–viii	Contents		
VI: 1–10 [1]	The histology of the island of Reil	Herbert C Major MD	Medical Director West Riding Asylum
VI: 11–26 [2]	The weight of the brain in the insane	Crochley Clapham LRCP Lond etc.	West Riding Asylum
VI: 27–42 [3]	On classification and nomenclature in nervous disorders	A H Rabagliati MA MD	Bradford
VI: 43–64 [4]	Calorimetric observations upon the influence of various alkaloids on the generation of animal heat	W Bevan Lewis LRCP Lond, MRCS	Pathologist and Assistant Medical Officer, West Riding Asylum
VI: 65–84 [5]	Hyoscyamine in the treatment of some diseases of the insane	Robert Lawson MB	Assistant Medical Officer, West Riding Asylum

(continued)

Table 6.1 (continued)

Reference	Title	Author(s) and qualifications	Affiliation(s)
VI: 85–107 [6]	The climacteric period in relation to insanity	John Merson MD	Assistant Medical Officer, West Riding Asylum
VI: 108–119 [7]	Cases on the borderland of insanity	Henry Sutherland MD MRCP	Lecturer on Insanity to the Westminster Hospital School of Medicine
VI: 120–149 [8]	Clinical notes on conditions incidental to insanity	Robert Lawson MB	Assistant Medical Officer, West Riding Asylum
		W Bevan Lewis LRCP Lond	Pathologist and Assistant Medical Officer, West Riding Asylum
VI: 150–169 [9]	The cranial outline of the insane and criminal	Crochley Clapham LRCP Lond	West Riding Asylum
		Henry Clarke LRCP Lond	Surgeon, West Riding Prison
VI: 170–231 [10]	Notes on the pathology of general paresis of the insane	James-Crichton Browne [*sic*, with hyphen] MD FRSE	Lord Chancellor's Visitor of Lunatics
VI: 232–253 [11]	A case of epilepsy (under the care of Dr Crichton-Browne [*sic*, with hyphen])	Medical Officers of the West Riding Asylum	–
VI: 254–265 [12]	Notes on the therapeutics of some affections of the nervous system	J Milner Fothergill MD MRCP	Assistant Physician to the West London Hospital, etc
VI: 266–309 [13]	On epilepsies and on the after effects of epileptic discharges (Todd and Robertson's hypothesis)	J Hughlings Jackson MD FRCP	[No affiliation given]

NB: The volumes are designated with Roman numerals, both here and throughout the text, as per the title pages of each volume. The titles of some articles differ between the tables of Contents and the title page of the paper. [With additions and silent corrections from Larner (2023b), Supplementary Table S1.]

[a]*Sic*. This nomenclature, used in the affiliation for four of Jackson's five publications in *WRLAMR* (III:175–195; III:315–349; IV:24–29; V:105–129), may be confusing. The Hospital in Queen Square where Jackson worked was at this time the "National Hospital for the Paralysed and Epileptic". A quite separate institution was the "Hospital for Epilepsy and Paralysis" located from 1873 in London's Regent's Park, a hospital with which Jackson had no connection, although Ferrier was "Physician for Out-patients" there from 1877 to 1880 prior to his move to Queen Square

Publications" appeared after the final paper in volumes III and IV, and eight pages in volume VI, but none in volume V.[27]

Inviting interested parties to subscribe to a publication is one tried and tested method to generate revenue up-front in order to fund, at least partially, a book or journal ahead of its publication. Some journals published a list of subscribers, but I have found none for *WRLAMR*.[28]

Structure and Contents of *WRLAMR*

WRLAMR was published as six annual octavo volumes between 1871 and 1876. Each of the six volumes ran to about 300 pages (in total 1838 pages) and contained from 12 to 15 articles of variable length and type (see Table 6.1 for complete listings). A total of 80 papers was published in all.[29]

In his analysis of *WRLAMR*, Viets divided these articles into several categories,[30] viz:

1. Papers reporting original research done at West Riding (62), these subdivided into (a) Clinical (24), (b) Therapy (12), (c) Pathological (14), (d) Experimental, human (8), and (e) Experimental, animal (4).
2. Papers read at West Riding (2).
3. Papers contributed to the *Medical Reports* (16).

In addition to these 80 papers, the meat of the journal, there were also some addenda. Each issue featured an epigraph (two in volume II) and a Preface by the editor. There were no additions after the last paper in volume I, but in

---

[27] In all three volumes containing these advertisements for "Smith, Elder, & Co.'s Medical Publications" John Galton's translation of Ecker's "*On the convolutions of the human brain*" (see Chap. 5) was included, priced at four shillings and sixpence. In volume VI, David Ferrier's (1876) monograph "*The functions of the brain*" appeared in the list of books advertised, price 15 shillings.

[28] *Contra* the statement of Sloffer (2023:32).

[29] Some authors have stated a total of 79 papers, although the reason(s) for this discrepancy is/are not clear to me. As far as I can ascertain this simple arithmetic error is first encountered in Bynum (1985:96; uncorrected in Bynum 1990:123) and is repeated by Oppenheim (1991:70) and by Pearce and Lees (2013:8). Whether each has independently miscounted, or simply abstracted their incorrect information from earlier authors, is not clear. Pearce and Lees cited neither Oppenheim nor Bynum; Oppenheim cited Bynum (at 332n52) but also Viets (1938) who gave the correct number (as did Finn 2012:80). Sloffer (2023:12) reported "nearly eighty" papers but later corrected (16, 19, 20, 33, 36, 37 Table 2). A case might actually be made for 81 papers if one shares Greenblatt's view (2022:174n83) that the two Appendixes (III:341–349) following Hughlings Jackson's second paper of 1873 "constituted a third, independent article".

[30] Viets (1938:483–487). A different classification was offered by Sloffer (2023:36–37, Table 2) but as with Viets this was essentially arbitrary.

volume II there was a listing of the members of the Asylum's Committee of Visitors (II:307) and the Resident Medical Officers (II:308) but these did not appear in subsequent volumes. *WRLAMR* never had a Correspondence section, perhaps because it was deemed unlikely to be of topical value in an annual, as opposed to a quarterly or weekly, publication. Limitations on page count might also have contributed to this decision, likewise to the absence of any indexing system.

Reprints or offprints of individual papers may have been available in some circumstances. For example, a reprint of Burman's paper on "On conia, and its use in subcutaneous injection" (II:1–40) was anonymously reviewed under the title of "Burman on conia" in *The British and Foreign Medico-Chirurgical Review*,[31] and the Wellcome Collection holds a reprint of William Browne's paper on "Impairment of language, the result of cerebral disease" (II:278–301).[32] In York and Steinberg's catalogue raisonné of the writings of John Hughlings Jackson, two items (A29, A33) are listed as reprinted from *WRLAMR*.[33]

Material to publish in *WRLAMR* does not seem to have been lacking. In the preface to the first issue Crichton-Browne noted that the limits originally assigned necessitated the "exclusion of several interesting articles" (I:v). Similarly, in the 1873 preface he reported that "Five very valuable essays, containing original observations made in the wards of the asylum, have ... been regretfully ... excluded" (III:iv), and in the 1874 preface five papers were said to have been excluded (IV:v). Some papers may have been specifically requested by Crichton-Browne, e.g. Allbutt's work on the obscurer neuroses of syphilis, which was prefaced by the author's comment: "When, in obedience to the kind insistence of my friend Dr. Crichton Browne, I undertook to write upon the present subject" (III:273). No criteria for selection or rejection were stated, likewise editorial policy on manuscript revision, or the provision of pre-publication proofs to authors. As previously noted (Chap. 5), one author retrospectively felt that his work was "so cut and mutilated for want of space that, when finished, I hardly recognised my own work".[34]

---

[31] *Br Foreign Med Chir Rev* 1873;51(102):444–445. Also *Dublin Journal of Medical Science* 1873;55:154–155 (reprint from *WRLAMR* vol II.).

[32] https://wellcomecollection.org/works/pr6abkbz/items (accessed 03/09/24). Printers' details: "Wakefield: R. Micklethwaite, Printer, Cheapside, Corn Market. 1872".

[33] York and Steinberg (2006:141) A29, 36-page pamphlet = III:315–349; A33, 23-page pamphlet = III:175–195. Printers' details: "London: Spottiswood and Co". The title page of a copy of the latter, autographed by Jackson to Kinnier Wilson, appeared as an illustration in Jellinek (2004:933, Figure 2), the original held in the library of the Royal College of Physicians of Edinburgh.

[34] Thompson (1874–1875b:579); he regretted the brevity of both of his *WRLAMR* articles (I:58–70 and II:302–306), which Wallis (2017b:300) takes to suggest that they were heavily edited. Certainly,

Many of the papers in *WRLAMR* related clinical histories and included patient details, such as initials, age, and date of admission, sometimes occupation and place of origin, and occasionally photographs, all of which would permit retrospective identification by reference to the original asylum case books (now held at West Yorkshire Archive Service; www.wyjs.org.uk). The concept of "patient consent" to publication did not exist at this time.

Dates of Publication of *WRLAMR*

The exact publication dates of the annual issues of *WRLAMR* are unknown. Crichton-Browne enclosed a copy of volume I with a letter to Charles Darwin dated 18th August 1871.[35] In his letter to Charles Darwin of 16th April 1873, Crichton-Browne seems to have anticipated that volume III would appear in July 1873,[36] and David Ferrier later stated that his paper therein (III:30–96) appeared "in the beginning of August".[37] This statement is corroborated by Harrington Tuke's Presidential address to the MPA on 6th August 1873 in which he reported that "Within the last few days, Dr. Crichton Browne … added a new remedy to our list, by his discovery of the value of nitrite of amyl in the treatment of epilepsy", footnoting the "last number of the West Riding Asylum Reports [*sic*]".[38]

Some inferences about publication dates can be made from both internal (limited) and external (more plentiful) evidence.

Internal evidence suggests a *terminus post quem* (a date after which) of 10th July 1871 for volume I, since that date is denoted as "the present time" by Churchill Fox (I:263); and 18th June 1872 for volume II, according to notes

---

Thompson's page allowance (2 papers, 18 pages) seems niggardly when compared to, say, Aldridge (3 papers, 103 pages). Whilst Thompson wrote of his first paper (13 pages) that "the space allotted to this paper is somewhat limited" (I:62), Aldridge's first paper filled 58 pages, and even when he had reportedly "exceeded the space allotted to me" (I:99) he managed to fill another 29 pages with potted case histories. On the other hand, with the benefit of hindsight, one might argue that ophthalmoscopy, the subject of Aldridge's papers, has proved a more durable innovation than sphygmography, the subject of Thompson's work.

[35] Darwin Correspondence Project, "Letter no. 7910," https://www.darwinproject.ac.uk/letter/?docId=letters/DCP-LETT-7910.xml (accessed 13/09/24). The copy of *WRLAMR* is in the Darwin Library, Cambridge University Library. I find no annotation regarding donation by Crichton-Browne or receipt by Darwin in the online copy.

[36] Darwin Correspondence Project, "Letter no. 8861," https://www.darwinproject.ac.uk/letter/?docId=letters/DCP-LETT-8861.xml (accessed 22/01/23).

[37] Ferrier (1874a:399).

[38] Harrington Tuke (1873:448). Also Harrington Tuke (1873–1874:332). Crichton-Browne's paper to which he was referring is III:153–174.

on two of Burman's patients (II:22n1 and II:24n1).[39] For volume V, Wallis included a patient who died on 25th July 1875 (V:265). Generally, it would seem that volumes appeared late in the year of publication or even, for the later issues, early the following year.

Hence, despite the publication date of 1876 for volume VI, internal evidence suggests a *terminus post quem* of, at best, early 1877.[40] Specifically, Robert Lawson's account of a general paralytic patient whose date of admission to WRA was recorded as 27th August 1876 included a footnote (VI:69) stating that "during 4 months which have elapsed since these notes were written". If "4 months" is correct, rather than just an estimate, then at minimum this footnote would date from 27th December 1876.[41]

Furthermore, Hughlings Jackson's paper (VI:266–309) contained a footnote (VI:287–288) referring to an article published by Charcot in the first issue of the *Revue Mensuelle de Médecine et de Chirurgie* dated January 1877.[42]

As regards external evidence, this is available in the form of published reviews of the volumes of *WRLAMR* (Table 6.2). The earliest review in the calendar year identified thus far is for the 1873 volume which appeared in the 3rd September 1873 issue of the *Medical Press and Circular*.[43] However, most reviews were published in the year following the date of the volume.

That the date of publication of *WRLAMR* may have become progressively later in each successive year is exemplified in the sequence of reviews for each of the six volumes which appeared in the *Journal of Mental Science* (one of only two journals in which, to my knowledge, all six volumes were reviewed, the other being the *American Journal of the Medical Sciences*;[44] Table 6.2) The October 1871 issue of the *Journal of Mental Science* noted the first volume of

---

[39] Volume II also has some May 1872 dates: the data on puerperal mania presented by Pedler covered a period up to 10th May 1872 (II:151); one of Burman's patients admitted in January 1872 was reported "up to the present (May 23rd)" (II:20; also II:21), others up to May 24th (II:23, 24, 26), and another was discharged 5th June 1872 (II:25n1).

[40] Cf. Finn (2012:90n291), who stated that: "The volume of the *Reports* that the paper [(VI:232–251)] appeared in came out in the summer of 1876, a few months after Crichton-Browne had left". The internal evidence presented here does not support this dating.

[41] That is, if and only if Lawson's notes were written on the day of admission. In this context, it is of note that an abstract of Lawson's paper (VI:65–84) appearing in *J Ment Sci* 1877–1878;23:368–372 (October 1877; Occasional notes of the Quarter) concludes "*West Riding Reports for 1877* [*sic*]".

[42] Greenblatt (2022:255n326). The paper in question is in fact Charcot and Pitres (1877), in which Hughlings Jackson was mentioned on p.4.

[43] Greenblatt (2022:168n38) inferred that *WRLAMR* for 1873 "appeared in the fall (October–November) of that year". The review in *Medical Press and Circular* cited here suggests it appeared at least one month earlier than Greenblatt suggested and, based on the comments of Crichton-Browne and Ferrier, possibly two or three months earlier.

[44] All six volumes were either noted as received (I, V, VI) or reviewed (II, III, IV) in the *Medical Press and Circular*.

Table 6.2 Contemporary reviews of *WRLAMR*

Volume 1 (1871)

[Anon]. The West Riding Lunatic Asylum Medical Reports. Edited by J. Crichton Browne, M.D., F.R.S.E. Vol. I. London: J. and A. Churchill, 1871.
Dublin Quarterly Journal of Medical Science 1871; 52(104): 439–440 (1st November 1871).
[Anon]. The West Riding Lunatic Asylum Medical Reports. Edited by J.C. Browne, M.D., F.R.S.E. London: J. and A. Churchill. 1871.
Journal of Mental Science 1871–1872; 17(80): 559–562 (January 1872).
[Anon]. Medical Reports of the West Riding Asylum.
British and Foreign Medico-Chirurgical Review 1872; 49(97): 25–46 (January 1872)
[This volume is also noted in *Lancet* 1872; 1: 83 (20th January; Reviews and Notices of Books) and mentions "Medical Reports of the West Riding Asylum".]
[Anon]. The West Riding Lunatic Asylum Medical Reports. Edited by J. Crichton Browne, M.D. Ed., F.R.S.E., Medical Director of the Asylum and Lecturer on Mental Disease, Leeds School of Medicine.
Indian Medical Gazette 1872; 7(11): 260–261.
"B.L.R." The West Riding Lunatic Asylum Medical Reports. Vol. 1. Edited by
J. Crichton Browne, M.D., F.R.S.E. pp. 265. London: J. & A. Churchill, 1871.
American Journal of the Medical Sciences 1872; 63(125): 180–190.

Volume 2 (1872)

[Anon]. West Riding Lunatic Asylum Medical Reports. Edited by J. Crichton Browne, M.D., F.R.C.S.E., [*sic*] &c. Vol. II. London: J. & A. Churchill.
Lancet 1872; 2: 564 (19th October; Reviews and Notices of Books).
[Anon]. The West Riding Lunatic Asylum Medical Report [*sic*]. Edited by J. Crichton Browne, M.D., F.R.S.E. Vol. II. London: Churchill, 1872.
The Practitioner 1872; 9: 362–365.
[Anon]. Dr. Crichton Browne's Reports (a). *Medical Press and Circular* 1872; 14: 537 (18th December).
[Anon]. The West Riding Lunatic Asylum Reports [*sic*]. Edited by J. Crichton Browne, M.D., F.R.S.E. Vol. II. London: J. & A. Churchill, 1872.
Birmingham Medical Review: A Quarterly Journal of the Medical Sciences 1872; 1: 265–269.
[Anon]. The West Riding Lunatic Asylum Medical Reports. Edited by J. Crichton Browne, M.D. Vol. 2. 1872.
Journal of Mental Science 1872–1873; 18(84): 583–586 (January 1873).
Erratum: *Journal of Mental Science* 1873–1874; 19(85): 168 (April 1873).
[Anon]. West Riding Asylum Reports.
British and Foreign Medico-Chirurgical Review 1873; 51(102): 337–344 (April 1873).
[Anon]. Pathological histology of the brain and spinal cord.
British and Foreign Medico-Chirurgical Review 1873; 51(102): 377–378 (April 1873)
"B.L.R." The West Riding Lunatic Asylum Medical Reports. Edited by J. Crichton Browne, M.D., F.R.S.E. Vol. ii. 8vo. pp. 306. London: J. & A. Churchill, 1872.
American Journal of the Medical Sciences 1873; 65(129): 204–209.
[Anon]. The West Riding Lunatic Asylum Medical Reports. Edited by J. Crichton Browne, M.D., F.R.S.E. Vol. II.
Dublin Journal of Medical Science 1873; 55: 425–429.

(*continued*)

Table 6.2 (continued)

[Anon].
Westminster and Foreign Quarterly Review 1873; 99(195): 297–298.

Volume 3 (1873)

[Anon]. The West Riding Lunatic Asylum Medical Reports (a). *Medical Press and Circular* 1873; 16: 218–219 (3rd September).
[Anon]. The West Riding Lunatic Asylum Reports [*sic*]. Edited by G.J. [*sic*] Crichton Browne, M.D., F.R.S.E. Vol. III. London: Smith and Elder, 1873.
The Practitioner 1873; 11: 285–288 [same errors in index, p.486].
[Anon].
Westminster and Foreign Quarterly Review 1873; 100(198): 492–493.
[Anon]. The West Riding Lunatic Asylum Medical Reports. Edited by J. Chricton [*sic*] Browne, M.D., F.R.S.E. Vol. III.
American Journal of Insanity 1873–4; 30: 286–290.
[Anon]. The West Riding Lunatic Asylum Medical Reports. by J. Crichton Browne, M.D. Vol. 3. Smith, Elder, and Co., 1873.
Journal of Mental Science 1873–1874; 19(88): 590–595 (January 1874).
[Anon]. West Riding Asylum Reports.
British and Foreign Medico-Chirurgical Review 1874; 53(105): 143–146 (January 1874).
"B.L.R." The West Riding Lunatic Asylum Medical Reports. Edited by J. Crichton Browne, M.D., F.R.S.E. Vol. III. 8vo. pp. vi., 349. London: Smith, Elder & Co., 1873.
American Journal of the Medical Sciences 1874; 68(135): 201–205.
[Anon]. The West Riding Asylum [*sic*] Medical Reports. Edited by J. Crichton Browne, M.D. (especially the papers by Ferrier, Hughlings Jackson, and Crichton Browne). London: 1873.
Glasgow Medical Journal 1874; 6(1): 101–113.

Volume 4 (1874)

[Anon]. West Riding Asylum Medical Reports (a). *Medical Press and Circular* 1874; 18: 383–384 (28th October).
[Anon]. The West Riding Lunatic Asylum Medical Reports. Edited by J. Crichton Browne, M.D., F.R.S.E. Vol. iv.
Journal of Mental Science 1874–1875; 20(92): 601–609 (January 1875).
[Anon]. The West Riding Lunatic Asylum Medical Reports. Edited by J. Crichton Browne, M.D., F.R.S.E. Vol. iv. London: Smith, Elder and Co. 1874.
British Medical Journal 1875; 1(739): 277–278. (27th February; Reviews and Notices)
[Anon]. The West Riding Lunatic Asylum Reports [*sic*]. Edited by J. Crichton Browne, M.D., F.R.S,E. Vol. IV. 1874. London: Smith, Elder, and Co.
Lancet 1875; 1: 476–477 (3rd April; Reviews and Notices of Books).
[Anon]. West Riding Asylum Reports [*sic*].
British and Foreign Medico-Chirurgical Review 1875; 56(111): 167–168 (July 1875).
[Anon.] The West Riding Lunatic Asylum Medical Reports. Edited by J. Crichton Browne, M.D., F.R.S.E.
Journal of Psychological Medicine and Mental Pathology (London) 1875; 1(1): 154.
[Anon]. West Riding Lunatic Asylum Reports [*sic*], Vol. iv. Edited by J. Crichton Browne, M.D.
Journal of Psychological Medicine and Mental Pathology (London) 1875; 1(2): 197–203.

(continued)

Table 6.2 (continued)

"B.L.R." The West Riding Lunatic Asylum Medical Reports. Edited by J. Crichton Browne, M.D., F.R.S.E. Vol. IV. 8vo. pp. 317. London: Smith, Elder & Co., 1874.
American Journal of the Medical Sciences 1875; 70(139): 194–199.
[Anon]. Recent works on psychological medicine. I. West Riding Lunatic Asylum Reports [*sic*]. Vol. IV. 1874.
Dublin Journal of Medical Science 1875; 60: 211–220.
[Anon]. The West Riding Lunatic Asylum Medical Reports. Edited by J. Crichton Browne, M.D., F.R.S.E. Vol. IV. London: Smith, Elder & Co. 1874. pp. 317.
Glasgow Medical Journal 1875; 7(2): 238–242.
[Anon]. The West Riding Lunatic Asylum Medical Reports. Edited by J. Crichton Browne, M.D., F.R.S.E. Vol. IV. London: Smith, Elder, and Co., 1874.
The Practitioner 1875; 14: 199–201.

Volume 5 (1875)

[Anon]. The West Riding Lunatic Asylum Medical Reports. Edited by J. Crichton Browne, M.D., F.R.S,E. Vol. V. London: Smith and Elder [*sic*].
Lancet 1876; 2: 224–225 (6th August; Reviews and Notices of Books).
[Anon]. The West Riding Lunatic Asylum Medical Reports. Edited by J. Crichton Browne, M.D., F.R.C.S.E. [*sic*] Vol. V. 1875.
Journal of Mental Science 1876–1877; 22(99): 458–464 (October 1876).
"B.L.R." The West Riding Lunatic Asylum Medical Reports. Edited by J. Crichton Browne, M.D., F.R.S.E. Vol. V. 8vo. pp. 292. London: Smith, Elder & Co., 1875.
American Journal of the Medical Sciences 1876; 72(143): 202–205.
[Anon]. III—The West Riding Lunatic Asylum Reports [*sic*]. The West Riding Lunatic Asylum Medical Reports. Edited by J. Crichton Browne, M.D., F.R.S.E. Vol. V. London, Smith, Elder & Co., 1875; 292 pages.
Journal of Nervous and Mental Disease 1876; 3(3): 470–475.
"T.W.F." The West Riding Lunatic Asylum Reports [*sic*].
Boston Medical and Surgical Journal 1876; 94: 636–638.
Atkins R. Report on nervous and mental disease.
Dublin Journal of Medical Science 1876; 61: 422–441 [at 426–8, 429–31, 436–9, 441].
[Anon]. The West Riding Lunatic Asylum Medical Reports. Edited by J. Crichton Browne, M.D., F.R.S.E. Vol. V. 1875. London: Smith, Elder & Co.
Glasgow Medical Journal 1876; 8(2): 224–229.
[Anon]. The West Riding Lunatic Asylum Medical Reports. Edited by J. Crichton Browne, M.D., F.R.S.E. Vol. V. 1875.
Edinburgh Medical Journal 1876; 21(8): 734–736.
de Boyer H. West Riding Lunatic Asylum medical [*sic*] Reports. vol. V. Edited by J. Crichton Browne. London: Smith, Elder and Co. *Le Progrès Médical* 1876; 4(19): 360–361 (6th May); 4(22): 422–423 (27th May); 4(23): 442–443 (3rd June).

Volume 6 (1876)

[Anon]. The West Riding Lunatic Asylum Medical Reports, Vol. vi., 1876. Edited by J. Crichton Browne, M.D., F.R.S.E., and Herbert C. Major, M.D.
Journal of Mental Science 1877; 23(103): 377–386 (October 1877).
"B.L.R." The West Riding Lunatic Asylum Medical Reports. Edited by J. Crichton Browne, M.D., F.R.S.E. and Herbert C. Major, M.D. Vol. VI. 8vo. pp. 309. London: Smith, Elder & Co., 1876.
American Journal of the Medical Sciences 1877; 74(147): 184–188.

(continued)

Table 6.2 (continued)

III—The West Riding Lunatic Asylum Medical Reports. The West Riding Lunatic Asylum Medical Reports. Edited by J. Crichton Browne, M.D., F.R.S.E., and Herbert C. Major, M.D. Volume VI. London, Smith, Elder & Co. 1876; 309 pages. *Journal of Nervous and Mental Disease* 1877; 4(4): 768–772.
"T.W.F." The West Riding Report [*sic*]. *Boston Medical and Surgical Journal* 1877; 97: 110–112.
[Anon]. The West Riding Lunatic Asylum Medical Reports. Edited by J. Crichton Browne, M.D., F.R.S.E., and Herbert C. Major, M.D. Vol. VI. London. 1876. *Glasgow Medical Journal* 1877; 9(3): 401–409.
[Anon]. The West Riding Lunatic Asylum Medical Reports. Edited by J. Crichton Browne, M.D., and Herbert P. [*sic*] Major, M.D. Vol. VI. London: 1876. *Edinburgh Medical Journal* 1878; 23(8): 736–739 (February 1878).

NB This does not claim to be a comprehensive listing

WRLAMR amongst books received and promised a review "in our next number",[45] which duly appeared in the January 1872 issue (the *Journal of Mental Science* was published quarterly, in January, April, July, and October). Likewise, Volume II was noted in the October 1872 issue with the assurance "Will be noticed in our next number",[46] which notice duly appeared in January 1873. Volume III was noted in the October 1873 issue[47] and reviewed in January 1874, and the review for Volume IV likewise appeared in the following January (1875) issue.[48] However, the reviews for *WRLAMR* Volumes V and VI did not appear until the following October issues of the *Journal of Mental Science*, i.e. 1876 and 1877 respectively (Table 6.2).

This of course risked some confusion, not least for *WRLAMR* authors themselves: for example, in the discussion following a presentation by a Dr. Duffin on Menière's disease given at the Clinical Society of London on 25th February 1876, David Ferrier's comments included a citation of his own

---

[45] *J Ment Sci* 1871–1872;17(October 1871):468 (Books, Pamphlets, &c., received for Review, 1871). As the *Journal of Mental Science* was a quarterly, the publication date of *WRLAMR* preceded this announcement. Receipt of this volume of *WRLAMR* was noted in the issue of 23rd August of *Medical Press and Circular* 1871;12:173 (Books, Pamphlets, and Medical Journals Received) but it does not appear to have been reviewed therein; and in the issue of 26th August of *Medical Times and Gazette* 1871;2:240 (Books Received), ditto.

[46] *J Ment Sci* 1872–1873;18(October 1872):473 (Books, Pamphlets, &c., received for Review, 1872). *Medical Times and Gazette* 1872;2:344 (21st September; Periodicals and Newspapers Received) noted receipt of "West Riding Lunatic Asylum Reports, vol.2"; *Medical Times and Gazette* 1872;2:466 (26th October; Medical Meeting at the West Riding Asylum, Wakefield) stated that Crichton-Browne "has been able to publish two volumes of Asylum Reports". The November 1872 issue of the *Edinburgh Medical Journal* (1872;18(5):480) noted this volume amongst "Publications received".

[47] *J Ment Sci* 1873–1874;19:489 (October 1873; Books received).

[48] *Medical Times and Gazette* 1874;2:436 (10th October; Books and Pamphlets Received) noted receipt of "West Riding Lunatic Asylum Reports, vol. iv". The review in the *Medical Press and Circular* appeared in the 28th October 1874 issue.

paper on the subject (V:24–39) as "West Riding Reports, vol. v, 1876 [*sic*]",[49] although *WRLAMR* volume V was dated 1875.

Further corroboration comes from the *Medical Press and Circular*, in which Volumes II, III and IV were reviewed, respectively, in the issues of 18th December 1872, 3rd September 1873, and 28th October 1874 (Table 6.2). Receipt of Volume V was noted in the issue of 19th January 1876 and of Volume VI in the issue of 16th May 1877.[50]

The *Lancet*, which only reviewed Volumes II, IV, and V, suggests a similar pattern, with reviews appearing in the issues of 19th October 1872, 3rd April 1875, and 6th August 1876 respectively (Table 6.2). Although this might be accounted for in part by tardiness on the part of the reviewer(s), the *Lancet* noted receipt of Volume VI of the "Medical Reports of the West Riding Lunatic Asylum" [*sic*] in the issue of 5th May 1877,[51] hence a similar date to that noted in the *Medical Press and Circular*. The very latest review of volume VI identified thus far appeared in the February 1878 issue of the *Edinburgh Medical Journal*.

Contributions to *WRLAMR*

In early 1874, after the first three volumes of *WRLAMR* had been published, Batty Tuke summarised their contents:

> The papers which compose the mass of the West Riding Reports [*sic*] are devoted to anatomy, physiology, pathology, general and morbid, and therapeutics, …[52]

---

[49] *BMJ* 1876;1:323 (11th March). Ferrier (1876:238) made the same dating error, "vol. v, 1876", with respect to Crichton-Browne's paper on the optic thalami (V:227–256). Commenting on Hughlings Jackson's paper (V:105–129), Greenblatt (2022:253n319) stated that "We do not know exactly when in the year 1875 this volume [V of *WRLAMR*] was published, but I agree with York and Steinberg (2006, p. 82), who make the reasonable assumption that it was later in the year, or maybe in early 1876." York and Steinberg 2006:82 in fact merely said "Volume dated 1875", but based on the evidence presented here I agree with Greenblatt's view that it was published "later in the year, or maybe in early 1876".

[50] *Medical Press and Circular* 1876;21:61 (19th January; Books, pamphlets, and medical journals received) and 1877;23:404 (16th May; Books, pamphlets, and medical journals received). The latter gave "West Riding Lunatic Asylum Reports". I could not find either of these volumes reviewed in issues of the *Medical Press and Circular* through to the end of 1878.

[51] *Lancet* 1877;1:669 (5th May; Books Etc. Received). Also *Br Foreign Med Chir Rev* 1877;60(119):249 (July–October 1877; "Books, pamphlets, &c., received for review"), later presumably because a quarterly publication.

[52] Batty Tuke (1874:109).

Here the contributions to the six volumes of *WRLAMR* are briefly summarised. Modifying Viets' categorisation,[53] these contributions are divided into clinical investigation and diagnosis; pharmacology and therapeutics; pathological anatomy; and experimental laboratory work, both animal and human (self-experimentation).

Clinical Investigation

Patient-related investigations described in *WRLAMR* included analysis of aggregate demographic data that could be obtained from the WRA case books, such as patients' weight change from admission (II:263), temperature (II:265–266), and the hourly distribution of mortality (IV:240–264), as well as clinical assessment of specific organ systems such as the heart (III:113–128 and III:216–257) and faculties such as colour perception (III:129–152). In an era before lumbar puncture for cerebrospinal fluid analysis, neurophysiology, and neuroimaging, the clinical investigations available were limited; for example, those mentioned in *WRLAMR* include dynamometry (II:17–18), pupillometry (II:223–253; IV:44, 313), and "urinology" (IV:63–93; Aldridge also examined the urine in his patients with epilepsy and general paralysis of the insane, I:92 and II:227, respectively[54]). Some data were presented as averages or percentages, but certainly the modern reader is struck by the total absence of any statistical analysis, reflecting the paucity or unawareness of techniques available at this time.[55]

As regards the investigation of disease, the application of new or emerging investigative technologies comprised a significant component of the contents of *WRLAMR*. Perhaps the most notable of these was the use of the ophthalmoscope.

---

[53] Viets (1938:483–487).

[54] A later WRA AMO, Ernest Birt (1886–1887), returned to the subject of urinology in the 1880s, without reference to his predecessors.

[55] Although some French physicians, including Pinel, had advocated use of the "calculus of probability" (Murphy 1981), this does not seem to have permeated to WRA. The transition of statistics to a specialised mathematical discipline inspired by Francis Galton and Karl Pearson did not begin until the end of the century (Magnello 2002). Magnello characterised the use of averages and percentages as "vital statistics" deriving ultimately from the ideology of Aristotelian essentialism, in contrast to the mathematical statistics based on significance tests deriving ultimately from Darwinian ideas about populations of species.

Ophthalmoscopy

Clifford Allbutt (see Chap. 7) was making ophthalmoscopic observations on WRA patients as early as 1867. Following Allbutt's contributions to the nascent ophthalmological literature, application of the ophthalmoscope was most thoroughly explored at WRA by Charles Aldridge who had received some training from Allbutt in Leeds (see Chap. 5). In his three papers, Aldridge made observations "in mental and cerebral diseases" (I:71–128), "in general paralysis, after the administration of certain toxic agents" (II:223–253),[56] and "in acute dementia" (IV:291–304). Part of the rationale for this endeavour was the known relationship between the circulation of the retina and the brain:

> We may, therefore, take the ophthalmoscopic appearances of the retinal circulation as an index and guide to the condition of the cerebral, and from this basis we shall be able to make some interesting inquiries, and investigations into the influence of drugs upon the intra-cranial circulation. (I:90)[57]

This understanding was the basis for Aldridge's (audacious!) criticism of Hughlings Jackson's nomenclature of "epilepsy of the retina" for the retinal appearances in an epileptic observed during a portion of a fit (I:84).

Aldridge was unequivocal in his enthusiasm for the ophthalmoscope:

> In this instrument I believe we possess a most valuable agent for investigating the pathology of the multiform and obscure cerebral changes which go hand in hand with mental derangement. (II:224)

Other WRA clinicians also recognised this, for example, McDowall:

> by far the most important additions have been made to our knowledge of the functions of the retina since the introduction of the ophthalmoscope. (III:132)

---

[56] This paper was reviewed by Hughlings Jackson in *London Medical Record* 1873;1:22–23 (15th January) and 151 (12th March). I do not find these items included in the listings of Hughlings Jackson's published writings produced by York and Steinberg 2006 or Greenblatt (2022:473–502). For further details, see Larner (2025m).

[57] Also at II:233: "having shown elsewhere that various drugs produce certain well marked changes in the retinal circulation, I think we may fairly assume that in many cases, if not in all, these agents produce like effects in the cerebral vascular system."

Aldridge's ophthalmoscopic observations were also mentioned in other authors' papers,[58] for example in Milner Fothergill's essay on "cerebral anaemia" (IV:94–151) wherein the latter opined that the "ophthalmoscope lights up the pathology of cerebral conditions as regards the vascular system very distinctly" (IV:115).

Hughlings Jackson also contributed an ophthalmological report "On a case of recovery from double optic neuritis" (IV:24–29), illustrated with a chromolithograph, and urged the "necessity for the routine use of the ophthalmoscope". A demonstrating ophthalmoscope, rather than a hand-held device, was used by John Hunter Arbuckle in his experimental observations of retinal arteries and veins in rabbits over many hours as they were administered various pharmacological agents then in clinical use, such as nicotine, atropine, hydrate of chloral, nitrite of amyl, and morphia (V:130–148). Later clinical publications by Arbuckle included ophthalmological observations made on patients at WRA.[59]

Otolaryngoscopy

Otolaryngological studies were pursued at *WRLAMR* by Lennox Browne (V:149–159 and V:271–283) but these appear to have been opportunistic studies which were not followed up further. He noted that "the mirror was in all cases well tolerated, and not one case of retching due to reflex irritation occurred", explaining that "the tolerance with which the mirror is borne by general paralytics is due to diminution of sensibility of the pharynx" (V:273).

John C. Galton contributed "Notes on the condition of the tympanic membrane in the insane" (III:258–272) examining the membrane with "Troltsch's reflector—a concave mirror, three inches in diameter, and of six inches focal distance, mounted upon an ebonite handle, and resembling the reflector used in laryngoscopy in that it has at the centre a small circular space, free from amalgam backing, through which the observer looks" (III:264).

Sphygmography

Another novel technology which featured in several *WRLAMR* publications was the sphygmograph, a device which transcribed a patient's arterial pulse pressure on to paper. Invented and named by Karl Vierordt (1818–1884), the

---

[58] For example, Burman (1873).
[59] Arbuckle (1876a, c).

sphygmograph was later (1863) modified by Étienne-Jules Marey (1830–1904) to provide greater sensitivity and detail, such that the instrument was sometimes termed "Marey's sphygmograph".[60] Both Balthazar W. Foster and John Burdon Sanderson had written monographs on the subject of sphygmography in the late 1860s, and tracings had been illustrated by Lauder Brunton in his original work on nitrite of amyl in angina pectoris. Francis Anstie, later to lecture at the first medical *conversazione* at WRA (see Chap. 9), worked with Burdon Sanderson and gave two lectures on sphygmography at the Royal College of Physicians in 1867.[61] Hence, this was a highly topical subject.

At WRA, George Thompson (Chap. 5) championed the use of sphygmography (I:58–70 and II:302–306), using the modification to the device suggested by Anstie (I:59).[62] Tracings were also mentioned and/or illustrated in other *WRLAMR* papers, for example by Mitchell (I:48–49; these accredited to Thompson), by Milner Fothergill (III:126; also IV:117–118, tracings performed by Lauder Brunton; V:174), and by Benham in his experimental work examining the therapeutic effect of cold on the head (IV:152–178) and the actions of nicotine (IV:307, 315–317). Reference was also made to other contemporary studies using sphygmography (e.g. V:11 and V:174). Despite Thompson's evident enthusiasm, the value of sphygmographic recordings was not universally acknowledged at this time,[63] a skepticism born out by the failure of the sphygmograph to become established in clinical practice.

Bevan Lewis returned to the subject in 1881, when he was "Senior Assist. Med. Officer" at WRA, but his paper made no mention of Thompson nor his prior publications in *WRLAMR*.[64]

Clinical Diagnosis

Diagnosis presents a problem for the historian of medicine. Disease categories evolve over time, hence revisiting the diagnoses of yesteryear, perhaps with the

---

[60] Biographical material on Marey may be found in Silverman (1996/2003). For an account of sphygmography in asylum practice, see Wallis (2017b), wherein George Thompson's work is discussed (at 300, 302–303, 305).

[61] Foster (1866), Burdon Sanderson (1867) (see also Romano 2002:79–86), Lauder Brunton (1867) (see also Fye 1986:224), Anstie (1867). The sphygmograph was later adapted by Charcot for use at the Salpêtrière to record tremors (Goetz et al. 1995:114–115).

[62] Anstie (1868).

[63] Bartholow (1874:310) planned to make sphygmographic observations in his study of cortical excitability in a human subject, a study prompted in part by Ferrier's experimental animal work at WRA (Harris and Almerigi 2009:100).

[64] Bevan Lewis (1881–1882).

intention of diagnostic revision in light of new knowledge, is pointless,[65] particularly if one takes the Kuhnian view that old and new taxonomic structures and language express incommensurable ideas.[66]

Nineteenth-century county asylums housed a heterogeneous population of inmates. Whilst all suffered from what contemporary commentators called lunacy, or insanity,[67] this catch-all category might be subdivided into various forms, including melancholia, mania, dementia, idiocy and imbecility, as well as people with epileptic seizures (sometimes ostensibly and admittedly "sane"). In addition, forced incarceration of the mentally normal at the behest of their families, for example for pecuniary gain, was not unknown. It should also be remembered that general medical and surgical problems could sometimes supervene in patients whose primary problem related to mental health,[68] hence the employment of honorary physicians and surgeons by the Asylum (see Chap. 2).

This was an era predating the systematizing of Emil Kraepelin (1856–1926), although attempts at disease categorization were far from unknown.[69] A nosology promulgated by AMOAHI in 1842 encompassed mania, melancholia, monomania, moral insanity, dementia including imbecility, and congenital idiocy.[70] Of the clinical papers in *WRLAMR*, most addressed the catch-all category of "insanity" but some were devoted to specific conditions such as general paralysis of the insane, mania, dementia, or epilepsy. Diagnosis at WRA was largely clinical but new approaches facilitated by new technologies (*vide supra*) were sometimes pursued.

---

[65] But the attempt has, of course, been made. For an example pertinent to diagnoses made in a nineteenth-century asylum in northern England (Rainhill), see Parker et al. (1993).

[66] For example, Hacking (1998:87): "when an old classification collapses, we cannot translate the names for the old 'kinds' … into names for 'kinds' in the new system of classification." My thinking on retrospective diagnosis is summarised and exemplified in Larner (2025n, o), respectively.

[67] Crichton-Browne (1926:55) offered the following definition: "Insanity is a misfit of the mind to its environment, a disturbance of the harmony which should exist between the outer world and the order of consciousness."

[68] For example, *BMJ* 1875;1:345 (13th March; West Riding Asylum. Obstruction of the bowel by a biliary calculus. (Under the care of Dr. Crichton Browne)).

[69] Even Edward Jenner (1749–1823), the pioneer of smallpox vaccination, attempted a classification of "intellectual capacity" (see Larner (2003a); reprinted in adapted form in Larner (2019b:84–86)). As will be seen (Chap. 7), Crichton Browne (1875–1876b) criticised a contemporary classification of mental disease produced by David Skae.

[70] Digby (1985:135).

General Paralysis of the Insane; Syphilis

General paralysis of the insane (GPI), or just "general paralysis", was a common indication for admission to asylums in the nineteenth century. As it was, according to Aldridge:

> A disease, known to but few outside our asylum walls, it has devolved upon the alienist physician to record all that is known of its etiology, symptomatology, and pathological anatomy. (II:224)

The disorder was recognised clinically on the basis of its symptoms (e.g. I:65), both psychiatric (maniacal excitement, exalted ideas, delusions of grandeur) and neurological (gait disorder, sensory impairments, epileptiform seizures, dementia), and corroborative neurological findings (inequality of the pupils, tremulousness of the tongue, and alteration of gait). As a clinical diagnosis, however, it was vulnerable to diagnostic error, as Aldridge noted:

> one cannot help feeling that many cases are set down as general paralysis which have but little resemblance to it. (II:224)

A number of papers in *WRLAMR*, seven in all,[71] were explicitly devoted to the description or investigation of GPI, and of course patients with this condition featured in many other papers. By contrast, only one paper explicitly addressed syphilis (III:273–284); this was written by Allbutt, who had also published elsewhere on the subject.[72]

The interrelation between GPI, locomotor ataxy (this term originated with Duchenne de Boulogne in 1858[73]), and syphilis was not clearly defined at this time, but both Nicol (I:178–208) and Bevan-Lewis (V:85–104) noted the similarity of spinal cord lesions in GPI and locomotor ataxy. However, Aldridge reported that in 43 patients with GPI undergoing ophthalmological assessment "in two cases only was there any sign of syphilis" (II:227). Plaxton reported two cases from WRA in which tabes was followed by mental

---

[71] These seven were: I:129–151 (Burman: statistics); II:223–253 (Aldridge: ophthalmoscopy); III:113–128 (Milner Fothergill: heart sounds); IV:63–93 (Merson: urinology); V:85–104 (Bevan-Lewis: sciatic nerve histology); V:198–226 (Newcombe: epileptiform seizures); and V:271–283 (Lennox Browne: laryngoscopy). Hurn (1998:65n101) cited only four of these (Aldridge, Merson, Lennox Browne, Milner Fothergill). Finn (2012:127) stated that "between 1875–1876 … cases of general paralysis assumed a dominant place in the volumes" of *WRLAMR* but as the above listing of papers shows, whilst three dated from 1875 there was not one from 1876.

[72] Allbutt (1868e, 1872).

[73] Spillane (1981:320). See, for example, Ferrier (1876:49).

symptoms which were thought to be "simulating" GPI.[74] Burman's analysis of data from the Devon Asylum regarding the causes of GPI included only a single case of syphilis amongst 276 cases (I:141–142, Table VII) although venereal excesses were noted as a common cause elsewhere in his paper (e.g. I:148).

The prognosis of GPI was recognised to be extremely limited. Burman's analysis found only seven of 271 patients "survived admission for periods exceeding four years" (I:139) and of the patients examined with the ophthalmoscope by Allbutt at WRA Aldridge could find none surviving 4 years later (II:224–225).

The evolution of ideas regarding the relationship of GPI and syphilis involved many clinicians in the nineteenth century. Ashworth credited Steenberg in Denmark as having "demonstrated that general paralysis was due to syphilis" in 1860,[75] yet this name features not at all in other histories of GPI,[76] perhaps because Esmarch and Jessen had made the suggestion that syphilis caused GPI before this, in 1857. Fournier, in 1875, is sometimes credited as the first to suggest that syphilis might cause primary neural disease (a "neurosis"),[77] but it was not until 1905 that the causative agent, *Treponema pallidum*, was isolated by the dermatologist Erich Hoffmann and the zoologist Fritz Schaudinn. A year later the bacteriologist August von Wasserman developed a test to diagnose its presence in humans which still carries his name,[78] but it was not until 1913 that Noguchi and Moore showed syphilitic spirochaetes in the brains of patients with GPI.[79] It is probable that many of the patients labelled as having GPI at WRA did indeed have a syphilitic aetiology, what would now be considered the tertiary stage of syphilis, or neurosyphilis.[80] Of note, neurologists appeared to be more interested in tabes

---

[74] Plaxton (1878–1879).

[75] Ashworth (1975:33).

[76] For example, Quétel (1990), Pearce (2012), Ropper and Burrell (2019). Hurn (1998:94–95) noted that "Following Esmarch and Jessen, alienists in Scandinavia seized upon the link" but Steenberg is not mentioned by name.

[77] Fournier (1875).

[78] Quétel (1990), Ropper and Burrell (2019:115–117).

[79] Noguchi and Moore (1913).

[80] The difficulties of making this equivalence were addressed by Wallis (2017a:10–12). Of course, some authorities, such as Bruno Latour (2000), would not permit such reasoning, arguing that individuals cannot die of diseases before their characterization. Latour's example concerned the diagnosis of tuberculosis in the mummy of an Egyptian pharaoh, millennia before Koch's discovery of the tubercle bacillus in Berlin in 1882. To paraphrase Latour, *mutatis mutandi*, "*Treponema pallidum* have a local history that limits them to Berlin at the turn of the century. They may be allowed to spread to all the years that come *after* 1905 [date of the first microscopical identification of *T. pallidum* by Schaudinn and Hoffmann] … but … they cannot jump back to the years *before*." (italics in original). For counterarguments concerning retrospective diagnosis, see Larner (2025n).

dorsalis, as a disorder of sensori-motor function, than in GPI, possibly because those afflicted with the latter were more likely to find their way into the hands of alienists.[81]

Epilepsy

Aldridge observed that:

> Asylum wards present, perhaps, the best field for observations of this nature, for there a large number of epileptics are gathered together, and some of them are sure to have one or more fits in the course of every day. (I:81)

But, as Crichton-Browne affirmed, "Epilepsy is a generic term, and it includes many species and varieties" (III:166). The most serious of these, status epilepticus, when "consciousness was not fully recovered between the paroxysms" (III:171), was noted by Thompson to be "very common in lunatic hospitals" (II:303).

A number of papers in *WRLAMR*, nine in all,[82] were explicitly devoted to epilepsy or seizures or convulsions. Four of these were by Hughlings Jackson (for whom see Chap. 7) and focused mainly on theoretical issues related to localisation. Jackson's definition of epilepsy as "a sudden, occasional, excessive, and rapid discharge of grey matter of some part of the brain" was repeated by Wallis (V:269). Other papers related to investigation (see section "Sphygmography") and treatment (see section "Pharmacotherapies"), but two were clinical reports, one an extended case presentation (Patient EC, over the period from 26th September 1874 to 1st March 1876; VI:232–253),[83] the other a case series of 100 WRA patients with general paralysis (V:198–226).

In the latter paper, Newcombe confirmed the male preponderance of GPI (F:M = 1:4) and recorded seizures in 60 of the 100 patients. These seizures were classified as either "epileptiform", meaning "sudden attacks … characterised by a series of more or less severe involuntary muscular movements, with or without impairment or loss of consciousness"; or "apoplectiform", meaning "sudden impairment or loss of consciousness as occurs without convulsive phenomena" (V:199). The former preponderated (51/60). Newcombe

---

[81] Hare (1959).

[82] These were II:302–306 (Thompson: sphygmography); III:153–176 (Crichton-Browne: nitrite of amyl); III:175–195 (Jackson: convulsions); III:315–349 (Jackson: investigation); V:1–23 (Merson: diet); V:105–129 (Jackson: epileptic paroxysms); V:198–226 (Newcombe: seizures in general paralysis); VI:232–253 (Medical Officers: case of); VI:266–309 (Jackson: after effects).

[83] This paper was discussed by Finn (2012:89–90) as an example of the "methodology and practice" of the Asylum. Some clinical details of this patient also appeared in Bevan Lewis (1889:236).

attempted to compare his findings with those previously presented by Burman (no citation given, but presumably I:129–151) although these were based on observations made at the Devon Asylum. Both Hughlings Jackson and Ferrier's work in *WRLAMR* was also noted. The method of investigating the epilepsies advocated by Jackson was referenced (V:199, referring to III:175–195) and his explanation of seizure mechanism was included, amongst others: "Lastly, are we, with Dr. Hughlings Jackson, to consider epileptiform seizures as essentially dependent upon 'discharging lesions' of the cortical substance of certain convolutions of the cerebral hemispheres?" (V:208). Ferrier's experimental findings were also referred to: "Professor Ferrier's experiments upon rabbits and cats, in which he so successfully produced epilectic [*sic*] convulsions by applying electrodes connected with an induction apparatus to the surface of various parts of the hemispheres" were noted to contradict "the argument that the medulla is the sole seat of the lesion" (V:208) and indeed supported Jackson's views on "discharging lesions" in the hemispheres (V:212). Newcombe also observed a notable clinical phenomenon: "One of the most striking after-symptoms is the occurrence of unilateral paralysis, which follows in nearly every case of unilateral convulsion or of general convulsion more severe on one side than the other. Though the loss of power is in some cases so transient as to have passed away and left no trace in a very few hours' time, it may last for days or even weeks, and rarely, I might say very rarely, for months. In the latter cases the paralysis has all the character of that following extensive hemorrhagic [*sic*] apoplexy". Undoubtedly this is a description of the post-ictal paralysis described by Robert Bentley Todd in 1849 ("Todd's palsy") and later commented on by Jackson (VI:266–309).

Many other passing references to epileptic seizures or convulsions are to be found in *WRLAMR*. Treatment options mentioned for seizures included bromides, chloral hydrate, hyoscyamine, conia, and even chloroform.

Phthisis (Tuberculosis)

Many years after leaving Wakefield, Crichton-Browne reported that:

> When Medical Director of the West Riding Asylum I was struck by the number of patients received from the prison who laboured under a speedily developed phthisis, although it was, of course, impossible to say that it was of prison origin.[84]

---

[84] Crichton-Browne (1926:97). This observation prompted his request to Dyson Wood (or possibly Henry Clarke) for information on the effects of prison diet on body weight (see Chap. 5).

As one of the most prevalent clinical conditions of the nineteenth century, the relationship between phthisis (tuberculosis) and insanity was of interest to Crichton-Browne and his colleagues.

Clouston in Edinburgh had reported a higher rate of deaths due to tuberculosis in asylums compared to towns in Scotland, and also characterised a condition of "phthisical mania".[85] Nicol and Dove's examination of the data from WRA (I:233–251) did not support these conclusions: they found "a proportion of 15.6 deaths from phthisis to every 100 deaths in the asylum" (I:237) whereas "Over the whole kingdom, however, out of every one hundred deaths over five years of age, seventeen are ascribed to phthisis" (I:238). Their conclusion was that "It is not pretended that these arguments and facts prove that insanity does not depend on tubercle, any more than Dr. Clouston's facts and arguments can be said to prove that it does. This is a matter in which nothing is easier than to see that there is some causal connection, and nothing perhaps more difficult than to see what precisely is the order of the connection" (I:245). They also made the claim that "It is a fact, of which detailed proof might be offered, that with the careful regulation and improvement of the hygienic conditions in the Wakefield Asylum, a decided decrease of tubercle has been observed of late years" (I:249n).

Dementia and Mania

The term dementia was used somewhat generally at this time to denote any cognitive deficit, not only of senile or chronic origin but also "acute dementia".[86] The cause might be alcoholic, epileptic, infective (general paralysis of the insane, as dementia paralytica[87]), or traumatic. "Dementia" no doubt included conditions which might now be subsumed under the term psychosis (later characterised by Kraepelin as "dementia praecox"), characterised by hallucinations and delusions sufficient to compromise social and occupational functions,[88] as well as idiocy and imbecility, conditions which might now be termed mental deficiency or learning disability. Hence it is often difficult for

---

[85] Clouston (1863–1864).

[86] Both the papers in *WRLAMR* explicitly referring to dementia in their titles (IV:265–290; IV:291–304) specified "acute dementia". Andrews (2014) argued that it was only in the latter nineteenth century that "senile" became clearly defined as an association with dementia.

[87] Hare (1959).

[88] For example, Crichton-Browne (1920:218) stated that "I remember reporting the case of a young woman (S. W-) who had been a schoolmistress and who laboured under dementia praecox - or acute dementia as we then called it". I do not find this patient reported in Crichton-Browne's *WRLAMR* paper on acute dementia (IV:265–290).

today's clinician to know what to make of the patients reported in *WRLAMR* under the heading of dementia. Certainly, the nineteenth-century category did not inevitably carry the implication of progressive and irreversible deterioration, some patients no doubt suffering from depression, and possibly delirium. "Acute dementia" could also afflict children (IV:267–268).[89]

The term mania was generally used to denote episodes characterised by great motor excitement, sometimes with destructive behaviour to the self and/ or environment. If persistent, exhaustion and emaciation could ensue, in part because such patients could only be fed, and hence medicated, with difficulty. The treatment of mania "in use at the early part of the present [19th] century …, at the West Riding Asylum" was described by Pedler (II:147):

> The use of the sleeves (strait waistcoat) was almost universal in the management of the maniacal, whilst that method of treatment would seem in our time cruel and unjustifiable. Cold shower baths, general and local bleedings, of more or less severity were frequent, and the usual depletory remedies in general use for other diseases were used indiscriminately for mania of all kinds, under the general impression that insanity was the result of congestion or inflammation of the brain and its membranes.

Treatment options for mania explored during the Crichton-Browne era included bromides, cannabis, ergot, and conia, as well as removal to a padded room.

Pharmacology and Therapeutics

The mid-Victorian era saw the ascendancy of medical and moral treatment over psychological approaches in the management of asylum patients.[90] Neither psychotherapy nor hypnosis seems to have found any favour at WRA.[91] Indeed, from the outset Crichton-Browne was keen to explore pos-

---

[89] See, for example, data on admissions to St Lawrence's Hospital in Bodmin, Cornwall, between 1870 and 1875, where 32 patients were recorded as suffering a first attack of dementia under the age of 19 (Hill and Laugharne 2003).

[90] Clark (1981). Medical and physical treatments were commonly employed by Ellis at WRA and in other county asylums in the early nineteenth century (Smith 1999:194–207).

[91] The only reference to hypnotism and "Mr. Braid" that I find in *WRLAMR* is by Mitchell (II:91–92). Clark (1981:310n90) referred to the "comments of Dr Major" following a presentation by Hack Tuke "On the mental condition in hypnotism" to the Medico-Psychological Association in February 1883. Certainly "H.C. Major" was listed amongst those attending but I can find no comments from him in the published report, only by Wood and by Savage (*J Mental Sci* 1883–1884;29(April 1883):124–126). Hypnosis was used occasionally at Queen Square in the nineteenth century, for example by Charles Beevor, and indeed into the twentieth century by Charles Symonds (Shorvon and Compston 2019:111

sible medical treatments for insanity,[92] so it is not surprising that many of the papers in *WRLAMR* focus on this subject. For convenience, they are divided here into pharmacotherapies and physical therapies.

None of these studies was "controlled," rather than opportunistic, hence constituted therapeutic experiments rather than clinical trials. For example, Courtenay, examining the effect of opium on appetite, acknowledged that "the sceptic will say that all these results were *post hoc* and not *propter hoc*, but to him I can only answer that such results, even *post hoc*, are good" (II:263). However, an attempt at a crossover trial of different dietary regimens, farinaceous versus nitrogenous, in patients with epilepsy was attempted by Merson (V:1–23). Although George and Trimble have subsequently characterised this work as "based on older thinking",[93] Merson was in fact quite explicit that the direct stimulus to his study was the current thinking of Hughlings Jackson on the investigation of epilepsy, as detailed in one of his five *WRLAMR* papers (III:326–328). Of course, from our modern perspective the trial was subject to many observer and selection biases: small numbers (n = 24, 12 in each group), no randomisation, no blinding, brief trials (1 month on each diet, one group AB, second group BA), no wash-out period, subgroup analysis of those showing a "decided decrease" in the number of fits, etc.[94] Merson's conclusion that "the actual number of fits is less under a farinaceous dietary than under a nitrogenous" (V:22) cannot be considered robust.

Pharmacotherapies

Therapeutic experiments exploited a variety of medications available from the Asylum pharmacy, often for purposes other than those for which the medication was originally thought to be indicated ("repurposing" *avant le nom*!). Finn stated that 18 out of the 80 papers published in *WRLAMR* were directly concerned with tests and trials of the dispensary's supplies, on both patients and animals,[95] but gave no further breakdown. One presumes that many of these drugs, the *de facto* pharmacopoeia of WRA, appeared on the stalls dedicated to drugs and medicinal preparations at the annual medical *conversazione*

---

and n27). Ferrier and Hughlings Jackson had a patient with catalepsy hypnotised on several occasions at Queen Square between April and June 1881 (Riese and Gooddy 1955).

[92] Many potential treatments for "insanity" were available, see for example Anon (1874–1875).

[93] George and Trimble (1992:248).

[94] Merson's trial does not feature in an historical overview of methods to control selection bias in therapeutic experiments (Chalmers 2001). Adams (2010) considered Crichton-Browne's (1872a) work on conium as a (flawed) controlled evaluation of drug treatment.

[95] Finn (2012:112).

(Chap. 8). Some of these pharmacological agents, now briefly considered, had originally been used for purposes of anaesthesia.

Nitrous Oxide

Nitrous oxide (N_2O) was discovered by Joseph Priestley (1772) and investigated by Humphry Davy in the early nineteenth century. It had become a popular phenomenon as "exhilarating gas" or "laughing gas"[96] before its potential as an anaesthetic agent was realised.

At WRA, N_2O was researched by Samuel Mitchell (I:27–57 and II:73–96), not only in experimental animals (rabbits) but also, as per the example of Humphry Davy, in humans, not only himself but also friends and some melancholic patients. His conclusion was that N_2O did not modify their symptoms to any noticeable extent. Aldridge took advantage of Mitchell's studies to examine the effect of N_2O on the retinal circulation in two patients, finding dilatation of the arteries, similar to that he had observed with nitrite of amyl (I:98).

Ether

Known since the sixteenth century, and marketed as "sweet vitriol", ether (diethyl ether, $(CH_3CH_2)_2O$, or ethoxyethane) became established as an anaesthetic agent following William Morton's demonstration at the Massachusetts General Hospital in October 1846. It became quickly established in the United Kingdom.[97]

Ether was investigated at WRA by Samuel Mitchell (II:73–96), specifically in combination with nitrous oxide, his principal area of interest. The hope was that the slow onset of action but persistent effect of ether would complement the rapid onset of action yet brief effect of nitrous oxide. For want of anyone undergoing a surgical operation, Mitchell could only experiment on

---

[96] For example, "laughing gas" was known to Charles Dickens who mentioned it in *The Chimes* (1844; Second Quarter): "the grin upon his withered face expanding … as if he were inhaling laughing gas". For its possible use for the purposes of entertainment at the first (1871) WRA medical *conversazione*, see Chap. 8.

[97] Traditionally the earliest use of ether anaesthesia in the United Kingdom has been ascribed to Robert Liston at University College London in December 1846, but there are other candidates, such as Scott and Fraser in Dumfries, and Archer and Yankiewicz in Liverpool (Larner 2025p:204–205).

himself and some of his colleagues (II:77–79).[98] In Ferrier's animal experiments, either "ether or chloroform was administered" (III:35).

Chloroform; Chloral Hydrate

Chloroform ($CHCl_3$) was first synthesized in 1831,[99] and was in clinical use from 1847 following the self-experiments of James Young Simpson in Edinburgh.[100] It was applied in various clinical situations, not only anaesthesia. At WRA, Mitchell briefly explored its experimental use in combination with nitrous oxide (II:76, 79). Burman (III:62) mentioned use of chloroform for a patient with seizures. It appears to have been prescribed to a patient with melancholia (II:276). Wallis (V:259, 264, 266) also described its occasional use in epilepsy, noting that the effect of the inhalation was transient, seizures recurring after treatment was discontinued.

In Ferrier's animal experiments "ether or chloroform was administered" (III:35) and Benham noted that "The following further experiments were performed on the living animal, every care being taken to keep the animal well under the influence of chloroform during the whole operation" (IV:158). It was also used in his studies of nicotine (IV:308), likewise by Lawson (V:73) and by Arbuckle (V:132) in their experimental animal work.[101]

Chloral hydrate (CCl_3CHO), a compound related to chloroform, found various uses at WRA. Crichton-Browne reported that "experiments with chloral were commenced in this asylum, in February 1870" in his publication on its inconveniences and dangers which appeared in the *Lancet* in April 1871.[102] The following year, Burman, mentioning "similar cases already described by Dr Crichton Browne", reported two cases with chloral hydrate-associated rash from his time at the Devon County Lunatic Asylum, where he thought the treatment had been first tried in around 1869, and where he had observed the physiological effects of the drug on himself.[103] Reporting two cases of weakness affecting particularly the lower limbs in association with chloral hydrate treatment, Manning cited Crichton-Browne's experience with

---

[98] Crichton-Browne amputated the leg of a patient, Stephen Pickles, who was "sinking rapidly under caries of the bones of the ankle", on 11th January 1873, but his account in the Medical Director's Journal (as cited by Bolton 1928:610) gave no details regarding anaesthesia.

[99] Stratmann (2003).

[100] McCrae (2010).

[101] Stratmann (2003) does not mention use of chloroform in experimental physiology.

[102] Crichton Browne (1871c) (quote at 440).

[103] Burman (1872a).

the drug, namely of erythema in 19 out of 40 cases treated up to June 1870 and in one fatal case the patient staggered as if intoxicated.[104]

Only one *WRLAMR* paper was specifically devoted to chloral hydrate, Wallis's "On the therapeutic value of chloral hydrate in epileptic convulsions" (V:257–270), in which he quoted Crichton-Browne's opinion that "A river of chloral has flowed through the land, and all diseases have been indiscriminately immersed in it" (V:257).[105] Other examples of its use may be found in the pages of the journal. Aldridge examined the effect of chloral hydrate on the retinal circulation in epileptics (I:98–99) and Sutherland noted in passing a patient taken ill after a dose (I:225). Pedler reported it to be "a most valuable remedy" in puerperal mania (II:149), as had also been noted elsewhere by Madden.[106] Milner Fothergill noted that "chloral acts pronouncedly upon the vascular system, lowering the heart's action and lessening blood pressure very markedly" and included it, amongst others, as a "neurotic which diminishes cerebral activity" (V:184). It seems to have been the principal, but certainly not the only, medication given to patient EC during the long course of her seizure disorder (VI:232–253).[107] As evidenced by Wallis's account, the drug could be given *per rectum* and repeatedly if necessary.

Crichton-Browne later published experimental studies examining chloral hydrate.[108] Both Milner Fothergill and Lauder Brunton were involved in a discussion about the treatment of cholera by subcutaneous injection of chloral hydrate held at the Royal Medical and Chirurgical Society in October 1874.[109]

By 1876, Lawson opined that "In the actual practice of this Asylum, chloral has been found to be so free from disadvantages (and it has been used here to an extent and in such doses as has perhaps not been equalled in any other public institution) that it demands priority over all other drugs in the treatment of the status" (VI:67). Describing the treatment of a further patient with epileptiform seizures, Lawson and Bevan-Lewis (VI:131–132) stated that "chloral hydrate is perhaps the most useful medicine which has ever been employed in asylum practice. The benefits resulting from its use are so clearly

---

[104] Manning (1873:696). Data from Crichton Browne (1871c:440).

[105] Original in Crichton Browne (1871c:440).

[106] Madden (1871:485–486).

[107] Hughlings Jackson's patient "Z", known to posterity as "Dr. Z", in fact Dr Arthur Thomas Myers (1851–1894), was said to have died from an overdose of chloral hydrate (Jackson and Colman 1898). For Z/Dr. Z/Myers, and his distinction from Quaerens, another pseudonymous patient with epilepsy under Jackson's care, see Larner (2025q).

[108] Crichton Browne (1875a).

[109] *BMJ* 1874;2:569–570 (31st October).

and quickly perceptible, and the dangers resulting from the employment of a good preparation of it are so few, that it constitutes a most valuable item in the alienist's pharmacopoeia".[110]

Morphia, Opium

> morphia, the accursed drug with which these dark men [asylum keepers] in these dark places [private asylums] coax the reason away out of the head by degrees, or with a potent dose stupify [*sic*] the victim, then act surprise, alarm; and make his stupor the ground for applying medical treatment to the doomed wretch.[111]

Such was the popular reputation of morphia in the 1860s, despite which opiates found applications beyond simply analgesia in WRA practice. Many of the cases of "insanity" treated with hypodermic injections of morphia by Bywater Ward (I:152–163) had mania (chronic, puerperal) although most, if not all, of these patients were treated in Warwick Asylum rather than WRA.[112] Nevertheless, Pedler noted the use of morphia for puerperal mania at WRA (II:149). Some of Bywater Ward's patients had melancholia rather than mania. In his *WRLAMR* paper, Courtenay (II:254–277) reported on 91 melancholic patients, of whom 49 were treated with opium in the 15 months between 1st January 1871 and 25th March 1872, hence most cases predated his arrival at WRA. His conclusion was that opium in small doses ("Fifteen minims of the Tincture combined with an equal amount of Sulphuric Ether"; II:259) acted as a tonic by inducing hyperaemia to counteract the anaemic state of the brain which occurred in melancholia. In this context, Milner Fothergill noted opium amongst those medications described as a "neurotic which diminishes cerebral activity" (V:184).

---

[110] Some years later, Ernest Birt, a later AMO at WRA, reported that "It is a noteworthy fact that, in this Asylum, during the past seven years the only cases in which chloral has failed to arrest convulsions … have been those in which the patient had not been taking a bromide, continuously, for a long period" (Birt 1886–1887:372n1). Chloral hydrate is still available, as "Welldorm".

[111] From Charles Reade's *Hard Cash* (1863, chapter XLI).

[112] Hypodermic injection of morphia was also described in *BMJ* 1867;2:369; *J Ment Sci* 1878–1879;24(January 1879):623–626.

Ergot of Rye, Ergotine

Following Crichton-Browne's publication on the subject of ergot of rye in the treatment of mental diseases,[113] Churchill Fox (I:261–265) described six cases of "excitement", probably mania, of epileptic origin in two cases, in which symptoms had been ameliorated by ergot. He noted that "the liquid extract of ergot has now almost superseded the tincture in the practice of the West Riding Asylum" (I:261). He also reported that he had "seen it secure rapid recovery from that singular and obscure condition, the status epilepticus" (I:264). Crichton-Browne reported that in status epilepticus "Ergot or ergotine injections are not trustworthy" (III:167) but nevertheless ergotine injections were sometimes employed in this dire clinical situation (III:171, 172).

During its use in maniacal attacks, Aldridge was able to examine the effect of ergot of rye on the retinal circulation in patients (I:94–95) and noted that it caused "contraction of the minute arteries of the retina". He also noted that he had "seen aged patients take the drug for several weeks, with benefit to mental symptoms and no inconvenience to the general system" (II:230). The effects of subcutaneous injection of Ergotine proved identical to those of the liquid extract of ergot (II:243–244).[114]

Conia, Conium

Conia, the active principle of *Conium maculatum* (hemlock or poison hemlock), hence designated as a vegetable neurotic, was investigated by Crichton-Browne,[115] and also by Burman who showed that "when neutralised with Acetic Acid and dissolved in spirit and water, Conia, as a hypodermic [subcutaneous] injection, acts both quickly and in a powerful manner, ... with good effect in subduing the motor excitement in cases of mania" (II:4) although with less effect on the mental faculties.

Burman documented both animal and human experimental studies, including himself, as well as clinical usage.[116] Indeed, his starting point was Crichton-Browne's earlier publication on the use of conium in acute mania

---

[113] Crichton Browne (1871e).

[114] Ergotine acts as an agonist at some subtypes of serotonin receptor.

[115] Crichton Browne (1872a).

[116] The pharmacology was, of course, unknown at this time. Amongst the volatile alkaloids found in hemlock, one, coniine, has a structure similar to nicotine (Burman noted that one preparation had "a strong peculiar odour, resembling ... in my opinion, that of the pale and acrid nicotic juice which accumulates in the stem of an old pipe" (II:6)). Coniine binds to nicotinic acetylcholine receptors producing inhibitory effects in the CNS which can lead to respiratory collapse and death, hence the use of hemlock

which gave details of 12 cases admitted after 25th February 1871. Pedler later reported use of conia in puerperal mania to be of great advantage (II:149).

The latter part of Burman's paper addressed the combination of conia and morphia for the treatment of acute mania, as did a later paper.[117]

Nitrite of Amyl

Lauder Brunton (see Chap. 7) had reported the utility of nitrite of amyl in attacks of angina pectoris in 1867.[118]

In what we might now term "re-purposing", nitrite of amyl was investigated for different indications in patients at WRA. Its possible use in epilepsy was described by Crichton-Browne (III:153–174), who also described it causing yawning on inhalation in unconscious patients (reportedly also observed by Major).[119] This usage in epilepsy was prompted not because of an understanding of drug pharmacology but more probably because of the paucity of successful therapeutic agents then available. Crichton-Browne's rationale for its use in epilepsy hinged on the presumption that loss of consciousness was caused by "cerebral anaemia" as a "consequence of spasmodic contraction of the intra-cranial vessels", and that "the nitrite of amyl indisputably prevents contraction of vessels and cerebral anaemia during its inhalation" (III:158–159).

Aldridge's most particular examination of the effects of drugs used in the treatment of epilepsy on the retinal circulation was that involving nitrite of amyl, which produced increase in the size of the arteries (I:95–98). Its effects on the retinal circulation were also observed in experimental animals by Arbuckle (V:130–148). Later Clapham also tried it for the treatment of sea-sickness.[120]

---

for the purpose of execution, e,g, of Socrates. Motor weakness, sometimes to the point of paralysis, is also a symptom.

[117] Burman (1872b).

[118] Lauder Brunton (1867).

[119] Crichton Browne (1874b).

[120] Clapham (1875). Travelling by sea to Uppsala in August 1877, Crichton-Browne gave nitrite of amyl to a lady in a "state of complete collapse" whose husband reported that she had been "incessantly sick since we left Hull, and I fear she is dying", even though he had "never myself used it or seen it used in such a case". The effect was reported to be miraculous (Crichton-Browne 1926:166–168). I wonder if Crichton-Browne had seen or was aware of Clapham's paper.

Hyoscyamine, Hyoscine, Belladonna

Plants of the Solanaceae family such as deadly nightshade (*Atropa belladonna*) and henbane (*Hyoscyamus niger*) are sources of the crude drug belladonna from which alkaloids such as hyoscyamine, hyoscine (also known as scopolamine) and atropine may be derived. These compounds may have both sedative and stimulant effects, generally drying up physiological secretions, speeding the heart rate, and lowering blood pressure.[121]

Aldridge examined the effect of belladonna (II:235–236) and hyoscyamine (II:236) on the retinal circulation, finding both to cause hyperaemia. Pedler found hyoscyamine to be of little value in puerperal mania (II:149). Belladonna was tried by Courtenay for melancholia without evident effect (II:271) but, according to Milner Fothergill, "Belladonna, Dr. Crichton Browne tells me, is only useful in the early stages of emotional melancholia, where it is eminently beneficial" (IV:148). The effects of hyoscyamine on experimental animals (V:40–84) and in therapeutics (VI:65–84) were researched extensively by Robert Lawson.[122] He found it to be hypnotic, diuretic, mydriatic, drying up oral/salivary secretions, with a biphasic effect on heart rate (initially slowing, then increasing). His clinical experience encouraged him to use the drug in various forms of mania and excitement.[123]

Physostigma

Derived from the Calabar bean (*Physostigma venenosum*), physostigmine was discovered by Robert Christison (1797–1882) in Edinburgh in 1846 and its medical applications were suggested by Thomas Richard Fraser (1841–1920) in a thesis which won the Edinburgh gold medal in 1862.[124] Physostigmine

---

[121] The pharmacology was, of course, unknown at this time. Hyoscyamine is the levorotary isomer of atropine, an antagonist of muscarinic acetylcholine receptors, hence an anticholinergic.

[122] Also Lawson (1876b).

[123] Lawson's work on hyoscyamine as described in *WRLAMR* was still a topic for discussion in March 1879 when at the MPA meeting in London George Savage presented on "Hyoscyamine, and its uses". Crichton-Browne, President, was in the chair and Sutherland and Clapham were among those participating in the discussion; Lawson does not appear to have been present (*J Ment Sci* 1879–1880;25(July 1879):300–303).

[124] According to Crichton-Browne (1937:32), Thomas Fraser "elucidated the mystery of the Calabar Bean". Fraser was later a co-author on two papers with Ferrier and Lauder Brunton in the *Journal of Anatomy and Physiology* (Fraser et al. 1871; Rutherford et al. 1872). In the first of these, Fraser's "Report" (389–396), which discussed nitrous oxide, chloral, chloroform, ether, nitrite of amyl, and atropia amongst other drugs, was separate from Brunton and Ferrier's Report (396–411); and likewise in the second (Fraser's report 490–502; Brunton and Ferrier's report 472–490). Hence these subsections appear to have been written independently.

promotes secretions, constricts the pupil, and slows the heart rate. Milner Fothergill classified Calabar bean as one of the "vegetable vascular depressants" (V:178) and recognised it as "the physiological antagonist of belladonna" (V:186).[125]

Thompson (I:67) noted Fraser's work on Calabar bean and that "This drug has been used extensively by Dr. Crichton Browne, in the treatment of general paralysis in this asylum, and has been recommended by him as a valuable means of exercising a favourable influence on the course of the disease". Furthermore, "I do not exaggerate when I say that in every case very marked improvement has followed the use of the drug" (I:70). The subsequent spat between Thompson and Crichton-Browne about the value of Calabar bean in general paralysis has already been noted (Chap. 5).[126]

Mitchell also referred to Fraser's work on the Calabar bean (II:82).

Merson reiterated Crichton-Browne's recommendation of Calabar bean in general paralysis (IV:91) and Fothergill (IV:111) noted that "Conditions of cerebral anaemia are now deliberately induced by the use of agents which depress and slow the heart's action, as for instance the Calabar bean, in states of cerebral hypervascularity; and for this purpose Dr. Crichton Browne has used the physostigma to control the wild outbreaks of general paralysis".[127]

Nicotine

Benham (IV:306–317) found, contrary to previous researchers, that nicotine caused cessation of respiratory effort in experimental animals long before cardiac pulsations ceased, its cardiac action thus contrasting with that of the Calabar bean as reported by Thomas Fraser, although both had the same effect on the pupil (constriction; IV:313–315).[128]

---

[125] The pharmacological action of physostigmine, not known at this time, is due to reversible acetylcholinesterase inhibition which indirectly stimulates nicotinic and muscarinic acetylcholine receptors, hence it is a cholinomimetic, with effects opposite to the anticholinergic actions of atropine-type compounds such as hyoscyamine.

[126] Documented in Thompson (1874–1875b) and Crichton Browne (1875–1876a).

[127] See also Fothergill (1874:78). In 1934, physostigmine by injection was demonstrated to be the first effective treatment for myasthenia gravis by Mary Broadfoot Walker (1888–1974), a native of Wigtown in Dumfries and Galloway (Larner 2025p:206).

[128] The pharmacology of nicotine extends beyond agonism at nicotinic acetylcholine receptors to promoting the release of many CNS neurotransmitters, such that low doses have stimulating effects, such as tachycardia, which are reversed at higher doses.

Bromides

Bromides, the first partially effective medication for epilepsy, came into general use in the early 1860s,[129] in part based on the comments of Sir Charles Locock, a gynaecologist, made in 1857, and the studies of the physician Samuel Wilks.[130] Their use in asylum practice had also been reported, not least by Crichton-Browne,[131] who described bromide of potassium as "the head and front of all systems of treatment of epilepsy in recent years" although he found it "worse than useless during the status" (III:167).

At WRA, bromides found various uses, not only in patients with seizures. For example, Pedler found it one of the most valuable remedies in puerperal mania (II:149–150) since it "seems to have great power in controlling the lewd discourse and errotic [*sic*] desires of the puerperal maniac".[132] Courtenay found it to be without effect in melancholia (II:271). Adverse effects were also noted: for example, Milner Fothergill stated that "A condition of cerebral anaemia with its consequences, psychical and physical, is not uncommonly produced by the administration of remedial agents, especially by the large doses of bromide of potassium now in vogue" (IV:111). Elsewhere he described it as a "neurotic which diminishes cerebral activity" (V:184).[133]

Cannabis

Cannabis indica seems to have been used on an occasional basis at WRA for the treatment of mania (e.g. I:264, II:21). Lauder Brunton noted that "cannabis indica … calms excitement, but when taken in large doses by a healthy man seems to completely destroy all inhibitory power, the person having all sorts of ideas running through the brain without the power to direct them, and performing all sorts of antics without being able to stop, although perfectly aware of the foolish nature of his actions" (IV:221).[134]

---

[129] Crichton-Browne (1878–1879:365) spoke of "the years subsequent to 1862—in those years, in fact, in which the bromide of potassium came into general use".

[130] Eadie (2012). Wilks was later (1887) President of the Neurological Society of London.

[131] Crichton Browne (1865). Also by Clouston (1868–1869), Kesteven (1869–1870). See also Wallis (V:259).

[132] Churchill Fox (I:264) also mentioned its use in a patient with chronic mania, along with cannabis indica, but "ultimately it lost its effect".

[133] The pharmacological mechanism of action of bromides may be related to movement of the ion through neuronal chloride channels facilitating increased gamma-aminobutyric acid (GABA) inhibition through cell membrane hyperpolarization.

[134] Could this be a report of self-experimentation?

Strychnia

Milner Fothergill (VI:264) noted that "In most cases of convalescence after asthenia strychnia will be found a useful adjunct to the other medicinal agents" but little evidence for its use at WRA is to be found elsewhere in *WRLAMR*. Mitchell reported that "Strychnia acts by destroying the power of the tissues and fluids, to absorb oxygen and exhale carbonic acid" (II:83) whilst Milner Fothergill thought that "Strychnine and belladonna have a similar general action, while they dilate the blood-vessels of the cerebro-spinal system; belladonna selecting the meso-cephalic vessels, while the action of strychnine falls rather on the spinal blood-vessels" (IV:147).[135] Bevan-Lewis examined its effect on the generation of animal heat (VI:53–55).

Physical Therapies

Some of the approaches described here may now seem odd, even bizarre, but it should be remembered that in the contemporary context the idea of "counter-irritation" appeared highly plausible.[136] Indeed, Crichton-Browne himself had applied the method, according to his contribution to a discussion on general paralysis of the insane at a meeting of the MPA held in January 1871:

> Guided by some successful experiments in the treatment of acute hydro-cephalus carried out, if he remembered correctly, in the Children's Hospital in Edinburgh, he had two years ago applied counter-irritation by means of croton-oil, liniment or tartar emetic ointment, to the shaven scalps of four patients in whom the symptoms of general paralysis, bodily and mental, were well pronounced; small doses of biniodide of mercury, and iodide of potassium being at the same time administered. The results obtained in these four cases, although the counter irritation was only maintained for a short time—about a month—were assuredly such as to encourage further experiment in the same direction. Of the four patients thus treated, three were still alive, while all the other inmates of the asylum, noted as having been at exactly the same stage of the disease at the same time, had died long ago. The one man treated by counter-irritation who had died, displayed a singular improvement in intelligence after being thus treated. … In the other three men submitted to counter-irritation the rancour and speed of the disease have been remarkably moderated.[137]

---

[135] Pharmacologically strychnia is an antagonist of glycine and acetylcholine receptors.

[136] Counter-irritation and ice bags were used at Queen Square in the nineteenth century: Shorvon and Compston (2019:111).

[137] *J Ment Sci* 1871–1872;17(April 1871):148–149.

Baths

Balneotherapy featured occasionally in the treatment regime; as noted (Chap. 3), Turkish baths were erected at WRA in 1871, and their use was mentioned (I:259). For example, "free use of the warm bath, whereby the whole secretory system is stimulated, and the blood becomes of normal constitution" was described by Pedler for puerperal mania (II:143; also II:148).

The "surprise bath" does not seem to have been used at WRA. Pedler described it thus: "This consisted of a perfectly dark room, with a trap in the floor. The patient being turned loose into this chamber wandered about excitedly until the floor suddenly seemed to give way under his feet, and he was immediately in cold water up to his arm-pits. The attendants, waiting at the door, were ready, as soon as this happened, to come to the assistance and rescue of the terrified patient. The recoveries under this system of treatment must have been few and the deaths numerous" (II:147).

Nevertheless, a cold shower or bath was advocated by Crichton-Browne in patients with "acute dementia":

Cold, which is so hazardous to acute dements when they are for any length of time exposed to it, may conduce to their recovery when it is properly employed. Suddenly and momentarily applied to the skin it is an effectual tonic to the vessels, and thus the shower or plunge bath, or free sponging with cold salt water, may shorten the duration of the disease which we have been considering. I give a decided preference to the shower-bath, as the best method of applying cold in this disease. It administers a healthy mental as well as a cutaneous shock, and is sometimes a powerful emmenogogue [stimulant of menstrual flow], and I am sure I have seen patients roused promptly out of their lethargy by a short series of shower-baths. As a tonic a shower-bath should not exceed ten seconds in duration, and should be followed by brisk friction." (IV:288)

Cooling, Ice

Cooling of the head was used on occasion,[138] sometimes in the form of an ice cap. However, Benham's cadaveric experiments found this produced absolutely no change in brain temperature (IV:152–178) and Crichton-Browne

---

[138] In the eighteenth century, John Wesley (1703–1791), the founder of Methodism, had prescribed for the treatment of "Raging Madness" either "cloths dipt in *cold water*" or to "set the patient with his head under a great *water-fall*, as long as his strength will bear: or, pour water on his head out of a tea-kettle" (1960:19, 87), [spelling and italics as in original]. (I thank Dr. Mari Huws-Edwards for bringing this book to my attention, October 2023.)

thought it had no beneficial effect in acute maniacal attacks (IV:176), although Milner Fothergill was of the opinion that "The application of cold to the head will also be found useful in most cases" of cerebral hyperaemia (V:185).[139] In status epilepticus, Crichton-Browne noted "ice to the spine, although very valuable, cannot be pronounced curative" but that "ice to the neck and spine sometimes does unmistakable good" (III:167, 170); presumably this was considered to be a stimulant.

Sinapism

Sinapisms, or mustard plasters, were applied to the legs and feet in some cases of status epilepticus (III:170, 171), presumably as a stimulant to rouse the patient. Burman suggested their use in cases of overdosing with conia, applied to the sides of the chest to stimulate respiratory movements (II:35).

Electrotherapy

The application of electricity as galvanism or faradism was a common approach to the diagnosis and treatment of neurological disease in the latter part of the nineteenth century.[140] Indeed, the possible use of electricity in the treatment of "lunacy" dated to the eighteenth century.[141] Hence Allbutt's suggestion of "electric treatment of the insane" based on his knowledge of the subject of electrotherapy[142] was not surprising, prompting the study reported in *WRLAMR* (II:203–222).[143] Lowe examined the electro-muscular contractility

---

[139] Another nineteenth-century example of treatment of presumed psychiatric disease with the application of icepacks to the head may be found in Hacking (1998:140). It may also be noted here that cooling improves transmission at the neuromuscular junction, hence its use, in the form of the "ice pack test", in patients with suspected myasthenia gravis, a disorder of neuromuscular transmission; improvement in ptosis in this situation has both high sensitivity and specificity for a diagnosis of myasthenia gravis (Larner 2004).

[140] Shorvon and Compston (2019:123–126), discussed the use of electrical therapy at the National Hospital in the nineteenth century. Armand de Watteville, later editor of *Brain*, was physician to the electrotherapeutic department at St. Mary's Hospital, London, and in 1878 published *A Practical Introduction to Medical Electricity* (Larner and Triarhou 2025b).

[141] John Wesley (1960:87) had listed "*electrify*" amongst his suggested treatments for lunacy; he also stated that "I am firmly persuaded, there is no remedy in nature, for nervous disorders of every kind, comparable to the proper and constant use of the *electrical machine*" (Wesley 1960:91) [italics in original]. (I thank Dr. Mari Huws-Edwards for bringing this book to my attention, October 2023.)

[142] Allbutt (1871b).

[143] Todd and Ashworth (1991:394) later credited this study as prefiguring the work of Cerletti which eventually led to the development of electroconvulsive therapy (ECT), but Allbutt's "electrotherapy" was not inducing epileptic seizures, hence its omission from the history of "shock therapy" by Shorter and

to faradisation in several conditions, finding impairment or absence in patients with general paralysis, locomotor ataxy "in which the power of locomotion was affected to such an extent as to prevent the patient walking without assistance", and in progressive muscular atrophy (III:196–215).

Diet; Feeding

Regimen had been a feature of medical advice since antiquity and remained so in the nineteenth century. For example, Herbert Major was of the opinion that "taking the nerve cells for example, we know that the great cause of their disease and destruction is a deficient or vitiated nutritive supply" (IV:224), although only one paper in *WRLAMR* was devoted expressly to diet, namely that of John Merson (V:1–23), specifically in patients with epilepsy.[144] Mayhew recommended for acute delirious melancholia "Animal broths, jellies, milk, and farinaceous liquids, frequently in small quantities" (I:260).

Food refusal by patients at the Asylum was no small problem, often resulting from melancholic inertia or delusions of poisoning,[145] hence the topicality of Lawrence's paper on the subject in *WRLAMR* (I:209–217). Various feeding methods were described therein, including persuasion, spoon or feeding-jug, and catheter, but evidently the most frequently used method at WRA was the stomach pump. The favoured position for the patient was supine upon a bed, rather than upright, apparently without any incidence of choking. Rather than using the standard wooden gag, "In the West Riding Asylum the mouth is always opened by one of the screw keys … In this way the greatest freedom is afforded in passing the oesophageal tube, and the finger may be inserted to give the tube the necessary inclination, and guide it over the root of the tongue into the oesophagus, should there be any difficulty in passing it" (I:215). As for the specific treatment, "The most convenient articles for administration with the stomach pump are a pint of new milk with a flipped egg, and a glass

---

Healy (2007) is entirely understandable. Strangely, this paper by Allbutt was not referenced by Rolleston (1929) in his biography, perhaps because of Allbutt's implication that the work was actually done by others. It was mentioned in the history of electricity in the treatment of mental illness in the nineteenth century by Beveridge and Renvoize (1988:159).

[144] This study by Merson was referenced by Bevan-Lewis (1889:220) as "based upon too limited a number of instances, to warrant final acceptance". It was also recalled many years later by Crichton-Browne (1895:75, 1927:41) in a lecture on dreamy states.

[145] Selected cases requiring artificial feeding reported in *WRLAMR*: WM (I:180); MC (II:105); AE (II:269); AB (II:271); patient with "acute dementia" (VI:147–148); EC (VI:238). Nicol and Dove (I:246) noted that "those who are depressed, refuse their food, either habitually or now and again. If artificial feeding is resorted to, the effects can hardly be expected to be the same as when the nutriment is naturally ingested". See also Crichton-Browne (1926:95).

of sherry in it; or an equal quantity of beef tea, thickened with arrow-root; but the diet as well as the medicine which it is proper to give must vary with the nature of the case, and at the discretion of the medical officer" (I:216–217). Incidentally, beef-tea seems frequently to have been resorted to (e.g. I:255, 257; II:26, 140, 180; IV:35, 287; V:264, 266, 270; VI:209, 213, 238) as an item of extra diet for strengthening the patient, sometimes as an enema.

It is evident from comments made elsewhere in *WRLAMR* that other WRA clinicians also used this method of artificial feeding, for example Aldridge reported that in patients with acute dementia "we require to feed the patient by means of that most valuable instrument, the much maligned stomach-pump" (IV:294; also IV:295), and Pedler reported that the treatment of patients suffering from puerperal mania "is altogether incomplete unless great care is taken that they have sufficient food. Should it be refused, it must be administered in liquid form by the stomach tube" (II:150). Patient EC required to be "fed by the oesophageal tube" (VI:238). The subject of "forcible feeding" was also later addressed by Henry Sutherland (see Chap. 5) based on his experience at WRA.[146]

Alcohol

Contrary to the situation reported in 1766, it seems unlikely that Wakefield in 1866 suffered from the strange want of ale-houses wanting customers.[147] Certainly, some contributors to *WRLAMR* felt it had therapeutic value, for instance Mayhew recommended "Wine and other stimulants" for acute delirious melancholia, acting by "tranquillising the agitated nervous centre, at the same time that they sustained strength and vigour" (I:259). "Wine and brandy" were given in many cases of puerperal mania (II:156). Brandy was frequently mentioned as a treatment (e.g. I:73, 123, 183, 255, 257; III:172; IV:33, 35; V:264, 266, 270; VI:71, 213, 234, 238, 244). Aldridge observed the effects of alcohol on ophthalmoscopic appearances (II:230–231). Milner Fothergill thought that for instances of cerebral hyperaemia "Alcohol with opium at bedtime, rest in bed, nutritive food, &c, are the measures which contain the most promise in these cases" (V:183).

---

[146] Sutherland (1872). He also published on artificial feeding of the insane (Sutherland 1875a) and, many years later, on prognosis in cases of food refusal (Sutherland 1883–1884), as well as the entry in Tuke's *Dictionary of Psychological Medicine* (Sutherland 1892).

[147] Coote (1986:40). This, to my reading, is the only direct reference to Wakefield in Oliver Goldsmith's 1766 novel *The Vicar of Wakefield*. I suspect that Goldsmith had little, if any, personal knowledge of Wakefield.

Others were against alcohol. Major believed that alcohol excess played a large part in the causation of insanity[148] and eventually discontinued beer at WRA, as did John Merson when superintendent at Hull (see Chap. 5), although he had administered it to patients in his studies of "urinology" at WRA (IV:78–80, 83, 92).

Pathological Anatomy

As discussed in Chap. 4, almost from the outset of his superintendency Crichton-Browne was keen to appoint a "competent pathologist … to secure complete and reliable post mortem examinations",[149] no doubt with a view to explore the pathological anatomy of insanity in general, and probably general paralysis in particular. The first appointee, McDowall, published no pathological material from WRA, either in *WRLAMR* or elsewhere, but the pathological tradition at WRA once established, principally by Major, far outlasted Crichton-Browne's superintendency, being carried on by both his successors, Major and Bevan-Lewis, and others.[150]

Pathological work was both macroscopic and microscopic. The former category included gross observation, as in Sutherland's report on arachnoid cysts (I:218–232) and Crichton-Browne's on general paralysis of the insane (VI:170–231). The latter category featured some measurements of brain weight in the insane, as also performed by Crochley Clapham (III:285–298 and VI:11–26), who also made measurements of the cranial outline with Henry Clarke (VI:150–69).

However, it was the microscopical work, especially by Major and Bevan-Lewis, that was of particular note. These studies examined the histology of the brain in humans (Major: III:97–112; IV:223–239; VI:1–10) and animals (dog, horse, cat; Major: V:160–170), and of human peripheral (sciatic) nerve (Bevan-Lewis: V:85–104). Sankey (V:188–197) published on histological methods for human brain tissue, but it is doubtful whether this work took place at WRA. In addition to the microscopic work, Major used his tephrylometer to examine the thickness of grey matter in four brains, from patients dying of various causes, a total of 220 measurements for each brain (II:157–176).

---

[148] *Medical Press and Circular* 1878;25:530 (26th June; The West Riding Pauper Lunatic Asylum).

[149] *BMJ* 1867;2:186–187 (31st August; Lunatic Asylum reports).

[150] See Wallis (2017a). Also Larner 2026d.

Experimental Laboratory Work on Animals

Experimental animal work, vivisection, is the sphere in which *WRLAMR* is most likely to be remembered, principally as a consequence of the work of David Ferrier in the dedicated laboratory at WRA in 1873, the facilities of which had been offered to him by Crichton-Browne. Whilst Ferrier was perhaps the chief beneficiary of these facilities, a reading of *WRLAMR* indicates that he was certainly not alone in pursuing experimental work with animals. There appears to have been some, brief collaborative work with Crichton-Browne, a "rabbit rendered artificially epileptic by Professor Ferrier" being treated with nitrite of amyl. Crichton-Browne later repeated the experiment himself (III:162–163) and his further experimental researches also involved rabbits, dogs, guinea pigs, and cats.[151]

Animal experimentation was described in *WRLAMR* papers by several different authors: by Mitchell using rabbits (I:34–38 and II:73–77); Burman (II:1–40) using cats, dogs, rabbits, pigeons, frogs, guinea-pigs, and a sheep; by Aldridge (II:238–242, 244) using cats and rats; by Lawson (IV:40–84) using cats, rabbits, dogs, pigeons, and guinea-pigs; by Benham (IV:152–78 and IV:305–317) using dogs, rabbits, pigeons, frogs and guinea pigs; by Lauder Brunton (IV:198–199) using kittens; and by both Arbuckle (V:130–148) and Bevan-Lewis (VI:43–64) using rabbits.

Burman reported "great difficulty in getting dogs" whereas "a good supply of [rabbits] one can always procure" (II:10), perhaps as a consequence of the relatively rural location of the Asylum, whilst Aldridge bemoaned the fact that "some large rats were the only animals I could obtain" (II:241). Nowhere do mice appear as experimental subjects, nor monkeys. Ferrier's cerebral localisation studies on monkeys, although commenced in 1873 and mentioned in a footnote in his first *WRLAMR* paper (III:89n2), were undertaken in London with funding obtained from the Royal Society.[152] Nevertheless, non-human primates, or at least their brain tissues, were available at the WRA laboratory since Herbert Major's 1875 thesis, *Histology of the brain in apes*, was based on work done at Wakefield (NB Major used the term "apes" in a manner different from current usage).[153] Experimental animal work undertaken in the

---

[151] Crichton Browne 1875a.

[152] *Lancet* 1873;2:788.

[153] Monkey brain was also amongst the pathological specimens displayed at the 1872 WRA medical *conversazione* according to the printed programme, WYAS C85/1382, "West Riding Asylum, Wakefield. Medical Conversazione, 15th October, 1872". Also in 1875 (see Fig. 8.2).

WRA laboratory was also published elsewhere than in *WRLAMR*, for example Crichton-Browne's experimental investigations appeared in the *BMJ*.[154]

The details of the experimental animal work reported in *WRLAMR* can sometimes make for harrowing reading and are reflective of contemporary practices which inadvertently served to provoke and energise the members of the growing anti-vivisection movement. Ferrier's work in particular served to shape the thinking of the anti-vivisectionists,[155] which culminated in a Royal Commission on Vivisection in 1875[156] and the passage through Parliament of the Cruelty to Animals Act in 1876.[157] Ferrier was later (1881) to be targeted, unsuccessfully, for attempted legal sanction for his experimental work on monkeys under the terms of this Act but this did not relate to his work at WRA.[158] Evidently, however, Ferrier was alive to the possibilities of criticism even in 1873: in his first *WRLAMR* paper, based on studies of pigeons, fowls, guinea-pigs, rabbits, cats, and dogs, he "mentioned here, once for all, that before and throughout all the following experiments, ether or chloroform was administered" (III:35),[159] words which Crichton-Browne quoted in a defence of vivisection and of Ferrier in a letter to the *Times* following the appearance of an advert for the Society for the Abolition of Vivisection.[160]

Human Experimentation

One of the principal concerns of the anti-vivisectionists was that animal experimentation might be the top of a slippery slope which would eventually culminate in scientists undertaking experiments on humans, specifically involving patients. No such activity occurred at WRA, although one may argue that any clinical trial is equivalent to human (therapeutic) experimentation, and this may have been particularly the case in an era when no conception of informed patient consent actuated clinical practice. Here, comment is confined to self-experimentation by members of the WRA staff.

---

[154] Crichton Browne 1875a.

[155] Finn and Stark (2015).

[156] Hornsby (2019).

[157] Ozer (1966); French (1975).

[158] Bone and Larner (2024).

[159] May one perhaps detect a certain weariness in Ferrier's "once for all" suggesting that this was not the first time he had emphasized his use of these agents in animal experiments, or faced criticism from those opposed to vivisection?

[160] Reprinted in *BMJ* 1875;2:180 (7th August; Vivisection).

No doubt in the tradition of Humphry Davy (1778–1829) who had self-experimented with nitrous oxide,[161] Samuel Mitchell administered the drug to himself (I:45–48) and to some of his friends (I:44). Likewise, in his work with ether and nitrous oxide, after limited animal experiments (on rabbits), Mitchell "proceeded to experiment on myself, and on such of my friends as were willing to join me in the investigation" (II:77).[162] Burman injected himself and other medical officers (Wood, Courtenay, Mitchell) with conia (II:16).[163] Benham applied dilute nicotine to his own eyeball three times to observe the effects on the pupil (IV:313) but "found so much difficulty in getting volunteers to take this very nauseating drug, even in minute quantities, that I have only been able to administer it to seven persons who are non-smokers" (IV:315).

Was Crichton-Browne aware that his Medical Officers were experimenting on themselves? His Cavendish Lecture of 1895, describing Mitchell's work on nitrous oxide, makes clear that he was,[164] although I have found no convincing evidence that Crichton-Browne himself was ever a subject of such self-experimentation.

Contemporary Critical Reception of *WRLAMR*

It has rightly been said that "There are difficulties for the historian making the attempt to map or quantify the influence of any periodical".[165] This is certainly true of *WRLAMR*: nothing is known of its circulation, or whether or not there were subscribers. It is barely mentioned in a review of psychiatric journals of the nineteenth century.[166] That there was a market for such material might be suggested by Crammer's report that the *Journal of Psychological Medicine and Mental Pathology* "had a steady circulation of about 400, far in

---

[161] Another role model may have been Lauder Brunton (see Chap. 7) who had self-experimented with digitalis. Does his account of the effects of cannabis (IV:221; *vide supra*) suggest personal experimentation?

[162] Is it possible that the number of Mitchell's friends had declined since his earlier experiments? Or had there been unwillingness on the part of his (erstwhile?) friends, overt or covert, to take part in the initial experiments? Of note, another, later self-experimenter with nitrous oxide was Victor Horsley (Horsley, 1883–1884; discussed in Adan and Larner 2025:512).

[163] As mentioned earlier, Burman had previously self-experimented with chloral hydrate, prior to his time at WRA (Burman 1872a).

[164] Crichton-Browne (1895:73).

[165] Richardson and Bynum (1992:96).

[166] Shepherd (1992:201).

excess of all the institutions for the insane at the time".[167] But some indirect indices exist by which the impact of *WRLAMR* might be judged. Potential measures of influence which can be tracked include both published reviews of the journal (Table 6.2) and citations (independent, rather than self-citation) of papers published in the journal (Table 6.3).[168]

A number of reviews of the volumes of *WRLAMR* were published in the contemporary medical press (Table 6.2). The first volume of *WRLAMR* was noted in at least two British medical journals, the *Journal of Mental Science* (the forerunner of the *British Journal of Psychiatry*) and the *British and Foreign Medico-Chirurgical Review*. The reviewer in the latter journal stated that "We believe the volume of Asylum Reports under review to be the first of its kind. It inaugurates a new era in psychological literature, and the originators may be congratulated on their enterprise." The reviewer in the *Journal of Mental Science* had a different, more guarded, perspective: "Although it would be untrue to say that this is a valuable contribution to science, yet that it is an important addition to medical literature no one will deny."

The inaugural volume of *WRLAMR* was also noted internationally: the *Indian Medical Gazette* opined that "As the first report of the kind, in addition to its intrinsic merits, this volume deserves notice". In the *American Journal of the Medical Sciences* the reviewer, "B.L.R.", noted "The design is praiseworthy, and the execution, so far, very commendable". The impression gained from these contemporary reviews is that commentators thought that something new and potentially important if not valuable was being attempted in *WRLAMR*.

Subsequent volumes were likewise reviewed in both national and international journals of varying degrees of prestige, suggesting a wide dissemination of the research findings at WRA. The domestic medical journals included both general and specialist publications: the former included the *Lancet, British Medical Journal, Glasgow Medical Journal* and *Edinburgh Medical Journal* (the two forerunners of the *Scottish Medical Journal*), *Medical Press and Circular, British and Foreign Medico-Chirurgical Review*, and the *Dublin Journal of Medical Science*; the latter comprised the *Journal of Mental Science* and the *Journal of Psychological Medicine and Mental Pathology*. In addition, brief notices also appeared in a general interest publication, the *Westminster and Foreign Quarterly Review*. Foreign medical journals reviewing *WRLAMR* included the *Boston Medical and Surgical Journal* (forerunner of the *New*

---

[167] Crammer (1996:216).

[168] Here I deal with published reviews, rather than general comments such as those of Batty Tuke (1874:109) mentioned previously.

Table 6.3 Some contemporary citations of *WRLAMR* papers

WRLAMR paper (Author: title)	Contemporary citations (Author. Reference)
I;58–70 Thompson: The sphygmograph in lunatic asylum practice	Bigelow HR. *Medical Record* 1874;9:231 ["West Riding Reports"]
I:71–128 Aldridge: The ophthalmoscope in mental and cerebral diseases.	Fisher. *Boston Med Surg J* 1873;88:112, 113 [misdates "West Riding Reports" as 1872 at 111]. Swanzy. *Dublin Journal of Medical Science* 1877;63:27.
I:152–163 Ward: On the treatment of insanity by the hypodermic injection of morphia.	Diarmid. *J Ment Sci* 1876–1877;22(April 1876):18. Bodington. *BMJ* 1876;2:143.
I:164–177 Pedler: Mollities ossium and allied diseases.	Anon. *J Ment Sci* 1874–1875:20(April 1874):164.
I:218–232 Sutherland: Arachnoid cysts.	Ringrose Atkins. *Dublin Journal of Medical Science* 1875;59:497.
II:1–40 Burman: On conia, and its use in subcutaneous injection.	Harrington Tuke. *Lancet* 1873;2:448.
II:177–202 Nicol: The mental symptoms of ordinary disease.	Laycock. *Lancet* 1874;1:49.
II:203–222 Allbutt: The electric treatment of the insane.	Anon. *J Ment Sci* 1874–1875:20(April 1874):106. Anon. *J Ment Sci* 1874–1875:20(July 1874):232 (review of chapter in Bucknill & Tuke's *Psychological Medicine*, 3rd edition).
II:223–253 Aldridge: Ophthalmoscopic observations in general paralysis, and after the administration of certain toxic agents	Hughlings Jackson. *London Medical Record* 1873;1:22–23 (15 January) and 151 (12 March).
II:278–301 Browne: Impairment of language, the result of cerebral disease.	Laycock. *J Ment Sci* 1875–1876;21(July 1875):167.
III:30–96 Ferrier: Experimental researches in cerebral physiology and pathology.	Hughlings Jackson. *London Medical Record* 1873;1:275–276 (7 May). Hughlings Jackson. *Lancet* 1873;2:840. Anon. *Dublin Journal of Medical Science* 1873;56:374–6. Thompson Dickson. *J Ment Sci* 1873–1874;19(October 1873):376–377. Anon. *British and Foreign Medico-Chirurgical Review* 1875;55:345–7. Anon. *British and Foreign Medico-Chirurgical Review* 1876;57:278–280. Brown-Séquard. *Lancet* 1876;2:281. Charcot & Pitres. *Revue Mensuelle de Médecine et de Chirurgie* 1877;1:4.

(continued)

Table 6.3 (continued)

WRLAMR paper (Author: title)	Contemporary citations (Author. Reference)
III:97–112 Major: Observations on the histology of the brain in the insane.	Mickle. *BMJ* 1875;2:756.
III:153–174 Crichton Browne: Nitrite of amyl in epilepsy.	Harrington Tuke. *Lancet* 1873;2:448. Harrington Tuke. *J Ment Sci* 1873–1874;19(October 1873):332. Thompson Dickson. *J Ment Sci* 1873–1874;19(October 1873):385. Smith. *Dublin Journal of Medical Science* 1874;57:145–6. Anon. *Le Progrès Médical* 1874;2:579. Swanzy. *Dublin Journal of Medical Science* 1877;63:28 [incorrectly cites pagination as "53–174"].
III:216–257 Burman: Heart disease and insanity.	Mickle. *BMJ* 1875;2:756.
III:285–298 Clapham: The weight of the brain in the insane.	Anon. *BMJ* 1877;1:165. Mickle. *J Ment Sci* 1875–1876;21(January 1876):573
IV:30–62 Ferrier: Pathological illustrations of brain function.	Charcot. *Le Progrès Médical* 1874;3:283. Anon. *British and Foreign Medico-Chirurgical Review* 1876;57:275.
IV:63–93 Merson: The urinology of general paralysis.	Ashe. *J Ment Sci* 1876–1877;22(April 1876):89.
IV:94–151 Fothergill: Cerebral anaemia.	Thorowgood. *BMJ* 1874;2:817.
IV:179–222 Lauder Brunton: On inhibition, peripheral and central.	Anon. *Lancet* 1875;1:312–3. Ferrier, 1876:18, 283. Obersteiner. *Brain* 1878–1879;1(4):452.
IV:223–239 Major: Observations on the histology of the morbid brain.	Mickle. *BMJ* 1875;2:756. Ringrose Atkins. *Dublin Journal of Medical Science* 1877;63:46, 52.
V:24–39 Ferrier: Labyrinthine vertigo. Menière's disease	Sutherland. *London Medical Record* 1876;4:68–9. Gowers. *BMJ* 1877;1:287.
V:105–129 Hughlings Jackson: On temporary mental disorders after epileptic paroxysms.	Coats. *BMJ* 1876;2:649. Anon. *BMJ* 1877;1:431–2.
V:188–197 Sankey: A new process for examining the structure of the brain. With a review of some points in the histology of the cerebellum.	Anon. *BMJ* 1876;1:51. Ringrose Atkins. *Dublin Journal of Medical Science* 1877;63:44.

(continued)

Table 6.3 (continued)

WRLAMR paper (Author: title)	Contemporary citations (Author. Reference)
V:227–256 Crichton Browne: The functions of the thalami optici.	Bevan Lewis. *Lancet* 1876;2:503. *Medical Times and Gazette* 1876;2:489. Ferrier, 1876:238. Brown-Séquard. *Lancet* 1877;1:709 and 827.

NB This does not claim to be a systematic, far less a comprehensive, review, merely a narrative review to illustrate the point that *WRLAMR* papers were known and cited outside WRA during the period around the immediate lifetime of the journal

England Journal of Medicine), *American Journal of the Medical Sciences*, *American Journal of Insanity* (forerunner of the *American Journal of Psychiatry*), *Journal of Nervous and Mental Diseases*, as well as the aforementioned *Indian Medical Gazette*.

Whilst it may indeed be the case that, at this time, "the medical journals were generous in the space given to reviews of even the most trivial offerings",[169] nevertheless *WRLAMR* evidently gained widespread coverage in review columns. Although, then as now, one cannot read too much into the opinions of reviewers, nevertheless in general these were positive. The *Lancet* reviewer opined of the second issue (the first to be noted therein[170]) that "we think this instalment a decided advance on its predecessor" but gave no specific reason(s), and the *Westminster Review* noted that "instead of long-winded psychological discussions we have brief pointed essays on practical subjects, which, hit or miss, at any rate have no ambiguity about them". However, the same volume was deemed by the *American Journal of the Medical Sciences* (again reviewed by "B.L.R.") "hardly equal in interest and value to its predecessor". The *Medical Press and Circular* judged the third volume to be "an era in the physiology of the nervous system, for in no other way can we adequately describe the impression which Professor Ferrier's essay and one or two of its companions are likely to create". Standards were apparently maintained, at least in the opinion of the critics: the *BMJ* reviewer found the fourth volume to be "in no respect inferior to its predecessors" and of the fifth issue the *Journal of Mental Science* stated "This volume is the largest and, on the whole, the best that has appeared". The final volume was described in the *Edinburgh Medical Journal* as "an admirable volume … which no one interested in the treatment of

---

[169] Shepherd (1980:44).

[170] Although the first volume was noted in *Lancet* 1872;1:83 (20th January; Reviews and Notices of Books), this appearing in a review of the January 1872 issue of the *British and Foreign Medico-Chirurgical Review*.

insanity … can safely neglect to read," and in the *American Journal of the Medical Sciences* ("B.L.R." again!) as an "extremely valuable and creditable contribution to cerebral physiology, pathology, and therapeutics".

A contemporary commentator from the field ("for 9 years I have been engaged in the management of an asylum"), wrote in 1876:

> I cannot do better than cite the *West Riding Asylum Reports* [*sic*]. Those admirable Reports may, I think, be taken as a fair and trustworthy expression of the leanings of the medico-psychological world at the present moment, and anyone familiar with them will, I feel sure, agree with me that they overflow with the records of investigations which tend to link most closely—nay, I will say to identify—mental disease with cerebral lesion, or disorder of cerebral function, and to establish the therapeutics of insanity on a thoroughly physiological basis.[171]

As regards citations of papers, it has been noted that "as late as the 1840s, the convention of the reference had not yet developed in English-language medical periodicals, and many papers had none, either in the text or in footnotes or endnotes".[172] This was still largely true in the 1870s: certainly, no *WRLAMR* article had a dedicated reference or bibliography section, at most merely occasional footnotes referring to other publications. Hence no citation analysis or impact factor can be developed for any individual *WRLAMR* paper; only a narrative account might be offered. Clearly Ferrier's work (III:30–96) generated significant interest and comment, even in the year of its publication.[173]

The End of *WRLAMR*

Despite the general sense of approbation expressed in the reviews, only six volumes of *WRLAMR* were published. The final volume appeared after Crichton-Browne's resignation and departure from WRA and was co-edited by Herbert Major, the new superintendent (compare the change in affiliations of both Crichton-Browne and Major between volumes V and VI: Table 6.1).

Secondary sources have stated that Crichton-Browne's "successor" (Major was not named) was not willing to continue with the journal,[174] and certainly the unsigned preface to the final volume (which I take to be the work of

---

[171] Bodington (1876:141).
[172] Burnham (1992:172).
[173] Larner (2023c, 2025j).
[174] Critchley and Critchley (1998:157), Shorvon and Compston (2019:291).

Major) consists of a single, perfunctory sentence. Although the precise reasons for discontinuation are unknown, it is possible that the ever-growing patient population at WRA, the burden of administrative duties, a failure to recruit suitable assistant medical officers and clinical assistants, all may have contributed to Major's decision. It was certainly in keeping with the Lunacy Commissioners policy of discouraging superintendents from undertaking research that might distract them from administrative duties.

Another possibility is that Crichton-Browne intended the journal to end with his departure. According to Oppenheim, Crichton-Browne had "persuaded Churchill, the London medical publisher, to bring out the first two volumes and lined up Smith, Elder for the last four",[175] a wording which might suggest that he foresaw only six volumes. If so, Major may justifiably have felt no obligation to continue. However, research efforts did continue at WRA after Crichton-Browne's departure, particularly during the long superintendency of Bevan-Lewis (1884–1910).[176]

Another factor of potential significance was the passing of the Cruelty to Animals Act in 1876 (39 & 40 Vict. c.77). This required amongst its stipulations that premises on which animal experimentation took place be registered, a requirement which some institutional authorities were unwilling or refused to meet.[177] The burden of this registration would have fallen to Major. He may have been concerned that continuing animal experimentation at the Asylum might generate fears in the locality of experimentation on patients.

WRLAMR as the Precursor of *Brain: A Journal of Neurology*

That *WRLAMR* had fulfilled a need and had found a niche in the market, such that its demise left a gap, is perhaps evidenced by the prompt appearance of another journal devoted to similar topics: *Brain: a journal of neurology*.

Whilst the *Journal of Mental Science* might perhaps have taken up the mantle of the defunct *WRLAMR*, its then editor, Henry Maudsley, had no laboratory experience nor any evident taste for experiment, contrary to important strands in the content of *WRLAMR* and subsequently in *Brain*.[178] Certainly,

---

[175] Oppenheim (1991:70).

[176] This period is discussed by Wallis (2017a:passim).

[177] French (1975:194).

[178] Rollin (2003) opined that *WRLAMR* was "far more prestigious than the dull *Journal of Mental Science*, the official journal of the Medico Psychological Association". Maudsley relinquished the editorship of the *Journal of Mental Science* in 1878.

many *WRLAMR* authors also published in the *Journal of Mental Science* (*vide infra*) but Maudsley himself contributed neither to *WRLAMR*[179] nor to *Brain*.[180]

The origins of *Brain* are, regrettably, obscure: apparently no records of its founding and operations for its first 25 years are extant.[181] However, intimations of a new journal were already apparent in late 1877, when the *BMJ* reported:

> We understand that a new quarterly journal of mental diseases, entitled *Brain*, will be issued early next year by Messrs. Macmillan. The editors will be Dr. J.C. Bucknill, F.R.S., Dr. Crichton Browne, Dr. Hughlings Jackson, and Dr. Ferrier, F.R.S.[182]

This notice proved to be true in most particulars, with the exception of the reported focus on "mental diseases".

The title page of the first issue of the first volume of *Brain*, dated April 1878, listed the editors (in alphabetical order) as J. C. Bucknill, J. Crichton-Browne (*sic*, with hyphen), D. Ferrier, and J. Hughlings-Jackson (*sic*, with hyphen). Three members of this quadrumvirate were, as already discussed, closely associated with *WRLAMR*, the exception being John Charles Bucknill (1817–1897).[183] Although Bucknill did not publish in *WRLAMR*, he had

---

[179] Some possible speculations to account for this fact include, but are not limited to, Maudsley's antipathy to asylum medicine, and a commitment to publish in the *Journal of Mental Science*, which his editorship had helped to fashion into something different from Bucknill's initial conception of the *Asylum Journal*. In view of his clinical experience at WRA in 1857 (see Chap. 2), I doubt Maudsley had any particular antipathy to the institution per se; he cited cases from Crichton-Browne in his Gulstonian Lectures of 1870 (Maudsley 1870a:47, 49; b:610). Many years later, in 1920, Crichton-Browne gave the first Maudsley Lecture, in which he stated that "I made Maudsley's personal acquaintance at the table of that gracefully-refined and highly-gifted physician and philanthropist, Dr. John Conolly," hence before 1866, and that "I was never estranged from him by quarrel or misunderstanding, and the admiration and esteem in which I held him never for a moment paled" (Crichton-Browne 1920:199, 200).

[180] Turner (1988:170) phrased it thus: "Maudsley never wrote for—or his articles were never accepted for?—this particular journal". As there are apparently no records for *Brain* in this period (*vide infra*), it is unlikely that we shall ever know.

[181] This is according to a personal communication from Professor Alastair Compston, then Editor of *Brain*, dated October 2011, to Samuel Greenblatt (2022:263n34). See also https://guarantorsofbrain. org/history/ (accessed 08/09/2024). Compston's dedicated history of *Brain* is keenly awaited. Some details are available on the adoption of *Brain* as the official organ of the Neurological Society of London in 1887 (Larner 2026a).

[182] *BMJ* 1877;2:772 (1st December). Hence this was within 1 year of the appearance of the last *WRLAMR* (*vide supra*, "Dates of Publication" section).

[183] Bucknill is discussed in Chap. 9. Biographical material may be found in Scull et al. (1996:187–225). For his association with *Brain*, see Larner and Gardner-Thorpe (2023) (reprinted in adapted form in Larner 2025r). Holmes (1938:520) omitted Bucknill's name from the founders of *Brain*; likewise Young (1970:238n4), and O'Connor (1991:485). In this context, Finger (2000:167) wrote "Bucknell".

lectured at WRA, at the medical *conversazione* of November 1874. But was *Brain* indeed a collaborative venture, or was there a prime mover in this new undertaking?

Of the four candidates, a good case could be made for Bucknill taking the lead. He was the senior of the quadrumvirate, and considerably so: he was almost 20 years older than the next eldest (Hughlings Jackson) and more than 25 years older than the youngest (Ferrier). Furthermore, he had prior editorial experience, having been at the helm of the *Asylum Journal* (later to become the *Journal of Mental Science*) from its inception in 1853 until 1862 when he was appointed Chancery Visitor in Lunacy (the post taken up by Crichton-Browne on his departure from Wakefield in 1876). This journal was later credited with helping to establish the profession of asylum medicine as a credible branch of medical science.[184] Later commentators have also nominated Bucknill as the key figure in the new venture, opining that he resigned from the Visitorship "in 1876 … to edit the newly established journal, *Brain*"[185] and that he "had time … to found a new journal, *Brain*, in 1870 [*sic*]".[186]

A case can also be made for Crichton-Browne, since he too had founded a journal, *WRLAMR*, and had more recent editorial experience than Bucknill. Hence some have taken the view that Crichton-Browne was the "leading spirit",[187] "did most of the editorial work",[188] or that he was "probably the prime mover in establishing *Brain* in 1878".[189] It has also been claimed that Crichton-Browne edited *WRLAMR* "with the assistance" of Jackson, Ferrier and Bucknill and that "Sir James encouraged the editorial group to remain with him and founded the present-day journal *Brain*"[190] but this assertion does not withstand examination since there is no evidence for such an "editorial group" at *WRLAMR*.

As for Hughlings Jackson, it has been stated that *Brain* was largely his initiative.[191] Early in his career he had worked as a medical reporter for the

---

[184] Russell (1988:299), who also stated that the *Asylum Journal* was the private initiative of Bucknill.

[185] Beveridge (1998:54). The misdating with respect to *Brain* casts doubt on the validity of this claim. None of the other editors was mentioned. Hurn (1998:67) also stated that *Brain* was "founded in 1876" but the reference cited is 1878.

[186] Tyrer and Craddock (2012:2). A typographical error, perhaps? If not, the misdating casts doubt on the validity of this claim.

[187] Henson (1978).

[188] Critchley and Critchley (1998:157).

[189] Reynolds and Broussolle (2022:293).

[190] Snaith (1998:456).

[191] Shorvon and Compston (2019:131). They also included in their claim, for which they cite no source(s), the founding of the Neurological Society of London (see Chaps. 7 and 8).

Medical Times and Gazette, but editing other people's work was surely not his metier.

In his obituary of Ferrier, Sherrington stated that:

> On the suspension of the West Riding Medical Reports [*sic*], writes Sir James Crichton-Browne, referring to the changes consequent on his own retirement from Wakefield, it was Ferrier who urged that the work which the Reports had begun, should be in some form continued. It then came to be agreed that a "Neurological Journal" should be started in London, and thus "Brain" was launched in 1879 [*sic*].[192]

Written fully 50 years after the event, it is not clear what credence may be accorded to this account, doubts possibly compounded by the error in the stated launch date of *Brain*.[193]

However, that Ferrier was indeed involved in the early workings of *Brain* may be suggested by his citation of four papers in the journal in the footnotes of his book publication of the 1878 Gulstonian Lectures delivered to the Royal College of Physicians of London.[194] The "Prefatory Note" of this book was dated October 1878, some months after the first appearance of *Brain* (April 1878), whereas the four *Brain* citations are not found in the individual lectures themselves, delivered in March 1878, as published in the *BMJ*; indeed only two of the four papers are mentioned therein.[195] In two of the four *Brain* citations, a date of 1877 was given, referring to papers which appeared in the first and second issues of the journal (these happen to be the two not mentioned in the *BMJ*). The explanation for this dating error is not clear—it seems odd that a simple, uncorrected typographical error in the manuscript should occur twice. Could it be that *Brain* was originally anticipated to appear in 1877?[196]

---

[192] Sherrington (1928:xv). Sherrington's account may have been the source for Spillane (1974a:702, 1981:388) who wrote that "According to Crichton Browne it was Ferrier who urged that the work which the reports [*sic*] had begun should be continued in some form".

[193] I speculate that this misdating might stem from the fact that the first volumes of *Brain* overlapped 2 years (as mentioned below) and hence the first volume was dated 1878–1879. The 1879 dating was repeated by Spillane (1974a:702), verbatim with Sherrington ("*Brain* was launched in 1879") which I take to be Spillane's source. Of note, Spillane (1981:388) later corrected this error ("*Brain* was launched in 1878").

[194] Ferrier (1878a:67n1, 82n4, 94n2, 96n1), referring respectively to works by Haddon (*Brain* 1878;1(2):250–5), Gowers (*Brain* 1878;1(3):388–90), Mac Cormac (*Brain* 1878;1(2):256–60), and Duret (*Brain* 1878;1(1):29–47).

[195] Haddon in Ferrier (1878b:475–6); Gowers in Ferrier (1878c:516).

[196] In this context, Young (1970:198), writing of Hughlings Jackson, stated that "he was the founder (along with Ferrier and others) of the first English journal devoted exclusively to his field of interest: *Brain* (1877–)" [*sic*].

Brain was initially published in London by Macmillan and Co., in quarterly instalments appearing in April, July, October, and January, such that each volume overlapped 2 years (as was the case for the *Journal of Mental Science*). Issues varied only slightly in length, all around 144 pages. Hence the total pagination for each of the early volumes of *Brain* was approximately twice that of *WRLAMR* (ca. 576 vs. ca. 300). The extra space permitted the contents of *Brain* to be presented under a number of subheadings, viz.: Original articles; Critical Digests and Notices of Books; Clinical Cases; and Abstracts of British and Foreign Journals.[197] The initial retail price of *Brain* was 3 shillings and sixpence per issue, or an annual subscription of 14 shillings (hence no discount),[198] whereas the final volume of *WRLAMR* cost 9 shillings and sixpence. The relative costs per page were therefore approximately 3½d for *Brain* and 2¾d for *WRLAMR*.

Unlike *WRLAMR*, the first issue of *Brain* had no editorial preface, but launched directly into the first paper, Jonathan Hutchinson's "Notes on the symptom-significance of different states of the pupil" (*Brain* 1878;1(1):1–13). However, a "News" item in the April 1878 issue of the journal *Mind* might be deemed to serve as *Brain's* manifesto:

> The Journal will … include in its scope all that relates to the anatomy, physiology, pathology and therapeutics of the Nervous System. The functions and diseases of the nervous system will be discussed both in their physiological and psychological aspects; but mental phenomena will be treated only in correlation with their anatomical substrata, and mental disease will be investigated as far as possible by the methods applicable to nervous diseases in general.[199]

The end-papers of volume 1 of *Brain* included an unpaginated statement from the Editors, the text of which overlapped with that appearing in *Mind*.[200] Appended to this was a list of 58 names, described in the text as "supporters"

---

[197] The demise of the *British and Foreign Medico-Chirurgical Review* in 1877 (Anon 1877) may have been no more than coincidental, but might have suggested a need for, and hence inclusion of, "Abstracts of British and Foreign Journals" in *Brain*. Abstracts of foreign literature had been a feature of the *Journal of Mental Science* from the time (1863) of the editorship of Lockhart Robertson and Maudsley (Turner 1988:159).

[198] See https://guarantorsofbrain.org/history/ (accessed 08/09/2024). Did the price differential perhaps reflect in some way the costs of a metropolitan versus a provincial publisher? Most nineteenth century medical journals were published in London (Bynum and Wilson 1992:34).

[199] *Mind* 1878;3:295.

[200] The shared wording was: "but mental phenomena will be treated only in correlation with their anatomical substrata, and mental disease will be investigated as far as possible by the methods applicable to nervous diseases in general". Hurn (1998:67) cited this passage, referencing it as "*Brain: A Journal of Neurology*, 1878, 1, Introduction". I have examined a number of copies of volume 1 of *Brain*, both physical and virtual, and have found no initial "Introduction" or "Preface" or manifesto of any kind, merely

of *Brain* but in the page heading as "contributors", of whom eight had published in *WRLAMR* (Aldridge, Allbutt, Lauder Brunton, Clapham, Fothergill, Lawson, Bevan-Lewis, Rabagliati).[201]

Of the 38 authors who contributed to *WRLAMR*, no less than 15 subsequently contributed to *Brain* in its first six volumes (Table 6.4).[202] Of WRA resident staff, former or current, and excluding Crichton-Browne, only six subsequently contributed to *Brain*: Aldridge, Clapham, Galton, Lawson, Bevan-Lewis, and Newcombe. Of these, Aldridge and Galton contributed only to the Critical Digests and Notices of Books and/or Abstracts of British and Foreign Journals sections, rather than a substantive clinical or research paper, and Newcombe contributed only a case report. The remaining eight *WRLAMR* authors who subsequently contributed to *Brain* were non-resident staff, either visiting clinicians and/or external contributors to *WRLAMR*: Allbutt, Lauder Brunton, Henry Clarke, Ferrier, Milner Fothergill, Hughlings Jackson, Rabagliati, and H.R.O. Sankey (see Chap. 7). Of these, Rabagliati was the only one not to contribute a substantive clinical or research paper.

Four *WRLAMR* contributors published in the first issue of *Brain* in April 1878: Allbutt (pp. 60–78), Bevan-Lewis (79–96), Crochley Clapham (97–100), and Ferrier (101–108), these contributions accounting for about one third of the total page content of the first issue. Several other *WRLAMR* contributors appeared in first volume of *Brain* (1878–9): Aldridge, Lauder Brunton, Clarke, Crichton-Browne (who had permission to access WRA records for his later publications), Milner Fothergill, Galton, Hughlings Jackson, Lawson, Rabagliati, and Sankey, a total of 14 in all.[203] Newcombe published in the second volume.

Certainly, many *WRLAMR* authors (13/38) also published in the *Journal of Mental Science* in the period 1871–1883 (Table 6.5), of whom nine were WRA resident staff, former or current, and including Crichton-Browne. The remaining four were non-resident (W.A.F. Browne, Henry Clarke, Milner Fothergill, Hughlings Jackson) but, unlike the situation with *Brain*, only the latter two were physicians.

---

the first paper by Jonathan Hutchinson. The note from the Editors of "Brain" appeared in the unpaginated end-papers.

[201] I wonder if the designated "supporters" of *Brain* might possibly overlap with Sloffer's (2023:32n47) "subscribers" to *WRLAMR*.

[202] Larner (2023b:4443) was therefore in error when giving a total of 14, this lapse occasioned by the omission of Aldridge, as a consequence of an over-reliance on the journal contents as listed in the *Brain* online archive rather than examining hard copy journals.

[203] This number differs from that reported by Todd and Ashworth (1991:416) who stated that "nine of the contributors to the first volume [of *Brain*] had had papers published in the *Medical Reports*" but they gave no further details which might permit clarification of this discrepancy.

Table 6.4 Authors (listed alphabetically) common to both the six volumes of *WRLAMR* (1871–1876) and the first six volumes of *Brain* (1878–9 to 1883–4) (compare with Table 6.5)

Author	Publications in *WRLAMR* Title. Year;volume:pages.	Publications in *Brain* Title. Year;volume(issue):pages.
Aldridge, Charles	The ophthalmoscope in mental and cerebral diseases. 1871;I:71–128. Ophthalmoscopic observations in general paralysis, and after the administration of certain toxic agents. 1872;II:223–53. Ophthalmoscopic observations in acute dementia. 1874;IV:291–304.	Abstracts of British and Foreign Journals. 1878–1879;1(3):422–4.
Allbutt, T. Clifford	The electric treatment of the insane. 1872;II:203–22. On the obscurer neuroses of syphilis. 1873;III:273–84.	On brain forcing. 1878–1879;1(1):60–78. Critical Digests and Notices of Books. 1879–1880;2(1):95–9. Critical Digests and Notices of Books. 1879–1880;2(3):385–90. Case of epileptiform migraine. 1883–1884;6(2):246–9.
Brunton, T. Lauder	On inhibition, peripheral and central. 1874;IV:179–222.	Reflex action as a cause of disease and means of cure. 1878–1879;1(2):143–54. On the position of the motor centres in the brain in regard to the nutritive and social functions. 1882–1883;4(4):431–40. Reviews and Notices of Books. 1883–1884;6(2):263–6.
Clapham, W. Crochley S.	The weight of the brain in the insane. 1873;III:285–98. The weight of the brain in the insane. 1876;VI:11–26. The cranial outline of the insane and criminal. 1876;VI:150–69. [with H Clarke]	On skull mapping. 1878–1879:1(1):97–100. Abstracts of British and Foreign Journals. 1879–1880;2(4):591–2.

Clarke, Henry	The cranial outline of the insane and criminal. 1876;VI:150–69. [with WCS Clapham]	The effects of seclusion on the body weight. 1878–1879;1(2):210–4. Heredity and crime in epileptic criminals. 1879–1880;2(4):491–527.
Crichton-Browne, James	[Preface. 1871;I:iii–v.] Cranial injuries and mental diseases. 1871;I:1–26. [Preface. 1872;II:iii.] Cranial injuries and mental diseases. 1872;II:97–136. [Preface. 1873;III:iii–iv.] Nitrite of amyl in epilepsy. 1873;IV:153–74. [Preface. 1874;IV:v.] Acute dementia. 1874;IV:265–90. [Preface. 1875;V:vi.] The functions of the thalami optici. 1875;V:227–56. Note on chronic mania. 1875;V:284–92. Notes on the pathology of general paresis of the insane. 1876;VI:170–231.	Critical Digests and Notices of Books. 1878–1879;1(2):215–9. Abstracts of British and Foreign Journals. 1878–1879;1(2):279–81. Critical Digests and Notices of Books. 1878–1879;1(3):379–82. Critical Digests and Notices of Books. 1878–1879;1(3):386–7. On the weight of the brain and its component parts in the insane. 1878–1879;1(4):504–18. On the weight of the brain and its component parts in the insane. 1879–1880;2(1):42–67. Abstracts of British and Foreign Journals. 1879–1880;2(2):290–1. Critical Digests and Notices of Books. 1880–1881;3(1):111. Critical Digests and Notices of Books. 1880–1881;3(1):112. A plea for the minute study of mania. 1880–1881;3(3):347–62. Critical Digests and Notices of Books. 1880–1881;3(4):528–31. Critical Digests and Notices of Books. 1881–1882;4(3):392–8. Reviews and Notices of Books. 1883–1884;6(1):120–4. The pulmonary pathology of general paralysis. 1883–1884;6(3):317–41.

(continued)

Table 6.4 (continued)

Author	Publications in *WRLAMR* Title. Year;volume:pages.	Publications in *Brain* Title. Year;volume(issue):pages.
Ferrier,[a] David	Experimental researches in cerebral physiology and pathology. 1873;III:30–96. Pathological illustrations of brain function. 1874;IV:30–62. Labyrinthine vertigo. Menière's disease. 1875;V:24–39.	Critical Digests and Notices of Books. 1878–1879;1(1):101–8. Critical Digests and Notices of Books. 1878–1879;1(2):229–31. Critical Digests and Notices of Books. 1878–1879;1(2):239–49. Clinical Cases ("Note by Dr. Ferrier"). 1878–1879;1(2):259–60. Pain in the head in connection with cerebral disease. 1878–1879;1(4):467–83. Vomiting in connection with cerebral disease. 1879–1880;2(2):223–33. Abstracts of British and Foreign Journals. 1879–1880;2(2):286–9. Critical Digests and Notices of Books. 1879–1880;2(3):400–2. Critical Digests and Notices of Books. 1880–1881;3(1):85–99. Crural monoplegia—limited cortical lesion of opposite hemisphere. 1880–1881;3(1):128–31. Abstracts of British and Foreign Journals. 1880–1881;3(2):286–8. Critical Digests and Notices of Books. 1880–1881;3(3):365–73. Critical Digests and Notices of Books. 1880–1881;3(3):383–95. Abstracts of British and Foreign Journals. 1880–1881;3(3):417–27. Cerebral amblyopia and hemiopia [*sic*]. 1880–1881;3(4):456–77. Critical Digests and Notices of Books. 1881–1882;4(1):111–2. Abstracts of British and Foreign Journals. 1881–1882;4(1):136–8. The localisation of atrophic paralyses. 1881–1882;4(2):217–32. Critical Digests and Notices of Books. 1881–1882;4(2):246. Abstracts of British and Foreign Journals. 1881–1882;4(2):270–6. The localisation of atrophic paralyses. 1881–1882;4(3):303–24. Abstracts of British and Foreign Journals. 1881–1882;4(3):428–30. Critical Digests and Notices of Books. 1881–1882;4(4):517–9. Abstracts of British and Foreign Journals. 1881–1882;4(4):554–62. The brain of a criminal lunatic. 1882–1883;5(1):62–73. Glioma of the right optic thalamus and corpora quadrigemina. 1882–1883;5(1):123–7. Abstracts of British and Foreign Journals. 1882–1883;5(2):288. Case of allochiria. 1882–1883;5(3):389–93. Abstracts of British and Foreign Journals. 1882–1883;5(3):429–32. Hemiplegic muscular atrophy of peripheral origin. 1882–1883;5(4):521–8. Observations on a case of cerebral cortico-medullary glioma. 1883–1884;6(1):67–77.

Fothergill, J. Milner	The heart sounds in general paralysis of the insane. 1873;III:113–28. Cerebral anaemia. 1874;IV:94–151. Cerebral hyperaemia. 1875;V:171–87. Notes on the therapeutics of some affections of the nervous system. 1876;VI:252–65.	The neurosal [*sic*] and reflex disorders of the heart. 1878–1879;1(2):195–209.
Galton, John C.	Notes on the condition of the tympanic membrane in the insane—Part I. 1873;III:258–72.	Abstracts of British and Foreign Journals. 1878–1879;1(2):277–79. Critical Digests and Notices of Books. 1878–1879;1(3):382–6. Abstracts of British and Foreign Journals. 1878–1879;1(3):418–20. Abstracts of British and Foreign Journals. 1878–1879;1(4):577–9. Abstracts of British and Foreign Journals. 1880–1881;3(3):413–5.
Jackson,[b] John Hughlings	Observations on localisation of movements in the cerebral hemispheres, as revealed by cases of convulsion, chorea and "aphasia". 1873;III:175–95. On the anatomical, physiological, and pathological investigation of epilepsies. 1873;III:315–49. On a case of recovery from double optic neuritis. 1874;IV:24–29. On temporary mental disorders after epileptic paroxysms. 1875;V:105–29. On epilepsies and on the after effects of epileptic discharges (Todd and Robertson's hypothesis). 1876;VI:266–309.	Abstracts of British and Foreign Journals. 1878–1879;1(2):285–286. On affections of speech from disease of the brain. 1878–1879;1(3):304–30. Auditory vertigo. 1879–1880;2(1):29–38. On affections of speech from disease of the brain. 1879–1880;2(2):203–22. Note on Dr. J. Hughlings-Jackson's [*sic*] case of auditory vertigo in April No. of "Brain". 1879–1880;2(2):274. On affections of speech from disease of the brain. 1879–1880;2(3):323–56. On right or left-sided spasm at the onset of epileptic paroxysms, and on crude sensation warnings, and elaborate mental states. 1880–1881;3(2):192–206. Abstracts of British and Foreign Journals. 1880–1881;3(2):266–8. On temporary paralysis after epileptiform and epileptic seizures; a contribution to the study of dissolution of the nervous system. 1880–1881;3(4):433–51. Abstracts of British and Foreign Journals. 1880–1881;3(4):554–5. Remarks by Dr. Hughlings-Jackson. 1881–1882;4(2):263. Abstracts of British and Foreign Journals. 1881–1882;4(2):276–82. Critical Digests and Notices of Books. 1881–1882;4(4):519–24. Localised convulsions from tumour of the brain. 1882–1883;5(3):364–74. Critical Digests and Notices of Books. 1882–1883;5(3):382–8.

(continued)

Table 6.4 (continued)

Author	Publications in *WRLAMR* Title. Year;volume:pages.	Publications in *Brain* Title. Year;volume(issue):pages.
Lawson, Robert	On the hourly distribution of mortality in relation to recurrent changes in the activity of vital functions. 1874;IV:240–64. On the physiological action of hyoscyamine. 1875;V:40–84. Hyoscyamine in the treatment of some diseases of the insane. 1876;VI:65–84. Clinical notes on conditions incidental to insanity. 1876;VI:120–49 [with W Bevan Lewis]	On the symptomatology of alcoholic brain disorders. 1878–1879;1(2):182–94. Abstracts of British and Foreign Journals. 1879–1880;2(1):148. Abstracts of British and Foreign Journals. 1879–1880;2(3):446–8. Abstracts of British and Foreign Journals. 1879–1880;2(4):592. Abstracts of British and Foreign Journals. 1880–1881;3(1):143–4.

Lewis, William Bevan	On the histology of the great sciatic nerve in general paralysis of the insane. 1875;V:85–104.	On the comparative structure of the cortex cerebri. 1878–1879;1(1):79–96.
	Calorimetric observations upon the influence of various alkaloids on the generation of animal heat. 1876;VI:43–64.	Application of freezing methods to the microscopic examination of the brain. 1878–1879;1(3):348–59.
	Clinical notes on conditions incidental to insanity. 1876;VI:120–49 [with R Lawson]	Notes on certain lesions of the nervous tissues of frequent occurrence in the brain of the insane. 1879–1880;2(3):364–72.
		Methods of preparing, demonstrating, and examining cerebral structure in health and disease. 1880–1881;3(3):314–36.
		Methods of preparing, demonstrating, and examining cerebral structure in health and disease. 1880–1881;3(4):502–15.
		Methods of preparing, demonstrating, and examining cerebral structure in health and disease. 1881–1882;4(1):82–99.
		Critical Digests and Notices of Books. 1881–1882;4(2):238–46.
		Methods of preparing, demonstrating, and examining cerebral structure in health and disease. 1881–1882;4(3):351–60.
		Critical Digests and Notices of Books. 1881–1882;4(3):377–80.
		Methods of preparing, demonstrating, and examining cerebral structure in health and disease. 1881–1882;4(4):441–66.
		Histological notes on a case of tabes with ophthalmoplegia externa. 1882–1883;5(1):41–55.
		Methods of preparing, demonstrating, and examining cerebral structure in health and disease. 1882–1883;5(1):74–88.
		Critical Digests and Abstracts from Journals. 1883–1884;6(2):278–86.
		On posterior spinal sclerosis, consecutive to disease of blood-vessels: microscopical examinations of the cord [with T Buzzard]. 1883–1884;6(4):461–86.
		[WBL "Report of microscopical examination of the spinal cord" 467–80]
		Abstracts of British and Foreign Journals. 1883–1884;6(4):569–76.
Newcombe, Charles F.	Epileptiform seizures in general paralysis. 1875;V:198–226.	Case of locomotor ataxy. 1879–1880;2(1):134–8.

(continued)

Table 6.4 (continued)

Author	Publications in *WRLAMR* Title. Year;volume:pages.	Publications in *Brain* Title. Year;volume(issue):pages.
Rabagliati, A. H.	On classification and nomenclature in nervous disorders. 1876;VI:27–42.	Abstracts of British and Foreign Journals. 1878–1879;1(3):424–32. Critical Digests and Notices of Books. 1878–1879;1(4):529–44. Critical Digests and Notices of Books. 1879–1880;2(2):234–50. Critical Digests and Notices of Books. 1881–1882;4(1):100–11. Critical Digests and Notices of Books. 1881–1882;4(2):233–8. Critical Digests and Notices of Books. 1882–1883;5(1):105–9. Reviews and Notices of Books. 1883–1884;6(3):404–13. Abstracts of British and Foreign Journals. 1883–1884;6(4):561–7.
Sankey, H R Octavius	A new process for examining the structure of the brain. With a review of some points in the histology of the cerebellum. 1875;V:188–97.	Two cases of microcephalic idiotcy [*sic*] in one family—convulsions of mother during pregnancy. 1878–1879;1(3):391–9.

With additions and silent corrections from Larner (2023b), Supplementary Table S2. The deficiencies therein resulted from the author's over-reliance on the contents listed in the *Brain* online archive, rather than examining hard copy journals

[a]For more detail on Ferrier's publications, the author is currently preparing a catalogue raisonné

[b]For Jackson's publications, I have followed the listing given by Greenblatt (2022:473–502) rather than the catalogue raisonné by York and Steinberg (2006)

Table 6.5 Authors (listed alphabetically) common to both the six volumes of *WRLAMR* (1871–1876) and the six contemporaneous and the six subsequent volumes of the *Journal of Mental Science* (1871–1872 to 1882–1883, volumes 17–28 inclusive) (compare with Table 6.4)

Author	Publications in *WRLAMR* Title. Year;volume:pages.	Publications in *Journal of Mental Science* Title. Year;volume(issue):pages.
Benham, William T.	On the therapeutic value of cold to the head. 1874;IV;152–78. The actions of nicotine. 1874;IV:305–17.	The result of a post-mortem examination on a hydrocephalic idiot (congenital). 1874–1875;20(July 1874):259–62.
Browne, William A. F.	Impairment of language, the result of cerebral disease. 1872;II:278–301.	The perception, &c., of time as a feature in mental disease. 1873–1874;19(January 1874):519–32. Necrophilism. 1874–1875;20(January 1875):551–60.
Burman, J. Wilkie	A contribution to the statistics of general paralysis; with remarks. 1871;I:129–51. On conia, and its use in subcutaneous injection. 1872;II:1–40. Heart disease and insanity. 1873;III:216–57.	On larceny, as committed by patients in the earlier stages of general paralysis. 1872–1873;18(January 1873):536–43. Four departmental asylums in the north-west of France. 1873–1874;19(January 1874):541–52. Four departmental asylums in the north-west of France. 1874–1875;20(April 1874):74–81. Some further cases of general paralytics committed to prison for larceny; with remarks. 1874–1875;20(July 1874):246–54.
Clarke, Henry	The cranial outline of the insane and criminal. 1876;VI:150–69. [with WCS Clapham[a]]	Embolism of the cerebral arteries—softening of the pons Varolii. 1878–1879;24(January 1879):617–22.
Crichton-Browne, James	[Preface. 1871;I:iii–v.] Cranial injuries and mental diseases. 1871;I:1–26. [Preface. 1872;II:iii.] Cranial injuries and mental diseases. 1872;II:97–136. [Preface. 1873;III:iii–iv.] Nitrite of amyl in epilepsy. 1873;III:153–74. [Preface. 1874;IV:v.] Acute dementia. 1874;IV:265–90. [Preface. 1875;V:vi.] The functions of the thalami optici. 1875;V:227–56. Note on chronic mania. 1875;V:284–92. Notes on the pathology of general paresis of the insane. 1876;VI:170-231.	Notes on epilepsy, and its pathological consequences. 1873–1874;19(April 1873):19–46. Correspondence. 1875–1876;21(April 1875):152. Skae's classification of mental disease. A critique. 1875–1876;21(October 1875):339–65. Presidential address, delivered at the Royal College of Physicians, London, on Friday, July 26th, 1878. 1878–1879;24(October 1878):345–73.

(continued)

Table 6.5 (continued)

Author	Publications in *WRLAMR* Title. Year;volume:pages.	Publications in *Journal of Mental Science* Title. Year;volume(issue):pages.
Fothergill, J. Milner	The heart sounds in general paralysis of the insane. 1873;III:113–28. Cerebral anaemia. 1874;IV:94–151. Cerebral hyperaemia. 1875;V:171–87. Notes on the therapeutics of some affections of the nervous system. 1876;VI:252–65.	The mental aspects of ordinary disease. 1874–1875;20(October 1874):387–409.
Jackson,[b] John Hughlings	Observations on localisation of movements in the cerebral hemispheres, as revealed by cases of convulsion, chorea and "aphasia". 1873;III:175–95. On the anatomical, physiological, and pathological investigation of epilepsies. 1873;III:315–49. On a case of recovery from double optic neuritis. 1874;IV:24–29. On temporary mental disorders after epileptic paroxysms. 1875;V:105–29. On epilepsies and on the after effects of epileptic discharges (Todd and Robertson's hypothesis). 1876;VI:266–309.	Two cases of intra-cranial syphilis. 1874–1875;20(July 1874):235–43. Nervous symptoms in cases of congenital syphilis. 1874–1875;20(January 1875):517–27. On syphilitic affections of the nervous system. 1875–1876;21(July 1875):207–25.
Lawson, Robert	On the hourly distribution of mortality in relation to recurrent changes in the activity of vital functions. 1874;IV:240–64. On the physiological action of hyoscyamine. 1875;V:40–84. Hyoscyamine in the treatment of some diseases of the insane. 1876;VI:65–84. Clinical notes on conditions incidental to insanity. 1876;VI:120–49 [with W Bevan Lewis]	The epilepsy of Othello. 1880–1881;26(April 1880):1–11.

Lewis, William Bevan	On the histology of the great sciatic nerve in general paralysis of the insane. 1875;V:85–104.	A case of disseminated cerebral sclerosis. 1877–1878;23(January 1878):564–5.
	Calorimetric observations upon the influence of various alkaloids on the generation of animal heat. 1876;VI:43–64.	The physiological action of alcohol in its relationship to animal heat, and its influence upon the vaso-motor nervous system. 1880–1881;26(April 1880):20–31.
	Clinical notes on conditions incidental to insanity. 1876;VI:120–49 [with R Lawson]	Teachings of the sphygmograph in general paralysis of the insane. 1881–1882;27(April 1881):1–11.
Major, Herbert C.	On the minute structure of the cortical substance of the brain, in a case of chronic brain wasting. 1872;II:41–52.	Note on the histology of the human brain. 1875–1876;21(July 1875):276–7.
	A new method of determining the depth of the grey matter of the cerebral convolutions. 1872;II:157–76.	Observations on the brain of the Chacma Baboon. 1875–1876;21(January 1876):498–512.
	Observations on the histology of the brain in the insane. 1873;III:97–112.	Case of paralytic idiocy with right-sided hemiplegia; epilepsy; atrophy with sclerosis of the left hemisphere of the cerebrum and of the right lobe of the cerebellum. 1879–1880;25(July 1879):161–5.
	Observations on the histology of the morbid brain. 1874;IV:223–39.	Atrophy and sclerosis of the cerebellum occurring in a case of epileptic imbecility. 1882–1883;28 (January 1883):532–5.
	On the morbid histology of the brain in the lower animals. 1875;V:160–70.	
	The histology of the island of Reil. 1876;VI:1–10.	

(continued)

Table 6.5 (continued)

Author	Publications in *WRLAMR* Title. Year;volume:pages.	Publications in *Journal of Mental Science* Title. Year;volume(issue):pages.
McDowall, T.W.	On the power of perceiving colours possessed by the insane. 1873;III:129–52.	Asylum notes on scarlet fever. 1871–1872;17(July 1871):210–20. A medico-legal case. Reduction of will—George Pagan v. Janet Pagan or Ford and others. Abstract of the case, with remarks. 1871–1872;17(January 1872):590–613. American psychological literature. 1872–1873;18(April 1872):129–147. Cases in which mental derangement appeared in patients suffering from progressive muscular atrophy. 1872–1873;18(October 1872):390–7. 1. French retrospect. 1872–1873;18(October 1872):431–45. 2. American psychological literature. 1873–1874;19(April 1873):142–57. 2. American psychological retrospect. 1873–1874;19(July 1873):304–7. Antiquarian scraps relating to insanity. 1873–1874;19(October 1873):386–98. 2. French retrospect. 1873–1874;19(January 1874):618–9. 2. American retrospect. 1874–1875;20(April 1874):145–56. 2. French retrospect. 1875–1876;21(April 1875):118–39. 1. American psychological literature. 1876–1877;22(April 1876):142–51. I. French retrospect. 1876–1877;22(January 1877):614–28. Two cases of bearded women. 1877–1878;23(April 1877):86–8. 2. French retrospect. 1877–1878;23(April 1877):128–34. Annales Médico-Psychologiques, for 1876 and part of 1877. 1878–1879;24(April 1878):133. Extracts from 31st Report of the Commissioners in Lunacy. 1878–1879;24(July 1878):329–33. French retrospect. 1878–1879;24(January 1879):665–75. Erysipelas in asylums. 1878–1879;24(January 1879):694–7. French retrospect. 1879–1880;25(October 1879):418–29. Diffused cerebral sclerosis. 1879–1880;25(January 1880):490–4. 2. French retrospect. 1880–1881;26(July 1880):312–21. 2. French retrospect. 1880–1881;26(October 1880):422–28. Chorea in an aged person. 1881–1882;27(July 1881):201–3. 1. French retrospect. 1881–1882;27(January 1882):595–601. 2. French retrospect. 1882–1883;28(April 1882):112–24. 3. Italian retrospect. 1882–1883;28(October 1882):428–34.

Sutherland, Henry	Arachnoid cysts. 1871;I:218–32.	The asylums of Paris, in 1872. 1873–1874;19(April 1873):87–92.
	Menstrual irregularities and insanity. 1872;II:53–72.	Two cases of delusion as a premonitory symptom—in the one case not followed by insanity, and in the other followed by symptoms necessitating the detention of the patient in an asylum. 1877–1878;23(July 1877):248–9.
	The change of life, and insanity. 1873;III:299–314.	
	Cases on the borderland of insanity. 1876;VI:108–19.	
Thompson, George	The sphygmograph in lunatic asylum practice. 1871;I:58–70.	Clinical memoranda. 1873–1874;19(January 1874):565.
	The sphygmograph in epilepsy. 1872;II:302–6.	Clinical memoranda. A case of apoplectiform congestion of the brain. Death. Autopsy. 1874–1875;19(April 1874):94–6.
		On the physiology of general paralysis of the insane, and of epilepsy. 1874–1875 20(January 1875):579–86.
		On the physiology of general paralysis of the insane and of epilepsy. 1875–1876;21(April 1875):67–74.

[a]Crochley Clapham, a contributor to *WRLAMR*, also appeared as subject, but not author, of an anonymous "Notes and News" article in the *Journal of Mental Science* ([Anon.] The noble forehead. *J Ment Sci* 1881–1882; 27 (January 1882): 623–624). This publication was erroneously ascribed to Clapham by Harrington (1987:299)

[b]For Jackson's publications, I have followed the listing given by Greenblatt (2022:473–502) rather than by York and Steinberg (2006)

Only six authors contributed to all three journals (*WRLAMR*, *Brain*, and the *Journal of Mental Science*): Crichton-Browne, Hughlings Jackson, Milner Fothergill, Bevan-Lewis, Lawson, and Henry Clarke.

Unlike the first volume of *WRLAMR*, the first volume of *Brain* was reviewed in the pages of *The Practitioner*, which concluded that *Brain* "will afford pleasant reading and many suggestions both for speculative thought and clinical practice".[204]

Brain was adopted as the official journal of the Neurological Society of London in 1887.[205] As Crichton-Browne noted in his Presidential Address to the Society on 2nd February 1888, "the journal *Brain* had passed into their hands".[206] *Brain* has now survived for nearly 150 years and continues to rank amongst the most significant journals in the clinical neurosciences.

Discussion

As has been pointed out for other medical journals of the nineteenth century, so for the *West Riding Lunatic Asylum Medical Reports*, "…the daily routine which actually produced the finished product remains a mystery".[207] It would seem likely that, as for the other aspects of his superintendency of WRA (Chap. 3), Crichton-Browne had complete control as editor, in terms of commissioning, reviewing, rejecting, and publishing the papers therein, and hence why the journal folded immediately upon his departure from WRA. The visiting and/or collaborating staff who were invited to contribute to *WRLAMR* were mostly physicians, in contrast to the resident staff who were exclusively asylum doctors. Moreover, the visiting and invited contributors shared an orientation to a scientifically-based understanding of brain function and dysfunction (Ferrier, Milner Fothergill, Hughlings Jackson, Lauder Brunton). The published material often attempted the presentation of aggregate data rather than case reports (single, extended) or series, putting it (anachronisti-

---

[204] *The Practitioner* 1878;20:438–439 (Brain: a Journal of Neurology), quote at 439.

[205] See https://guarantorsofbrain.org/history/ (accessed 08/09/2024). Bynum (1985:96) stated: "In 1866 [*sic*], *Brain* passed over to the control of the Neurological Society of London, founded that year under the presidency of Hughlings Jackson". The date given was evidently a typographical error for 1886, the foundation date of the Neurological Society of London under the presidency of Hughlings Jackson (NB 15 years after first WRA medical *conversazione*) but it was not until the following year, 1887, that the Society took over the publication of *Brain* under the editorship of Armand de Watteville. Jellinek (2005:430) also erred with "The four handed over the tenth volume of *Brain* in 1889 [*sic*] to the new London Neurological Society [*sic*]".

[206] *Lancet* 1888;1:325–326 (18 February; Neurological Society of London); quote at 326.

[207] Bynum and Wilson (1992:44).

cally) higher in the hierarchy of evidence; certainly, the journal amounted to more than simply a "collection of anatomical researches".[208]

The naming of the journal merits some consideration. "*West Riding Lunatic Asylum Medical Reports*" was purely descriptive, and certainly not a catchy or necessarily very memorable name. Being a mouthful, the journal has been liable to misnaming, not only by posterity but also by contemporary reviewers and authors, even those publishing in it (see Table 6.6, wherein the word "lunatic" seems to be the element most often omitted; admittedly some of these writers may have been simply abbreviating). Of note, all but one of the contributors from the resident staff, be they currently in post or previously so, listed their affiliation as "West Riding Asylum," the sole exception ("West Riding Lunatic Asylum") being Merson (IV:63; but not in his other *WRLAMR* papers: V:1 and VI:85), although "lunatic asylum" was used in the title of one paper (Thompson, I:58). Perhaps there was some effort to avoid the use of the term "lunatic", possibly dictated by the editor, as it might be deemed pejorative. Certainly, the AMOAHI from the outset of its existence in 1841 had recommended abandoning the terms "Lunatic" and "Lunatic Asylum".[209] Hence the use of "Lunatic Asylum" in the name of the journal might seem paradoxical.[210]

Now defunct for approaching 150 years, it would not be surprising if many neurologists of today were unaware of *WRLAMR* and its relationship to *Brain*. Various opinions have been expressed regarding this relationship. For example, Oppenheim stated that "the earlier, little known journal paved the way for the later, famous one",[211] George and Trimble described *WRLAMR* as "little-known",[212] and George labelled it as "this obscure journal".[213] Ormerod stated that Ferrier's "publication was hidden in a journal that was virtually unknown to scientists".[214] Whilst it might be accepted that *WRLAMR* is little known to posterity, contemporary evidence suggests that, to the contrary, it was in fact well known in the field, with reviews appearing in many journals, both national and international (Table 6.2), and likewise citations of individual papers (Table 6.3). In this context, Ferrier's first *WRLAMR* article

---

[208] Russell (1983:283).

[209] Renvoize (1991:36).

[210] My speculation is that the journal's name was to some extent (i.e. "West Riding Lunatic Asylum") required by the Committee of Visitors if, as I think likely, they were involved in some way in the funding of the publication (disbursing money on behalf of the local ratepayers). See also, for a further example, the full title of each Annual *Report*.

[211] Oppenheim (1991:71).

[212] George and Trimble (1992:249).

[213] George (2020:278).

[214] Ormerod (2006:32).

Table 6.6 Some examples of misnaming of *WRLAMR* over 150 years

Year	Author	Incorrect journal title
1872	*Lancet* (1872;1:83)	*"Medical Reports of the West Riding Asylum"*
1873	Ferrier (1873a:457)	*"West Riding Asylum Reports"*
1873	*BMJ* 1873;1:541	*"Reports of the West Riding Asylum"*
1878	Ferrier (1878a:131)	*"West Riding Reports"*
1888	Leyland (1888;II:29,62)	*"West Riding Asylum Medical Reports"* and *"West Riding Lunatic Asylum Reports"* (but named correctly at 1888;II:63, 67).
1889	Bevan Lewis (1889:220, 229, 236, 262, 267, 286, 403, 471)	*"West Riding Asylum Medical Reports"* and *"West Riding Asylum Reports"*
1928	Sherrington (1928:ix and xv)	*"Reports of the West Riding Asylum"* and *"West Riding Medical Reports"*
1928	Bolton (1928:608)	*"West Riding Reports"*
1938	Easterbrook (1938:297)	*"West Riding Asylum Medical Reports"*
1939	Holmes (1939:520)	*"West Riding Asylum Reports"*
1960	Lennox and Lennox (1960:715)	*"West Riding Lunatic Asylum Report"*
1965	MacNalty (1965:249)	*"West Riding Asylum Reports"*
1985	Bynum (1985:96; also 1990:123)	*"Reports of the West Riding Asylum"*
1988	O'Connor (1988:192, 194)	*"West Riding Lunatic Asylum Reports"* and *"West Riding Asylum Reports [sic]"*
1992	Shepherd (1992:201)	*"Reports of the West Riding Asylum"*
1993	Sander et al. (1993:603 and 604)	*"Reports of the West Riding Lunatic Asylum"* and *"Rep West Riding Lunatic Asylum"*
1995	Goetz et al. (1995:356)	*"West Rinding [sic] Lunatic Asylum Medical Report"*
1996	Crammer (1996:220)	*"West Riding Annual Medical Reports"*
2004	Taylor/Walton (https://doi.org/10.1093/ref:odnb/34137)	*"West Riding Hospital Reports"*
2008	Bewley (2008:124)	*"West Riding Medical Reports"*
2009	Harris and Almerigi (2009:114)	*"West Riding Lunatic Asylum Reports, London"*
2010	Adams (2010:160)	*"Medical Reports"*
2013	Lazar (2013:97, 102)	*"West Riding Lunatic Asylum Reports"*
	Lazar (2013:101)	*"West Riding Lunatic Asylum Medical Report"*
2019	Shorvon and Compston (2019:133n12)	*"West Riding Lunatic Asylum Reports"* (but named correctly at 2019:140,291).
2022	Reynolds and Broussolle (2022:293)	*"Medical Reports of the West Riding Lunatic Asylum"*
	Reynolds and Broussolle (2022:294 Table 3)	*"Annual Reports of the West Riding Lunatic Asylum"*
2023	Sloffer (2023:9, 16, 19, 20 and n29, 32, 33, 55, 72)	*"West Riding Pauper Lunatic Asylum Medical Reports"*

NB: This does not claim to be a comprehensive listing (other examples may be seen in the titles of reviews in Table 6.2)

(III:30–96) gave the journal considerable profile. The same is probably also true of Hughlings Jackson's contributions.

One view of posterity is that *Brain* was similar to *WRLAMR* in its range of contents but was more international in outlook.[215] Finn's conclusion was that "The most obvious … legacy of the [West Riding] asylum's work … was the neurological journal *Brain*, which was essentially a continuation of the asylum's own *Reports*".[216]

Undoubtedly there were continuities between *WRLAMR* and *Brain*: as has been shown, many of the significant players in terms of editing and contributing played similar roles in both journals, and there was overlap of subject matter. But there were also important discontinuities. As has been shown, the content of *Brain* was more extensive and diverse than that of *WRLAMR*, in part because of the greater space available. But perhaps the most clearly manifest change was in the designation of *Brain* as "a journal of neurology", thus clearly distinguishing it from the constituency of asylum clinicians which *WRLAMR* had set out to serve. This point was also emphasized in the "News" item on the new journal which appeared in *Mind*. If Ferrier was, as per Sherrington's obituary account, the principal moving force in initiating *Brain*, then this emphasis may be easily explained. Thus, the opinion that "Ferrier, Crichton-Browne, John Bucknill and John Hughlings Jackson … rebranded *The West Riding Lunatic Asylum Medical Reports* [*sic*] into the journal *Brain*"[217] does not appear to be consistent with the evidence.

In the first volume of *WRLAMR*, having enunciated his plan to publish a volume annually, Crichton-Browne concluded his Preface:

in the fervent hope that the series may in some measure conduce to the relief of suffering, the advancement of science, and the credit of the medical profession. (I:v)

Over 150 years since its first publication, it might now be deemed reasonable to consider whether or not these aspirations were fulfilled.

The relief of suffering is extremely doubtful, unless viewed indirectly, since none of the treatments examined and advocated is still in clinical use, at least for the purposes espoused at WRA. As to the advancement of science, this certainly was fulfilled, both experimentally by Ferrier and clinically by Hughlings Jackson: their ideas regarding cortical localisation remain central

---

[215] Jellinek (2005:430).
[216] Finn (2012:193).
[217] George (2020:278).

to daily neurological practice and to neuroscientific research. (Admittedly Jackson's work was not pursued at WRA, and Ferrier's only initially so.) By this same token, one might argue that *WRLAMR* has contributed to the credit of the medical profession. In actuality, *WRLAMR* was a precondition for the emergence of *Brain*, the latter a consequence rather than merely a subsequence of the former, and hence a factor in the origins of British neurology.

WRLAMR was an avenue through which the work of WRA could be communicated to a national and an international audience. Other avenues to further this purpose were also available, at least in a more local manner: the dedicated medical meetings held at WRA, termed *conversazione*, which will be examined in Part IV.

7

Prosopography: Contributors to *WRLAMR*

The purpose of this chapter is to present an extended prosopography of the visiting and non-resident clinicians who contributed to *WRLAMR*, numbering ten in all. As for the resident clinical staff (described in Chap. 5), this approach presents an opportunity to examine the social origins, training, and subsequent career trajectories of these individuals (Table 7.1). Herein those who visited (or possibly visited) WRA to contribute to the work and/or research but whose principal appointments were elsewhere are considered. Those individuals who came only to lecture at the WRA medical *conversazione* are considered in Chap. 9; only two of these lecturers also contributed to *WRLAMR*, namely William Turner (III:1–29) and William Carpenter (IV:1–23). As in Chap. 5, the names used as headings for each section are those which appear in *WRLAMR* although one ("A.H. Rabagliati") is suspect, as addressed in the individual section (also Table 7.1).

Of the 38 contributors to *WRLAMR*,[1] the majority were from the resident clinical staff at WRA (26/38 = 68%) and of these some were amongst the most prolific contributors to the journal (viz. Crichton-Browne, Sutherland, Major, Lawson). Finn reported that 58/80 (= 73%) papers in *WRLAMR* came from officers or clerks of the asylum.[2] Of these contributors, all but one listed their affiliation to WRA, current or previous, as "West Riding Asylum", the exception being John Merson (IV:63) who used "West Riding Lunatic Asylum". The vast majority of contributions to *WRLAMR* were single author papers with only occasional exceptions, viz.: Nicol and Dove (I:233–251);

---

[1] Sloffer (2023:16).
[2] Finn (2012:80).

© The Author(s), under exclusive license to Springer Nature Switzerland AG 2026
A. J. Larner, *The West Riding Asylum and the Origins of British Neurology 1866-1876*,
https://doi.org/10.1007/978-3-032-12591-0_7

Table 7.1 Provisional "dating profile" of clinicians either contributing to *WRLAMR* and/or visiting WRA, 1867–1876 (compare with Table 5.1)

Name	Qualifications[a]	Dates at WRA	MPA	Papers in *WRLAMR* (Part III)	Attendance at *conversazione* (Part IV)[b]
Allbutt, Thomas Clifford	FRS 1880 FRCP 1884 FLS	1867, 1872, 1874, 1875	1896 (Hon)	II:203–222 III:273–284	1872, 1874, 1875
Browne, William A. F.		–		II:278–301	–
Ferrier, David	MD Edin 1870 FRS 1876 FRCP 1877	1873	1895 (Hon)	III:30–96 IV:30–62 V:24–39	1873
Milner Fothergill, J.				III:113–128 IV:94–151 V:171–187 VI:252–265	–
Jackson, John Hughlings	FRCP FRS 1878	–	1866 (Hon)	III:175–195 III:315–349 IV:24–29 V:105–129 VI:266–309	–
Brunton, Thomas Lauder	FRCP FRS 1874			IV:179–222	–
Browne, Lennox		1875		V:149–159 V:271–283	–
Sankey, H.R. Octavius		1875	1879	V:188–197	1875
Rabagliati, A.H. (?Andrea C. F. Rabagliati)	MB Edin 1869 MD Edin 1872 FRCSEd 1890	1875	–	VI:27–42	1875
Clarke, Henry	LRCP Lond	–	1879	VI:150–169	–

[a]Qualifications are as per entries in the *Medical Directory* 1867–1876 (rather than *WRLAMR* publications, which may differ); if no *Medical Directory* entry has been found, qualifications are as per details in notification of appointment in the medical press
[b]Only *conversazione* attendances with documentary confirmation are included (i.e. minimum attendance); no details on 1871 attendees available at time of writing

Lawson and Bevan-Lewis (VI:120–149); Clapham and Clarke (VI:150–169); and the "Medical Officers of the West Riding Asylum" (VI:232–251). The mechanics of co-authorship (i.e. specific contributions to authorship) are sometimes explicit, for example many of the eight sections in the paper by Lawson and Bevan-Lewis contain the first-person singular pronoun. This might also be the case with Nicol and Dove where a footnote (I:245), stated that "circumstances have prevented the writer [*sic*, singular] from completing at present this portion of the argument".[3]

One of Crichton-Browne's key innovations was to broaden the community of practitioners working at and/or associated with WRA by inviting external clinicians to work and/or lecture there. Many of these also published material in *WRLAMR*, numbering 12/38 contributors (= 32%) and 22/80 papers (= 27%), seven based on research undertaken at Wakefield.[4] Indeed, it is the contributions from the non-resident, external clinicians without staff appointments at WRA which have been deemed the most significant by posterity.[5] These individuals and their connections with WRA are now examined.

T. Clifford Allbutt (1836–1925)[6]

Thomas Clifford Allbutt was a Yorkshireman, born in Dewsbury, about 5 miles from Wakefield. One may therefore legitimately speculate that he had heard of or been aware of the asylum at Wakefield from his early years.[7] After his undergraduate career at Cambridge and his medical training at St. George's Hospital, London, he undertook postgraduate study in Paris in 1860–1861 with Duchenne de Boulogne[8] before returning to Yorkshire. By the mid-1860s, he was developing his career as a physician in Leeds, a few miles north-west of Wakefield, for example as Honorary Physician to the Leeds Public Dispensary (1864–1879).[9]

---

[3] My intimation here is that Nicol was the prime mover, based on the record of his other publications both in *WRLAMR* and elsewhere, and his interests in general medicine (see Chap. 5), whilst Dove was the junior partner; perhaps he collected data after Nicol's departure?

[4] Finn (2012:80).

[5] For example, George and Trimble (1992). I largely concur with this judgment, but unlike George and Trimble I would suggest that Ferrier's work is as significant in the domain of experimental physiology as was Hughlings Jackson's in the domain of clinical neurology, accepting that others may take a different view.

[6] For biographical material on Allbutt, there are to my knowledge two book-length biographies, by Rolleston (1929) and by Bearn (2007), as well as other shorter pieces, including: Leyland (1888:II:1–7), Underwood (1963), Cohen (1971), Todd and Ashworth (1991:394–396), Keynes and Butterfield (1993), Pearce (2003b), Rolleston, revised Bearn, https://doi.org/10.1093/ref:odnb/30382, Worboys (2007); Jacob and Larner (2013) (reprinted in adapted form in Larner (2019b:135–138)). Not all of these shorter publications mention his association with WRA.

[7] Wade (2016:125).

[8] Reynolds and Broussolle (2018).

[9] The Leeds Public Dispensary wall list of Chairmen, Honorary Physicians and Surgeons may be seen at the Thackray Museum, Leeds (author visit 17/01/2025).

Allbutt was perhaps the first non-resident "recruit", as opposed to "appointment", to WRA made by Crichton-Browne.[10] According to the latter's much later testimony, he first met Allbutt when "fresh from Cambridge and St. George's Hospital, he settled in Leeds": presumably the proximity of Leeds and Wakefield, and possibly co-attendance at local medical meetings in the West Riding, were the factors that brought Allbutt and Crichton-Browne together. Both men were then "young and eager, and so we joined forces and pushed on together. … I was able to afford him facilities for research".[11] Following Crichton-Browne's invitation, Allbutt attended patients at WRA "during the second half of 1867"[12] in order to undertake examinations with the ophthalmoscope. His stated purpose was to look for changes in retinal blood vessels in patients with general paralysis akin to those reported in the brain in patients dying with this disease. The ophthalmoscope was still a relatively new piece of equipment at this time, invented by Helmholtz in 1851,[13] and Allbutt, along with John Hughlings Jackson (*vide infra*) was one of the early advocates for its use in the assessment of patients. Furthermore, as George Thompson later noted, Allbutt's "not being resident in or near the asylum, and not, therefore, possessing a very intimate knowledge of the patients, their previous symptoms, and the effects of treatment", his observations could "only be regarded as a most valuable foundation upon which other observers may be encouraged to raise a superstructure" (I:72).[14]

Allbutt presented ophthalmological case material from WRA at a meeting of the Royal Medical and Chirurgical Society in London on Tuesday 25th February 1868, although the substantive paper published in the *Medico-Chirurgical Transactions* was reported to be "Received Dec. 4th 1867".[15] In this, and the related publications based on this presentation, Allbutt acknowledged making observations at WRA and thanked Crichton-Browne for his

---

[10] Viets (1938:478) erred in stating that Allbutt "had made his earliest studies at this same hospital a few years before Browne's [*sic*] time", referencing Allbutt (1868c). Jellinek (2005:428) stated that Allbutt was Crichton-Browne's "former Edinburgh near contemporary" but Rolleston's memoir of Allbutt has no mention of him being in Edinburgh in the late 1850s or early 1860s, indeed the only Edinburgh reference relates to Allbutt's visit to the Royal Medical Society in February 1906 (Rolleston 1929:175–176). Jellinek's description of a "former Edinburgh near contemporary" of Crichton-Browne would perhaps be more fitting for Ferrier or Lauder Brunton, although their times in Edinburgh did not overlap.

[11] Both quotations from Crichton-Browne (1931:242–243).

[12] Rolleston (1929:40). Probably based on Allbutt (1868a:100), where he stated that his "examinations were made at various dates during the second half of the year 1867".

[13] On Hermann von Helmholtz and the invention of the ophthalmoscope, see Sherman (1989), Larner (1994), Keeler (2002), Otis (2007a:124), Finkelstein (2013:123). On its possible arrival in Great Britain in 1852, see Larner (2025i).

[14] One might read this as an early acknowledgement of the importance of blinding in research assessments.

[15] Allbutt (1868a) was the substantive paper; Allbutt (1868b, c, d) are brief reports. Rolleston (1929:39) dated the meeting at the Royal Medical and Chirurgical Society as "February 22".

help. His results were presented in a series of tables, by diagnosis, and patients were identified by name, age, and disease status, alongside the ophthalmological findings. Allbutt "hoped that by means of the ophthalmoscope one more effort would be made finally to establish the study of insanity upon a positive basis"[16] and he was of the view that "A lunatic asylum is, in fact, a museum of cerebral diseases",[17] statements which were presumably music to the ears of Crichton-Browne who had "furnished the brief diagnostic remarks" to Allbutt. These studies contributed to Allbutt's monograph on the subject of ophthalmoscopy, published in 1871 and dedicated to Hughlings Jackson, in which he noted that "The number of physicians who are working with the ophthalmoscope in England may, I believe, be counted on the fingers of one hand".[18] Subsequently Charles Aldridge, Allbutt's pupil (Chap. 5), was to take up the cause of ophthalmoscopy at WRA (Chap. 6).[19] Their ophthalmoscopic observations in general paralysis were later referred to by Milner Fothergill (III:121; *vide infra*).

Allbutt's original description of syphilitic periarteritis of the cerebral arteries in a patient with general paralysis was published in 1868 and, as noted by his biographer,[20] this finding was based on a specimen sent to him from WRA by Crichton-Browne. However, it was not until over 50 years later (1921) that Allbutt publicly acknowledged the source of his pathological material.[21]

As he had already worked at WRA, it was perhaps inevitable that Allbutt would contribute to *WRLAMR* following its inception in 1871. He was the author of two papers. The first of these, "The electric treatment of the insane" (II:203–222), has a slightly apologetic air, Allbutt admitting that he suggested the idea originally but acknowledging that the clinical work had been done by

---

[16] At time of writing [2023] there is contemporary resonance with trying to establish the diagnosis of functional neurological disorders on a positive basis, rather than by a process of exclusion, although it is not entirely clear whether or not the latter inference was implied by Allbutt here.

[17] Allbutt (1868c:328). Also Allbutt (1868a:98), "a hospital for lunatics is, speaking generally, a museum of cerebral diseases". In an earlier review co-authored by Allbutt, published in January 1868, some comments on the value of ophthalmoscopy in insanity were made (Allbutt and Teale 1868:146–148).

[18] Allbutt (1871a) (quotation at 9). His monograph was reviewed in *The Practitioner* 1871;7:362; *Lancet* 1872;1:14–15; *Br Foreign Med Chir Rev* 1872;49:429–447; *Birmingham Medical Review* 1872;1:50–56.

[19] Aldridge repeated Allbutt's judgment, "that the number of physicians who are in the habit of using the ophthalmoscope can be counted on the fingers of one hand" (IV:291–292).

[20] Rolleston (1929:258). Allbutt (1868e) did not mention either WRA or Crichton-Browne, nor did a supplementary note on this paper which appeared 4 years later (Allbutt 1872).

[21] Allbutt (1921:182), wherein he stated "When in 1868 I first described syphilitic arteritis, with dispersed granuloma, in the brain, it was in a specimen sent to me by Dr. (Sir) Crichton-Browne from the Wakefield Asylum". Discussing the changes in capillaries and minute arteries in general paralysis of the insane, Thompson (I:63) did not reference Allbutt's 1868 paper.

resident officers at WRA, principally Herbert Major.[22] Allbutt found the results to be disappointing (others, working elsewhere, reported a more positive outcome in occasional patients[23]). Allbutt's second *WRLAMR* paper, "On the obscurer neuroses of syphilis" (III:273–284) was written "in obedience to the kind insistence of my friend Dr. Crichton Browne" and featured cases "taken entirely from my own books, with the exception of some few which have come before me at the [Leeds] Infirmary".[24] The "neuroses" discussed included "intellectual and emotional disorders", "sleeplessness", "motor defects" and "neuralgia".

Allbutt's association with Crichton-Browne and WRA persisted beyond his clinical work. For example, he is recorded as being present at the medical *conversazione* (see Chap. 8) held in October 1872, November 1874, and November 1875, and was probably present in 1873.[25] He was present at the banquet honouring Crichton-Browne on his departure from Wakefield, held in April 1876.[26] He later published works in *Brain*, including in the inaugural issue of April 1878 (Table 6.5).

Crichton-Browne was instrumental in Allbutt's appointment as a Commissioner in Lunacy in 1889,[27] in which context Allbutt gave evidence to the Committee of the London County Council initiated by Brudenell Carter (see Chap. 9) to investigate the possibilities of a hospital, as opposed to an asylum, for the treatment of insanity in London.[28]

Allbutt was elected a Fellow of the Royal Society (FRS) in 1880, Fellow of the Royal College of Physicians of London (FRCP) in 1883, and was appointed its Goulstonian Lecturer the following year. He was an original member of the Neurological Society of London (1886). His career culminated as Regius Professor of Physic in the University of Cambridge, appointed

---

[22] Allbutt's suggestion was perhaps prompted by his treatment of other conditions with electricity (e.g. *BMJ* 1871;1:642–643) and his review of "electro-therapy" published in July 1871 (Allbutt 1871b). The *WRLAMR* paper was not referenced by Rolleston (1929) in his biography.

[23] Williams (1873).

[24] This paper was mentioned by Rolleston (1929:64) and also in a review of Buzzard's (1874) book on syphilis in *Medical Times and Gazette* 1874;1:543 (16th May).

[25] For 1872: *BMJ* 1872;2:474–475 (26th October; Medical Conversazione at the West Riding Asylum). For 1874: *Medical Times and Gazette* 1874;2:609–610 (28th November; Annual Conversazione at the West Riding Asylum). For 1875: *BMJ* 1875;2:680 (27th November; The West Riding Asylum). For 1873: *Yorkshire Post and Leeds Intelligencer* 27th November 1873, p.3 (West Riding Asylum. Medical Conversazione).

[26] *BMJ* 1876;1:516 (22nd April; Dr. Crichton Browne). *Yorkshire Post and Leeds Intelligencer*, 19th April 1876, p.3 (Presentations to Dr. Crichton Browne).

[27] Rolleston (1929:95–97). See also: *Biographies of Medical Lunacy Commissioners 1828–1912*, http://studymore.org.uk/6biom.htm#M17 (accessed 09/12/2023).

[28] Shorvon and Compston (2019:342–344). Neither Rolleston (1929) nor Bearn (2007) mentioned this episode in their biographies of Allbutt.

in 1892. However, it was not until 1896 that he became an Honorary Member of the Medico-Psychological Association (MPA). He was editor of the eight-volume *A System of Medicine* which appeared between 1896 and 1899 which included amongst its contributors Bevan-Lewis (Chap. 5), Ferrier (*vide infra*), and Brudenell Carter (Chap. 9). He was an "enthusiastic advocate" of plans to develop the Diploma of Psychological Medicine at the University of Cambridge in the late 1900s.[29]

William A. F. Browne (1805–1885)[30]

One might speculate as to what combination of filial request and parental obligation prompted William Alexander Francis Browne, by then aged 67, to contribute to the second volume of *WRLAMR*, the moreso in light of the fact that he had reportedly lost his eyesight at the age of 65 as the consequence of a carriage accident.[31] Nevertheless, despite the necessity of resigning from his duties as a Lunacy Commissioner in Scotland, he still frequently contributed articles to the medical literature. His paper in the second volume of *WRLAMR*, published in 1872, may have been one of the first composed after his loss of vision.

After he qualified in medicine from Edinburgh, where he knew Charles Darwin during the latter's abortive medical studies, William Browne visited Paris in the summer and autumn of 1832 where he studied under Esquirol at Charenton and Pariset at the Salpêtrière. On his return to Scotland he became the superintendent of the Montrose Royal Lunatic Asylum, the first such institution to be founded in Scotland (first patient admitted in May 1782), and it was there in 1837 that he delivered the lectures which were later published as *What asylums were, are, and ought to be: being the substance of five lectures delivered before the managers of the Montrose Royal Lunatic Asylum.*[32] Thanks to the philanthropy of Elizabeth Crichton (1779–1862), William

---

[29] Crammer (1996:221). For possible links between Allbutt and the character of Dr. Tertius Lydgate in George Eliot's novel *Middlemarch*, see Schneck (1970), Larner (2025b).

[30] Biographical material on W.A.F. Browne may be found in his obituary in *J Ment Sci* 1885–1886;31(April 1885):149–150; also, Harper (1955), Williams (1989:19–28), Oppenheim (1991:54–57), Renvoize (1991:48–49), Scull et al. (1996:84–122); Scull, https://doi.org/10.1093/ref:odnb/46958.

[31] *J Ment Sci* 1870; 16(July 1870):247–249 (The Scotch Lunacy Commission: the resignation of Dr. W.A.F. Browne). This announcement directly followed an article by his son: Balfour Browne (1870–1871). His youngest son, Vincent De Paul, had died on 1st February 1870 in Liverpool, aged 22 (*BMJ* 1870;1:197). Whether this was relevant to his subsequent resignation is not apparent. Reference to his "failing sight" may also be found in *BMJ* 1870;1:557 (28th May; The Lunacy Board).

[32] Browne (1837).

Browne was enabled to put his principles into practice at the newly founded Crichton Royal Institution in Dumfries (where his son, James, grew up; see Chap. 5). He introduced occupational, recreational and social therapy (e.g. theatricals, concerts, and a monthly magazine produced by the patients[33]) at the Crichton in the 1840s. In 1857 he was appointed the first Medical Commissioner in Lunacy in Scotland and in 1866 was President of the MPA.

William Browne's paper in *WRLAMR* was entitled "Impairment of language, the result of cerebral disease" (II:278–301), hence not obviously related to the subjects for which he had made his name and reputation, although he had published on the subject of "Derangements of the faculty of language" in 1833.[34] Having been a committed phrenologist early in his career, both in Edinburgh and Montrose,[35] the resurgence of interest in cerebral localisation of function occasioned by Broca's 1861 report of "aphemia" (probably equivalent to the later nomenclature of "aphasia") as a consequence of a focal brain lesion was therefore likely to be of interest to Browne. Indeed, this was a "hot topic", pertinent to debates on cortical localisation which were shortly to become a matter for experimental investigation at WRA. Browne's phrenological sympathies were perhaps evident in his opening reference to Gall (II:278), and to publications in the *Phrenological Journal*, which was mentioned twice (II:288, 292), but he also referred to the work of "Darx" (presumably Marc Dax, and/or his son Gustave Dax, possible forerunners of Paul Broca in the cerebral localisation of language function to the left hemisphere[36]). Internal evidence from Browne's paper suggests that he may have seen patients at WRA, as therein he mentioned patients "in this hospital" (II:282) or explicitly "in the West Riding Asylum" (II:284, 293, 299).[37]

Browne concluded that:

---

[33] Tait (1972:182). Crichton-Browne (1926:225–226) recounted a story about an actor receiving a rapturous reception when performing at the Theatre Royal, Dumfries, only to be told that "the doctor at the neighbouring asylum takes a part of the house and these ladies and gentlemen who have given you so good a reception are all lunatics". I presume the doctor in question to have been William Browne.

[34] Browne (1833). This *Lancet* paper was footnoted "Condensed from the *Phrenological Journal*, June 1833", but I have not been able to find the latter.

[35] Cooter (1976a:5), although in his lectures (Browne 1837) he barely mentioned phrenology, as noted by Cooter (1976a:19).

[36] For accounts of Dax, *père et fils*, and their works, see Harrington (1987:45–47), Leblanc (2017:87–96).

[37] "… the following passage, taken down from the lips of a patient in the West Riding Asylum, 3rd December, 1868" (II:293) as an exemplification of the symptom of the "fabrication of new words, which are known in asylums as jargons" and "having a vague resemblance to Greek" was also reported by Crichton-Browne (1926:59–60) but the two transcriptions are not identical. The jargon also appeared, verbatim, in an article entitled "My friend the mad-doctor" published in Dickens's journal *All the year round* in September 1873 (Anon 1873:473). Horniblow, the titular "mad-doctor", has previously been identified as Crichton-Browne (e.g. Neve and Turner 1995:406; Finn 2012:1–2) but without reference to this particular passage, which I have suggested makes the identification certain (Larner 2025e).

It must be confessed that the physiological and pathological evidence as to the localization of an organ for such a faculty [language] is as yet incomplete or contradictory, although it may be admitted that the weight both of scientific research, and scientific opinion preponderate in favour of the conclusion that some part of the anterior lobes, and perhaps some part of the orbital region, are connected with the formation and expression of articulate signs of thought. (II:300)

William Browne was the most pre-eminent "name" yet to have contributed to *WRLAMR*, thereby broadening the range of contributors to what had hitherto been essentially a house journal, albeit one which had already been noted in various reviews in medical journals (see Table 6.2). His *WRLAMR* paper was later cited by Thomas Laycock.

Browne later loaned material to the WRA medical *conversazione* of 1872, which was also attended by his son, J.H. Balfour Browne, a barrister with interests in the legal aspects of insanity (Chap. 9). William Browne also loaned a number of drawings by insane patients for display at the WRA *conversazione* of 1875.[38] Browne's work on the mental condition of epileptics was cited by Hughlings Jackson (*vide infra*) in his final *WRLAMR* paper (VI:304).

David Ferrier (1843–1928)[39]

David Ferrier (Fig. 7.1) was 30 years old in 1873 when he went to WRA to undertake a programme of experimental animal research,[40] at which time he held the positions of Professor of Forensic Medicine at King's College London

---

[38] For 1872: *Medical Press and Circular* 1872;14:360 (23rd October; Conversazione and lecture by Professor Turner). For 1875: *Medical Times and Gazette* 1875;2:603 (27th November; Conversazione at the West Riding Asylum).

[39] To my knowledge there is no full-length biography of Ferrier but there are numerous shorter pieces, one dating to his lifetime: Leyland (1888:II:61–67); other sources include, but are not limited to, Spillane (1974a:701–706, 1981:387–399), Horwitz (1994); Wade (2000:v–vi), Pearce (2003c), Sherrington, revised Bevan, https://doi.org/10.1093/ref:odnb/33117, Lock (2007), Sandrone and Zanin (2014), Akkermans (2016), Shorvon and Compston (2019:139–145). This section is based in part on Larner (2023c, 2025j), and ongoing work by the author on a projected biography of Ferrier, e.g. Larner (2023d), (reprinted in adapted form in Larner (2025k)), (2024d, 2025l), Bone and Larner (2024), Larner and Griffiths (2025).

[40] Finn and Stark were in error when stating that "In March 1873, David Ferrier, a 26-year old physician" (2015:14). I am assuming here, like Finn and Stark, that Ferrier first went to WRA in 1873, although in a lecture on hemiplegic epilepsy delivered in 1881 Seguin spoke of "Ferrier's researches upon the cortex of the brain, made in 1872 and 1873" (Seguin 1881:50). I wonder if this reference to 1872 might be a consequence of the misdating of Ferrier's initial paper in the commentary by Bowditch (1873:79) as "British Medical Journal, 26th April, 1872 [*sic*]". Viets (1938:481) stated that "Ferrier … did his work at West Riding in the spring of 1875 [*sic*]", but I think it can be accepted that this was a typographical error

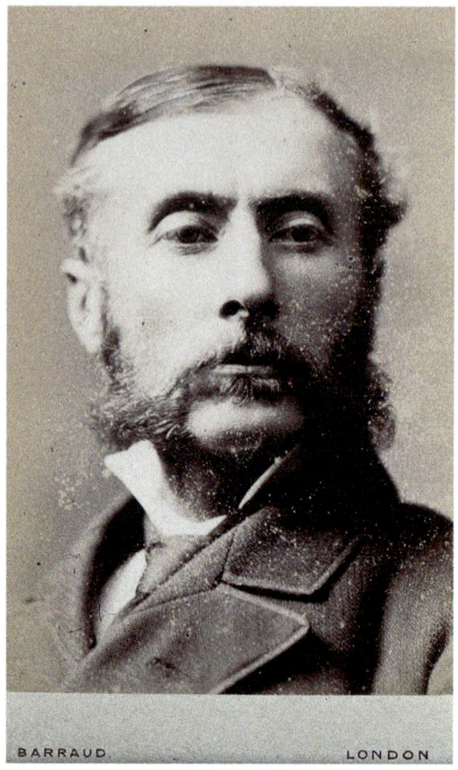

Fig. 7.1 David Ferrier

and Junior Physician to the West London Hospital, both appointments dating from 1872.[41]

His first university experience had been in his hometown of Aberdeen where he studied philosophy and classics (MA 1863)[42] and came under the influence of Alexander Bain (1818–1903).[43] He then spent some time in

---

as Viets also described Ferrier, correctly, as "a man of 30" and stated that "his famous paper, 'Experimental Researches in Cerebral Physiology and Pathology,' was published in the *Medical Reports* [*sic*] for that year, the third volume issued", hence evidently 1873.

[41] These appointments were noted respectively in *Medical Press and Circular* 1872;13:174 (28th February; Medical News), which called him "Dr. David Ferries [*sic*]"; and *Medical Press and Circular* 1872;14:428 (13th November; Appointments). Henry Maudsley was appointed physician to the West London Hospital in 1864 (Walk 1976:16) and "Consulting Physician to the West London Hospital, Hammersmith", in June 1873 (*Medical Press and Circular* 1873;15:524 (11th June; Appointments)). I have no information as to whether or not Ferrier and Maudsley ever interacted there.

[42] Johnston (1906:163).

[43] Bain's work also influenced Hughlings Jackson (VI:272). For Bain, see Young (1970:101–133).

Germany, at the University of Heidelberg,[44] possibly at Bain's suggestion, returning to study medicine at Edinburgh University (1865–1868). One of his teachers in physiology may have been William Rutherford (1839–1899).[45] After graduation with first class honours, Ferrier was assistant to Thomas Laycock, his notes being used for publications in the *BMJ* describing some of Laycock's treatments.[46] After a period in general practice with Dr William Edmund Image (1807–1903) in Bury St. Edmunds in Suffolk, which afforded him sufficient time to write an M.D. thesis ("The comparative anatomy and intimate structure of the corpora quadrigemina") which won the Edinburgh gold medal in 1870,[47] Ferrier moved to London where he worked with the experimental physiologist John Burdon Sanderson (1828–1905).[48] After a brief appointment at the Middlesex Hospital, Ferrier moved to King's College Hospital in 1871, initially as Assistant-Demonstrator of Practical Physiology in the Department led at that time by William Rutherford.[49] Early in his London career he became acquainted with John Hughlings Jackson (*vide infra*) and was influenced by his views on cerebral pathology.[50]

How and precisely when Ferrier became involved with WRA is, to my knowledge, unknown. Perhaps he knew Crichton-Browne through their Edinburgh links (although they did not overlap at the University[51]), or perhaps through Jackson, and/or through Laycock. Another possible conduit

---

[44] To my knowledge this biographical detail first appeared in Leyland (1888:II:61) and has been repeated in most subsequent biographical pieces. Leyland dated this visit as "1854", undoubtedly a typographical error for "1864".

[45] Rutherford (1873:392) described Ferrier as "my former pupil"; he was teaching classes in practical physiology in Edinburgh between 1865 and 1869.

[46] The publications are *BMJ* 1869;1:9 and *BMJ* 1869;2:8. Further details on Ferrier as Laycock's assistant as recalled by an Edinburgh contemporary may be found in Bramwell (1923:134, 145–146) (Bramwell's paper was reprinted in Ashworth (1986:61–77), Ferrier references at 62, 70).

[47] *Alphabetical list of graduates of the University of Edinburgh …*, 1879:37, 128.

[48] Ferrier described experiments performed with Burdon Sanderson in: *Medical Times and Gazette* 1871;2:229; *BMJ* 1871;2:223 (19th August); and *BMJ* 1873;1:429–430 (19th April). Burdon Sanderson also observed one of Ferrier's later monkey experiments (Ferrier 1875a:447). Hence the claim by Star (1989:57) that "Burdon-Sanderson [*sic*] hired Ferrier to come to London to do physiological experiments *after* his early work at the West Riding asylum" [my italics] is incorrect. Ditto Lazar (2013:96n2) with "John Burdon-Sanders (1829–1905)".

[49] Hence Ferrier was now Rutherford's "able colleague" (Rutherford 1873:392; see also Rutherford et al. 1872). Lauder Brunton (*vide infra*) referred to "My friend, Professor Rutherford" (IV:184). Like Ferrier, Lauder Brunton was a student of Laycock in Edinburgh according to Hollander (1921:405). Rutherford was not mentioned in the work on Laycock by James (1996).

[50] Ferrier (1892:884).

[51] *Contra* Sander et al. (1993:603) who claimed that "Crichton-Browne … qualified in Edinburgh with David Ferrier", despite also acknowledging that Ferrier qualified in 1868 and Crichton-Browne was appointed WRA superintendent in 1866! These authors also claimed that it was at "the West Riding Asylum in Wakefield where all three [Hughlings Jackson, Ferrier and Crichton-Browne] originally met" (Sander et al. 1993:602).

between Ferrier and Crichton-Browne was Milner Fothergill (*vide infra*). Various accounts have been published, and these are presented here chronologically.

According to Leyland, to my knowledge the only contemporary source, Crichton-Browne invited Ferrier to contribute a paper to *WRLAMR*, which began his experimental researches.[52] All the other accounts from those who knew Ferrier are retrospective. For example, in his obituary of Ferrier, Charles Sherrington (1857–1952) stated that:

> In March 1873, when he [Ferrier] was paying a visit to his friend and fellow Edinburgh graduate, Dr. (now Sir) James Crichton-Browne, then Director of the West Riding Asylum, Wakefield, conversation turned upon the excitability under galvanism of part of the cerebral surface of the dog as reported from the Continent by Fritsch and Hitzig [1870]. There followed, during the course of the spring and summer of 1873, in the laboratory recently founded at the Asylum … the memorable experiments with which Ferrier opened his detailed systematic exploration by faradic stimulation of all parts of the central nervous system in representative types of vertebrate from the lowest to the highest.[53]

Certainly, Ferrier had been aware of Fritsch and Hitzig's paper, in which they described galvanic stimulation of the dog cerebral cortex and showed that particular movements were associated with particular cortical locations (centres),[54] as early as 1871 since he had reviewed it in a publication in the *Journal of Anatomy and Physiology*[55] (he was presumably fluent in German as a consequence of his time in Heidelberg).[56]

It is also the case that Crichton-Browne had speculated on the nature of faradic stimulation prior to Ferrier's arrival at WRA:

---

[52] Leyland (1888:II:62).

[53] Sherrington (1928:ix). Sherrington's reference to the highest types of vertebrates might give the erroneous impression that Ferrier worked on primates at WRA, but this was not the case.

[54] Fritsch and Hitzig (1870). Peculiarly, Brazier (1961:6) dated this paper as "1871". Translations: Von Bonin (1960:73–96), Fritsch and Hitzig (1963, 2009). Commentaries: Wilkins (1963), Young (1970:224–233), Carlson and Devinsky (2009).

[55] Fraser et al. (1871:396). Lauder Brunton (*vide infra*) co-authored this part of the paper with Ferrier. This publication was noted by Lazar (2009) in his examination of the influence of the papers by Hitzig and by Ferrier on Anglo-American publications on cerebral physiology in the early 1870s. Greenblatt (2022:165) appeared unaware of Ferrier's 1871 publication since he wrote that "we would also like to know when he [Ferrier] knew about Fritsch and Hitzig, since he might have been a conduit for such information to Jackson, but there's no clear evidence for Ferrier's knowledge of it until the spring of 1873". The evidence is in fact clear that Ferrier had knowledge of the Fritsch and Hitzig paper in early 1871, 2 years earlier than Greenblatt stated.

[56] According to Purves-Stewart (1939:44), Ferrier had acquired a knowledge of German language and literature during his time there.

The nature of the change, which concussion, thus operating, induces in the vesicular neurine, can only be a subject of speculation, but it seems highly probable that it is analogous to that which the Faradic stimulus has been shown to establish in certain tissues, when it places them in a state of physiological activity. No structural alteration is effected; but a modification of condition and relation is introduced amongst the existing elements. (II:122)

Nearly 30 years after Ferrier's death, MacNalty stated that "The suggestion of this work came to Ferrier from that great pioneer in neurological research Sir James Crichton-Browne, as both Sir David Ferrier and Sir James informed me".[57] This was also nearly 20 after Crichton-Browne's death, so may be open to some doubts. Whilst I am inclined to give some credence to MacNalty's witness account, I doubt Crichton-Browne knew about Fritsch and Hitzig's paper,[58] whereas Ferrier certainly did. Moreover, Ferrier already had first-hand experience of laboratory research (with Burdon Sanderson) whereas there is no evidence that Crichton-Browne previously did. Perhaps Ferrier had discussed the paper with Crichton-Browne and his ideas to pursue similar research, time and place unknown, which then prompted Crichton-Browne to offer the resources of the WRA laboratory.

Modern commentators have slightly different accounts of how and when Ferrier found his way to WRA. For example, Millett stated that:

> Ferrier and Crichton-Browne had been classmates in Edinburgh, and saw each other regularly during the early 1870s, as Crichton-Browne organized a number of informal meetings or conversaziones at West Riding for the discussion of various neurological and physiological topics.[59]

However, they did not overlap at the University (Crichton-Browne 1857–1862; Ferrier 1865–1868)[60] and I know of no evidence (see Chap. 8) for Ferrier's attendance at the *conversaziones* of 1871 or 1872.

---

[57] MacNalty (1957:912).

[58] Finn (2012:139) stated of Fritsch and Hitzig that "it took a little while for their findings to spread around Europe, reaching Crichton-Browne's table only at a later date", i.e. unspecified. I would suggest that Ferrier may well have been the person who brought these findings to Crichton-Browne's "table".

[59] Millett (1998:286–287). Millett did not cite any primary source(s) to support this account. Lazar (2013:96) appears to have followed Millett's formulation. Barclay (1992:17) described Crichton-Browne as "a friend of David Ferrier from their medical student days in Edinburgh", an impossibility, as previously noted.

[60] I wonder whether the erroneous belief that Crichton-Browne and Ferrier were classmates, or qualified together (as per Sander et al. 1993:603), might have originated in descriptions of them as former fellow students of Dr. Laycock (Hollander 1921:406–407) or fellow Edinburgh graduates (Sherrington 1928:ix) or even simply as fellow Scotsmen.

Finger stated that:

The turning point in Ferrier's life occurred when *he decided* to visit Crichton-Browne in Yorkshire. The two physicians were eager to see each other and talked about many things, including the Fritsch and Hitzig experiments. Both Scots saw the work of the Germans on the motor cortex as a landmark, and both also saw several reasons to follow it up. Crichton-Browne then made Ferrier an offer he could not refuse. He told him that he would give him everything he needed if he would conduct the same sort of experimentation at his West Riding institution.[61]

Macmillan reported that Ferrier's reason for going to WRA was "because facilities for experimental physiological work throughout Britain, including those at King's, were then almost nonexistent". According to this account, "At the beginning of March 1873, scarcely 2 months after commencing his experiments, … Ferrier had mastered the method's very considerable technical difficulties".[62] Macmillan thus placed Ferrier at WRA from January 1873, *contra* Sherrington.

Finn stated that:

Late in 1872 [*sic*], when Crichton-Browne's good friend and fellow Scotsman Ferrier visited Wakefield for the annual conversazione, the two talked about many things, and Fritsch and Hitzig's results were chief among them. … Crichton-Browne … thus invited Ferrier back in March to conduct more electrical experiments in rooms of the asylum.[63]

Whether proactive or reactive, the accounts of Finger and of Finn are essentially speculative, in the absence of any citation of definitive evidence.[64] Likewise, there is no evidence to say whether Ferrier resided at WRA

---

[61] Finger (2000:162) [my italics]. Finger did not cite any primary source(s) to support this account.

[62] Macmillan (2000:183).

[63] Finn (2012:139). Finn referenced Finger (2000:162), and Young (1970:234–236), but I find no mention of Ferrier attending the 1872 *conversazione* in either of these sources. In the extant accounts of the 1872 WRA *conversazione* appearing in both the medical and local popular press, Ferrier's name does not appear (see Chap. 8), but of course absence of evidence is not necessarily evidence of absence. The "List of the gentlemen invited" published in the report of the *conversazione* which appeared in the *Leeds Mercury* (17th October 1872, p.8) did not include Ferrier's name. Sloffer (2023:9) repeated Finn's account and said it was "taken largely from Robert Young's description", referenced as Young (1970:238).

[64] I do not, of course, rule out the possibility that I have overlooked other sources confirming these accounts. For another (evidence-free) suggestion, is it possible that Ferrier might have heard about WRA from King's College graduates who had worked there, such as Charles Henry Mayhew or George Henry Pedler (see Chap. 5)? Certainly, Pedler was still in London, at Trevor Terrace, although this is about a 45-min walk from Ferrier's 1872 address at Portman Square.

throughout the Spring of 1873 or, as reported by Crammer, "came regularly to Wakefield (by train)".[65]

Suffice it to say that by March, or at the latest April, 1873 Ferrier was working in the laboratory at WRA, both according to his own first account of his work, published 26th April 1873,[66] and the contemporary notes of others. In a letter to Charles Darwin dated 16th April 1873, Crichton-Browne stated:

> Professor Ferrier of King's College has *just completed* an experimental investigation in my pathological laboratory which cannot fail to interest you and which must have an incalculable bearing on your views. By exposing the brains of living animals, under chloroform, and stimulating the cerebral grey matter by an electric current from Du Bois Reymond's [induction] coil he has discovered that every convolution of the brain is in direct relation with certain groups of muscles, and controls their actions. ... Professor Ferrier's researches which are to be published in the next volume of West Riding Asylum Medical Reports [*sic*] in July, will I believe constitute the most important advances yet made in cerebral physiology.[67]

Milner Fothergill, a colleague of Ferrier's (*vide infra*), stated in 1874 that Ferrier "commenced at Wakefield Asylum last Easter".[68] Thus, it appears that Ferrier spent in all only about 1 month at WRA pursuing his initial animal experiments.[69]

Whenever the exact starting date for Ferrier's work at WRA, the first published report of his findings, appearing in the *BMJ*, commenced thus:

> The opportunity kindly afforded me by Dr Crichton Browne, of experimenting on over thirty guinea-pigs, rabbits, cats, and dogs, in the pathological laboratory of the West Riding Asylum, Wakefield, has enabled me to arrive at certain results and conclusions which seem worthy of a brief preliminary notice, pending the publication of details of method, experiments, and illustrations, in the West Riding Asylum Reports [*sic*].[70]

---

[65] Crammer (1996:219).

[66] Ferrier (1873a).

[67] Darwin Correspondence Project, "Letter no. 8861," https://www.darwinproject.ac.uk/letter/?docId=letters/DCP-LETT-8861.xml (accessed 22/01/23) [my italics].

[68] Milner Fothergill (1874:77). Easter Day in 1873 fell on 13th April. Although Milner Fothergill might be referring to the Easter period, it is difficult to imagine that this could extend back to March, unless he meant the whole of Lent.

[69] Hence, I agree on this point with Finn (2012:161), as reflected in the title of Larner (2023c).

[70] Ferrier (1873a). Thornton (1976:28) erred when writing of "the experiments of David Ferrier made in the laboratory of the West Riding Lunatic Asylum where, working on rabbits, dogs and *monkeys* ..." [my italics]. Could Sherrington's account (1928:ix) have been the source for this error?

Listing 12 "important conclusions", and taking up less than a column of print, this paper summarised Ferrier's experimental findings which were subsequently reported in more detail in his *WRLAMR* paper (III:30–96), illustrated by WRA Clinical Assistant John Galton (see Chap. 5). There were further public presentations later in the year, including at the meetings of the British Medical Association in London (8th August)[71] and the British Association for the Advancement of Science in Bradford (19th September),[72] culminating at the WRA *conversazione* in November (Chap. 8);[73] also publications, for example in the *Journal of Anatomy and Physiology*.[74] The findings established the principle of cerebral localisation as physiological fact rather than, as previously, phrenological speculation and served to confirm the views of Hughlings Jackson on the pathology of epilepsy as a discharging lesion.[75]

Hughlings Jackson speedily responded to Ferrier's initial report, his publication appearing in the *BMJ* of 10th May,[76] and further responses from Jackson were to follow later in the year,[77] although his first reference to Ferrier's *WRLAMR* paper did not appear until December.[78]

By the time of his publication in *WRLAMR*, which appeared in late July or early August 1873,[79] the focus of Ferrier's experimental work had moved to

---

[71] *BMJ* 1873;2:241 (23rd August); *Medical Record* 1873;8:507 ("Experiments upon the brain").

[72] *Lancet* 1873;2:459 (27th September); *Lancet* 1873;2:503–504 (4th October); *Medical Press and Circular* 1873;16:275 (24th September); *Medical Times and Gazette* 1873;2:357–358 (27th September); *The Examiner* 1873;Issue 3426:966–967 (27th September); *Boston Medical and Surgical Journal* 1873;89(17):419 (23rd October [from *Dublin Medical Press and Circular*]).

[73] *Lancet* 1873;2:788 (29th November); *Medical Times and Gazette* 1873;2:625 (29th November).

[74] Ferrier (1873b). According to Greenblatt (2022:514) this paper was "published in 1874". For details of Ferrier's presentations and publications in 1873, see Larner (2023c, 2025j).

[75] Young (1970:234–248).

[76] Jackson (1873b). See also *BMJ* 1873;1:541–542 (Dr. Ferrier's researches on the functions of the brain). In his discussion of Hughlings Jackson's paper, Greenblatt (2022:166–168) surmised that it showed Jackson clearly had prior knowledge of Ferrier's primate results, suggesting that the two men were in contact at this time.

[77] These further comments by Hughlings Jackson on Ferrier's work appeared in Jackson (1873c), (III:175).

[78] Jackson (1873d), which speaks of "Ferrier's masterly article" (840). Most of Hughlings Jackson's 1873 responses to Ferrier's work are discussed in Larner (2025j).

[79] For this latter dating, see Ferrier (1874a:399). Lazar (2013:97n3) suggested June 1873, because of Ferrier's footnote (III:89n2; *vide infra*).

London[80] where he conducted similar experiments on monkeys.[81] These studies were undertaken with funding from the Royal Society, and in due course were reported there in Ferrier's Croonian Lectures for 1874 and 1875.[82] They were also mentioned in a footnote in the 1873 *WRLAMR* paper (III:89n2), where Ferrier reported that "I have now (June 14) ascertained the position of all these centres in the brain of the monkey, and therefore, by implication, their situation in man. These experiments will soon be published".[83]

However, Ferrier's connection with WRA was not at an end, as he published two further papers in *WRLAMR*: "Pathological illustrations of brain function" (IV:30–62) and "Labyrinthine vertigo. Menière's disease" (V:24–39). Of these, the first certainly involved, directly or indirectly, work at WRA since it was based on information contained in the separate case books

---

[80] Finn (2012:141) stated that Ferrier "was spurred on by the success of his work at Wakefield in 1873, as he returned to his London roles as Professor of Forensic Medicine at King's College, Professor of Practical Physiology at University College, and consultant to the National Hospital at Queen Square". Of these three listed roles, only the first is correct. Ferrier's appointment at Queen Square dated from 1880 and he never held a position at University College London. In the history of University College Hospital and its Medical School by Merrington, the only mention of Ferrier that I find (1976:107) relates to "Horsley's animal experimental work on the localization of brain function which often owed much to the pioneer work of Ferrier and Hughlings Jackson" (I thank Dr. Tom Hughes of Rhiwbina, Cardiff, for access to this book, 05/12/2024).

[81] Millett (1998:288) stated that these experiments were performed at the Brown Animal Sanatory Institution. Finn (2012:141 and n455) likewise stated that the experiments on the brains of macaques were "conducted at the newly built Brown Animal Sanatory Institution" and referenced Ferrier's notebooks held in the Royal College of Physicians of London. Whilst this may be true, the history of the Brown Institution by Wilson makes only a single, brief mention of Ferrier: "In 1870 he [Burdon Sanderson] hired a room over a stable in Howland Street and converted it into a pathological laboratory; brought Emanuel Klein, a histologist, over from Vienna; and worked with him, Lauder Brunton (later Sir Lauder), David Ferrier (later Sir David) and Edward Sharpey [*sic*] (later Sir Edward Sharpey-Schafer) on pathological problems" (Wilson 1979:172).

[82] Ferrier (1874b, c, 1875a, b). See Millett (1998), for an account of E.A. Waterlow's illustrations of the macaque brain.

[83] Lazar (2013:97n5) stated that "The early experiments with macaques took place between June 14, 1873 and September 5, 1873 at the Brown Institute" but he did not cite any primary source(s) to support this claim (possibly Millett 1998?). In fact, these dates come from both the unpublished manuscript of Ferrier's 1874 Croonian Lecture held in the Royal Society archives (AP/56/2) and from Ferrier (1874c:409). Hence there is a discrepancy between these dates and Ferrier's *WRLAMR* footnote (III:89n2) which stated that the positions were ascertained by this date (i.e. June 14). It seems implausible to suppose that all the localisations were confirmed in the first monkey Ferrier experimented upon. In this context, Lauder Brunton (1905:1087) erred with his statement that "it was only in the spring of 1874 [*sic*] that my friend Dr. D. Ferrier, by an inspiration of genius, began to use monkeys whose brains correspond so much more closely to the human brain than do those of dogs. He was thus able to localise the functions of the brain both sensory and motor in a way which, although it has undergone supplementation and correction, is still in the main both correct and complete"; ditto Jefferson (1953:69) with his statement that "In 1875 [*sic*] Ferrier … moved onto the monkey's cortex".

and post-mortem books of the Asylum.[84] In this paper, Ferrier attempted to correlate clinical and pathological findings in five patients in order "to show some of the clinical bearings of the experimental researches on the Functions of the Brain, published in the last number of these Reports" (IV:30 [capitals in original]). This information may possibly have been abstracted from the case books during his visit in the Spring of 1873, but there are later possibilities: he was in West Yorkshire in September 1873, presenting at the British Association for the Advancement of Science meeting in Bradford;[85] at WRA in November 1873 to present at the *conversazione* (Chap. 8); and in Leeds in March 1874, presenting at the Philosophical Hall.[86] The five patients selected had clinical diagnoses of epileptic insanity, epileptic mania (both with defects of memory), dementia, aphasia, and melancholia; all were associated with lesions of the hemispheres, either unilateral or bilateral. Of note, the right hemisphere tumour in the third patient was examined microscopically by Major (IV:39), yet it was Bevan-Lewis who later published further details of the case (VI:126) without acknowledging Major.[87]

After WRA, Ferrier was in the ascendant: a monograph on his studies, *The functions of the brain*, was published in 1876,[88] he was elected FRS in the same

---

[84] Finn (2012:124) pointed out "that for any doctor or clerk wishing to research the links between a patient's observed symptoms and their post-mortem appearance for purposes of research, they had to correlate two different volumes". In addition, specifically discussing Ferrier's "Pathological illustrations of brain function" (IV:30–62), Finn (2012:152) stated that Ferrier "was privy to the medical records at Queen Square", but I think this is unlikely since, as mentioned above, Ferrier did not hold an appointment at Queen Square until 1880. Finn also maintained (2012:151) that this was "a paper whose significance has escaped the attention of historians" although it had been discussed by Young (1970:236n3, n4; 237n11; 241n7; 242 and n2; 244 and n3, n4) who pointed out that "As soon as he [Ferrier] had reported his initial findings, he began investigating their clinical implications by interpreting some cases from the West Riding Lunatic Asylum" (Young 1970:244). See also Larner (2023c, 2025j).

[85] Reports in: *Lancet* 1873;2:459 and 1873;2:503–504; *Medical Press and Circular* 1873;16:275; *Medical Times and Gazette* 1873;2:357–8 and 1873;2:362–363; *Boston Medical and Surgical Journal* 1873;88:419. The substance of the lecture later appeared in *Nature* (Ferrier 1873c).

[86] *Leeds Mercury*, 18th March 1874, p.8.

[87] It is my presumption that Bevan-Lewis was the author of this section, devoted to "Voracious Appetite as an Initiatory Symptom of Brain Tumours", of the paper (VI:120–149) which was ascribed co-authorship by Lawson and Bevan-Lewis.

[88] Ferrier (1876). This work was dedicated to Hughlings Jackson (although aside from the dedication itself, he is referred to as "Hughlings-Jackson" throughout). John Galton's translation of Ecker's "*On the convolutions of the human brain*" was used by Ferrier (1876:297) to transpose, with caveats, cortical localisations in monkeys onto human brains (Ferrier 1876:298 (Fig. 59) and 302 (Fig. 61) for Ecker's images; 304 (Fig. 63) and 306 (Fig. 65) for transpositions). A second, much expanded edition of *The functions of the brain* appeared 10 years later (Ferrier 1886; reprinted in Wade 2000) again dedicated to Jackson; the Preface recorded that "grateful acknowledgments are due to Dr. Bevan Lewis, of the West Riding Asylum, for many beautiful sections and drawings illustrative of the structure of the brain and spinal cord". The copy of the second edition held at the Wellcome Collection in London is inscribed to "Sir James Crichton Browne/with the authors kind regards". There were also French and German translations of the 1876 edition, the latter including changes added by the translator, Heinrich Obersteiner (1847–1922), and

year, likewise a founder member of the Physiological Society.[89] He became FRCP in 1877 and the delivered the Goulstonian Lectures of the Royal College of Physicians (RCP) of London in 1878 on the subject of *The localisation of cerebral disease*.[90] He did not, however, entirely lose contact with WRA clinical staff: he introduced Robert Lawson when chairing a meeting at the Physiological Society in London on 15th February 1877,[91] and later communicated Bevan-Lewis's paper (co-authored with Henry Clarke) on cortical lamination to the Royal Society in January 1878.[92] As Lawson commenced at WRA in 1874 he might possibly have met Ferrier there, and been the link to Bevan-Lewis (they co-authored in *WRLAMR*: VI:120–149); alternatively Crichton-Browne might have introduced both separately to Ferrier.

Ferrier was appointed to the staff at the National Hospital for the Paralysed and Epileptic, Queen Square, London, in 1880. A possible set back occurred in 1881 when he was charged, at the instigation of members of the anti-vivisection movement, under the Cruelty to Animals Act of 1876 following the demonstration of two monkeys with experimental brain lesions at the International Medical Congress in London,[93] but he was acquitted.[94] This notoriety resulted in Ferrier becoming to a certain extent a public figure, referred to directly or indirectly in works of popular fiction either for or against vivisection.[95]

Ferrier was an original member of the Neurological Society of London in 1886 and became its President in 1894. A personal chair in neuropathology was granted by King's College London in 1889. However, it was not until 1895 that he became an Honorary Member of the MPA. He later published a long chapter on "The regional diagnosis of cerebral disease" in Allbutt's *A System of Medicine*, in both the first (1899) and second (1911) editions.[96] He

---

approved by Ferrier (1879; discussed by Macmillan 2000:267, 275–276). For the interactions between Obersteiner and Ferrier, see Larner and Triarhou (2025a).

[89] Sharpey-Schafer (1927:8).

[90] Ferrier (1878a). This work was dedicated to Charcot.

[91] Sharpey-Schafer (1927:43–44).

[92] Lewis and Clarke (1878). Discussed by Triarhou (2021:59–63).

[93] Finn (2012:159) erred in stating that both Ferrier and Goltz, his opponent in the debate, "each had a test animal to be … studied as their crucial experiment" since Ferrier exhibited two monkeys at the IMC (Larner and Griffiths 2025). Finn was perhaps referring to the animals (one dog, one monkey) sacrificed for pathological examination at the time of the demonstration.

[94] Bone and Larner (2024).

[95] See Pedlar (2003), Otis (2007b), Finn and Stark (2015:17), Larner (2023d) (reprinted in adapted form in Larner (2025k)).

[96] Ferrier (1899, 1911).

was President of the Medical Society of London in its 141st session (1913–1914).

The question of why Ferrier went to Wakefield to undertake experimental research remains unanswered. Why not pursue his studies at King's College, in Rutherford's department (as he later did when Gerald Yeo had become Professor of Physiology there)? Perhaps he was flattered by Crichton-Browne's invitation, and keen to initiate innovative work in a new purpose-built laboratory. Perhaps Jackson, and/or Laycock, encouraged him to take up the opportunity. Crammer has suggested that Ferrier's research "involved vivisection, then a very upsetting issue in London, and Ferrier may have been grateful for a quiet backwater like the Wakefield Asylum in which to do his research".[97] If so, Ferrier's prompt return to London, by June 1873, to pursue further experimental studies on monkeys would seem inexplicable.

Ferrier's work at WRA certainly attracted much attention, even in the year of publication,[98] not only because of its physiological importance but because of its clinical ramifications. It confirmed that clinico-anatomical correlation was feasible as the idiom of practice, at least in neurology,[99] and also had implications for possible surgical approaches to the central nervous system, later fully realised. Ferrier's work was referred to by other *WRLAMR* contributors (e.g. Hughlings Jackson, III:175, 176, 325; VI:283; Carpenter, IV:passim; Milner Fothergill, IV:106; Lauder Brunton, IV:199; Newcombe, V:208, 212; Crichton-Browne, V:227, VI:201, 225, 227).

J. Milner Fothergill (1841–1888)[100]

John Milner Fothergill was initially apprenticed to his father in the Westmoreland village of Morland before attending the Edinburgh Medical School (MD 1865)[101] where, like Ferrier, he was influenced by Thomas Laycock.[102] After some time in country practice with his father, he worked in

---

[97] Crammer (1996:219).

[98] Larner (2023c, 2025j).

[99] But not, as Crichton-Browne (1878–1879:355) had hoped, for "the anatomical substrata of subjective states".

[100] Biographical material on Milner Fothergill may be found in Leyland (1888:I:98–105) and Fye (1992/2003). The latter does not mention Fothergill's association with WRA. Also, Wallis, https://doi.org/10.1093/ref:odnb/9980.

[101] *Alphabetical list of graduates of the University of Edinburgh …*, 1889:38.

[102] James (1996:375–376).

Leeds[103] and then travelled to Vienna where he worked under the pathologist Carl von Rokitansky (1804–1878)[104] and wrote his first book, *The Heart and its diseases, with their treatment* (1872). Moving to London, he became Assistant Physician to the West London Hospital in Hammersmith where Ferrier had also had an appointment as a Junior Physician.[105] According to Sherrington's obituary of Ferrier,[106] Milner Fothergill shared accommodation in his early London years with Ferrier and Thomas Lauder Brunton, but this is not born out by their respective addresses in the *Medical Directory*, albeit after 1874 they were all living in close proximity to Portman Square.

Milner Fothergill contributed four papers to *WRLAMR* between 1873 and 1876. No affiliation was given for the first two papers; for third he was denoted as "Junior Physician to the West London Hospital" and for the fourth "Assistant Physician to the West London Hospital, etc." The first of these papers addressed "The heart sounds in general paralysis of the insane" (III:113–128), the second and third "Cerebral anaemia" (IV:94–151) and "Cerebral hyperaemia" (V:171–187) respectively. Consistent with his interest in therapeutics, his final paper was "Notes on the therapeutics of some affections of the nervous system", the penultimate paper in *WRLAMR* (VI:254–265).

It might be thought likely that Milner Fothergill's association with WRA and *WRLAMR* came about through Ferrier. However, the evidence suggests otherwise, in fact possibly the reverse. According to Leyland, Fothergill "paid repeated visits to the West Riding Asylum, at Wakefield, to familiarize himself with insanity; and contributed some notable papers to the *West Riding Asylum Reports* [*sic*]".[107] A contemporary source appears to corroborate the suggestion that he did attend WRA and see patients there:

---

[103] Finn (2012:105n342) stated that "Fothergill's links with Wakefield came about when he was a resident medical officer at the nearby Leeds Public Dispensary between 1869 and 1871" but he did not cite any primary source(s) to support this claim. I suppose it is possible that he may have met Crichton-Browne in Leeds during this period, perhaps through Clifford Allbutt who was Honorary Physician to the Leeds Public Dispensary at this time (*vide supra*).

[104] "Rokitanski" is mentioned at V:175 and n. He "first pointed out the connection betwixt cerebral apoplexy, with clot, and hypertrophy of the left ventricle with diseased vessels". Milner Fothergill's footnote stated that "The description is perfect; it was only left for clinical observers to explain the causation".

[105] Fothergill was appointed "Physician to the West London Hospital, vice Prof. D. Ferrier, M.D., appointed Assistant Physician to King's College Hospital." *Medical Press and Circular* 1874;18:233 (9th September; Appointments). [Ferrier's marriage was announced in the same column of the journal.] Also *BMJ* 1874;2:393 (19th September; Medical Appointments); *Medical Press and Circular* 1874;18:301 (30th September; Appointments) which specified "Junior Physician".

[106] Sherrington (1928:ix).

[107] Leyland (1888:I:99), but he did not say when these visits occurred. Perhaps this was the source of Finn's claim (*vide supra*) that Milner Fothergill's links with Wakefield dated from 1869 to 1871. James

At the recent meeting of the British Association at Bradford [September 1873], Dr. J. Milner Fothergill ... alluded to the facilities he had had to study his subject at this [Wakefield] asylum, where he found in fifty-five cases out of sixty-six evidences of an abnormal high-blood tension on the brain.[108]

Internal evidence from his *WRLAMR* publications is explicit:

In October last, when at the West Riding Asylum, Dr. Crichton Browne suggested to me to examine the hearts of several patients, who were the subject of general paralysis, ... (III:113)

Moreover, regarding the accentuation of the second heart sound detected in patients with general paralysis:

This accentuation was clear and distinct, and was as readily detected by Dr. Crichton Browne and Dr. Bell Pettigrew as by myself. (III:113).[109]

The October referred to is presumably 1872, and may have coincided with that year's medical *conversazione* at WRA since "Dr J.B. Pettigrew" of Edinburgh was amongst those invited and reportedly exhibited material on one of the stalls (see Chap. 8).[110]

Further evidence of Milner Fothergill's attendance at WRA may also be given:

Dr. Aldridge ... kindly examined for me some of the melancholics in the West Riding Asylum, who were being examined by me in order to illustrate several points in this paper. (IV:115)

(1996:376) said of Fothergill that "he was a frequent visitor to the West Riding Asylum" but he did not cite any primary source(s) to support this claim. Again, I wonder if this was based on Leyland.

[108] *The Wakefield Express, and Barnsley, Normanton, Pontefract, Ossett, Horbury & Dewsbury Advertiser* Volume 22, No, 1126, 29th November 1873, p.2, cols. 4–7 (Medical conversazione at the West Riding Asylum. Speech by Lord Houghton. Lecture by Dr. Carpenter). Milner Fothergill's paper to the British Association at Bradford was reported in *Lancet* 1873;2:468–469, and included comments by Ferrier (469). Milner Fothergill's paper published in the 1873 issue of *WRLAMR* in fact argued against arterial tension in general paralysis as "there is no distinct hypertrophy of the heart in general paralysis; and also there was an absence of the firm and sustained pulse, the hard pulse, in fact, of increased arterial tension, ..." (III:117). Perhaps the newspaper reference to "abnormal high-blood tension on the brain" corresponds to Fothergill's "increased vascular area above the aortic valves" (III:120).

[109] Todd and Ashworth (n.d.:131) stated that "Pettigrew assisted Fothergill in his researches at the Wakefield Asylum for his paper The Heart Sounds in General Paralysis". For Pettigrew, see Chap. 9.

[110] However, I do not find Fothergill's name recorded in any of the extant accounts of the WRA medical *conversazione*.

… extensive observations as to the condition of the circulation in various forms of insanity have been made by the writer in the wards of the West Riding Asylum. (IV:116)

By the courtesy of Dr. Crichton Browne, ample opportunities for observation have been furnished to the writer in the large institution under his supervision, and on such observations the following remarks are founded. (V:179)

During several lengthy visits to the West Riding Asylum, … (V:182)

Milner Fothergill also had other contacts with WRA. He was amongst those who received Ferrier's thanks at the end of his 1873 contribution to *WRLAMR* on cortical localisation (III:96) and he later judged Ferrier's paper on "The Localisation of Function in the Brain" read at the Annual Meeting of the BMA in Norwich in August 1874 to be "one of the most important of modern times".[111] He referred approvingly to papers by Allbutt (IV:146; VI:261), quoting from the former which had appeared in *WRLAMR*. At the Medical Society of London on 15th December 1873, Milner Fothergill presented "cases which had occurred in the practice of Dr. Crichton Browne" to illustrate the treatment of general paralysis of the insane with Calabar bean, some with apparent recovery.[112] This agent and Crichton-Browne's use of it for the treatment of general paralysis of the insane (e.g. I:67 and IV:91) was also referred to in Fothergill's paper on "The depressants of the circulation and their use", along with citation of one of Crichton-Browne's cases (E.W.) treated with nitrite of amyl for seizures.[113]

Milner Fothergill continued to write a variety of medical works after his contact with WRA. He published in both *Brain* and the *Journal of Mental Science*[114] (Tables 6.4 and 6.5 respectively). He died from complications of diabetes in 1888, aged 47.[115]

---

[111] *BMJ* 1874;2:289 (29th August).

[112] *BMJ* 1874;1:60 (10th January).

[113] Milner Fothergill (1874:77). The clinical details of Fothergill's "E.W." correspond to those of Crichton-Browne's "Eliza W." (III:161–162) and not to "Elizabeth W." (III:163–164), although the former is also named as "Elizabeth W." (III:162). For Crichton-Browne on the Calabar bean, see Crichton Browne (1874c), although he subsequently seemingly disavowed this paper (Crichton Browne 1875-1876a). See Chap. 5, section on George Thompson, for discussion.

[114] Milner Fothergill (1874–1875). Although the title is very similar to that of Nicol's *WRLAMR* paper of 1872 (II:177–202), the latter is not cited.

[115] Obituary: *BMJ* 1888;2:51–52 (7th July). There was no mention here of his association with WRA.

John Hughlings Jackson[116] (1835–1911)[117]

John Hughlings Jackson was 31 years old at the time of Crichton-Browne's accession to the superintendency at WRA in 1866. By this time, Jackson was already, as of 1862, Assistant Physician at the National Hospital for the Paralysed and Epileptic, Queen Square, London, and from 1863 Assistant Physician to the London Hospital and Lecturer in the Medical School.[118] These two hospitals, Queen Square and the London, were to remain his chief appointments throughout his professional life. He had published widely on epilepsy, aphasia, and chorea, as well as championing the use of the ophthalmoscope.[119] He had acquired the MD of the University of St. Andrews by examination in 1860, Membership and then Fellowship of the Royal College Physicians of London (1861 and 1868 respectively), become full physician at Queen Square (1867) and gave the Goulstonian Lectures at the RCP (1869). As early as 1866 Jackson had become a member of the MPA,[120] in contrast to Allbutt and Ferrier who had to wait until the 1890s before being elected as honorary members.[121] He was elected FRS in 1878.

---

[116] Professor Michael Swash of the Royal London Hospital has presented evidence that Jackson once made a request to the House Governor of the London Hospital (as it then was) in 1871 to the effect that "a slight dash betwixt my two names, so as to show that I use both" be used, hence Hughlings-Jackson (Swash 1986:982). The Critchleys (Critchley and Critchley 1998:177–9, 181) addressed "the saga of the inconsistent hyphen" and concluded with the hope that "the hyphenated name will not be reintroduced in the future in printed matter". Greenblatt (2022:165n20) also noted instances in which the hyphen was used, for example the title pages of *Brain* at its inception in 1878, until 1886–7. I have elected to retain the general usage of "Hughlings Jackson", not least because, as pointed out by the Critchley's (1998:179), "virtually all the world's literature shows Jackson to be indexed under 'J', not 'H'", a policy which is followed in the Bibliography here (a notable exception to this rule is found in Scott et al. (2012:275, 303)).

[117] Hughlings Jackson is the subject of two full-length biographies: Critchley and Critchley (1998), Greenblatt (2022). Following Greenblatt (2022:1n1), I shall generally refer to the former work as "The Critchleys". There are also many other shorter biographical pieces, for example: Critchley (1960), Swash (1986, 2005, 2015), Taylor, revised Walton of Detchant, https://doi.org/10.1093/ref:odnb/34137, Murray (2007), Shorvon and Compston (2019:130–139). The *ODNB* entry is marred by (at least) two errors: "in left-handed persons the speech centre is usually situated in the right hemisphere" [at 504] (the majority of left handers have the "speech centre" in the left hemisphere, as in right handers, although the overall percentage is less); and Hughlings Jackson "contributed many articles to … the *West Riding Hospital Reports* [*sic*]" [at 506].

[118] For Jackson at the London Hospital, see Swash (2024:183–192).

[119] For listings of Hughlings Jackson's published writings, see Broadbent (1903:356–366), York and Steinberg (2006), Greenblatt (2022:473–502). These may not be complete (e.g. Larner 2024e, 2025m).

[120] Jackson's election to MPA membership was confirmed at the MPA Annual Meeting in Edinburgh on 31st July 1866 (*J Ment Sci* 1866–1867;12(October 1866):422).

[121] Greenblatt (2022:55) stated that "presumably it was Laycock who recruited him [Jackson] to the Medico-Psychological Association *circa* 1866", which I think is a reasonable inference, although another influence might have been Daniel Hack Tuke (1827–1895), possibly one of Jackson's teachers during his time at the York Medical School, along with Laycock (Wetherill 1961; Dewhurst 1982:7; Greenblatt

How Hughlings Jackson came to be involved with WRA is, to my knowledge, unknown, but there are some suggestive possibilities. For example, there were shared influences with other personnel associated with the Asylum. Jackson's medical education at the York Medical School, around 1852–1855, had brought him into contact with Thomas Laycock before the latter moved to Edinburgh,[122] where, as previously described, Laycock influenced both Crichton-Browne and Ferrier, amongst others. Crichton-Browne may have known Jackson through the MPA: during Laycock's Presidency (1869–70), Crichton-Browne was on the Council and Jackson was Auditor (a role previously exercised by Crichton-Browne) and both men attended the annual meeting at York in August 1869.[123] Later authors have stated that Crichton-Browne was a "a life long friend" of Jackson.[124] Ferrier met Jackson soon after he moved to London in 1870.[125] Jackson shared with Allbutt an interest in developing the application of ophthalmoscopy in medical practice and was the dedicatee of the latter's monograph on the subject.[126] Individually or collectively, Laycock, Crichton-Browne, Ferrier, and Allbutt may have prompted or promoted Jackson's contact with WRA. As a Yorkshireman, born at Green Hammerton about 10 miles northwest of York, Jackson may have known of the Wakefield Asylum from an early age. Despite being based in London, it has been said that Jackson retained a deep affection for Yorkshire and visited his birthplace annually.[127]

Hughlings Jackson contributed five papers to *WRLAMR* between 1873 and 1876.[128] Of these, four related to epilepsy and the fifth was a single case

---

2022:12–13). Jackson was never subsequently elected an honorary member of the MPA (Dewhurst 1982:105).

[122] Both Reynolds (2020:711) and Greenblatt (2022:11) stated that Jackson was at York Medical School between 1852 and 1855; Critchley and Critchley (1998:26) stated that "In 1852 Hughlings Jackson became a student at York Medical School". Hence, Wetherill (1961:263) appears to have been in error in stating that he "entered the School in 1853".

[123] *J Ment Sci* 1869–1870;15:i, 462, 469, 474 (where Jackson's name is adjacent to Crichton-Browne's in a list of those present at the dinner). See also James (1996:64). Jackson's term as Auditor ended in 1871 (*J Ment Sci* 1871–1872;(October 1871):442). Crichton-Browne had been Auditor in 1866–1868 (e.g. *J Ment Sci* 1866–1867;12(October 1866):458; *J Ment Sci* 1867–1868;13(October 1867):i). Sander et al. (1993:602) claimed that it was at "the West Riding Asylum in Wakefield where all three [Hughlings Jackson, Ferrier and Crichton-Browne] originally met", thereby contradicting their later statement that "Crichton-Browne … qualified in Edinburgh with David Ferrier" (Sander et al. 1993:603); I suspect the former claim is unlikely to be correct, and the latter is definitely incorrect.

[124] Critchley and Critchley (1998:28). See also Dewhurst (1982:18).

[125] Ferrier (1892:884).

[126] Allbutt (1871a:v–vi). Jackson's ophthalmological work is mentioned in *WRLAMR* by Aldridge (I:84).

[127] Critchley and Critchley (1998:35). They suggested this story originated from James Taylor (*vide infra*).

[128] Dewhurst (1982:18) stated that Jackson was "the most prolific contributor to … *Asylum Reports* [*sic*]", which is incorrect: both Crichton-Browne (7) and Major (6) contributed more articles to *WRLAMR* than

report on "double optic neuritis" (IV:24–29) illustrating the clinical value of the ophthalmoscope.[129] Viets listed all five under "Papers contributed to the Medical Reports"[130] and certainly where details of patients are given in these papers they are from either the London Hospital or Queen Square. The four epilepsy papers were "Observations on localisation of movements in the cerebral hemispheres, as revealed by cases of convulsion, chorea and 'aphasia'" (III:175–195); "On the anatomical, physiological, and pathological investigation of epilepsies" (III:315–349); "On temporary mental disorders after epileptic paroxysms" (V:105–129);[131] and the very last paper in the final volume of the journal, "On epilepsies and on the after effects of epileptic discharges (Todd and Robertson's hypothesis)" (VI:266–309). The first of these was referenced in a later volume of *WRLAMR* (VI:135). All four subsequently appeared in James Taylor's posthumous selection of Hughlings Jackson's work.[132] George and Trimble, describing nineteenth-century views of epilepsy as reflected in the pages of *WRLAMR*, opined that "By far the most important writings in the *WRLAMR* are those by J Hughlings Jackson".[133] Greenblatt discussed all four papers, particularly the first two, in his biography of Jackson.[134]

The first of Jackson's *WRLAMR* papers began with an acknowledgement of Ferrier's work[135] as confirming Jackson's view that discharges of convolutions develop movements (III:175). Ferrier's experiments were also referred to by

---

Jackson (5), although on total printed page count Jackson (131) surpassed Major (86) but not Crichton-Browne (215). Ferrier also surpassed Major on page count (116) despite contributing fewer articles (3).

[129] With Crichton-Browne's permission "almost a verbatim reprint" of this paper and the accompanying chromolithograph appeared in *Royal London Ophthalmic Hospital Reports* 1875;8(Part 2):316–320 (A periscope of contemporary ophthalmic literature. Hughlings Jackson on recovery from severe double optic neuritis, in a case in which there was no defect of sight); also in an offprint, Jackson JH. A physician's notes on ophthalmology (2nd series). London: Harrison and Sons, 1875:1–5. The latter was referred to by Ferrier (1876:244), so presumably the author had given him a copy, but I do not find the offprint mentioned in the listings of Hughlings Jackson's published writings by York and Steinberg (2006) or Greenblatt (2022:473–502).

[130] Viets (1938:487).

[131] Jackson's handwritten annotations on this paper in a copy of *WRLAMR* he once owned have been reported (Larner and Swash 2024).

[132] Taylor et al. (1931 [1996]:77–89, 90–111, 119–134, 135–161). For James Taylor (1859–1946), see Triarhou and Larner (2024).

[133] George and Trimble (1992:248). On the subject of epilepsy, Borch (2018:184) noted "its neurologization [*sic*] at the close of the nineteenth century" but it is evident that this process was already in progress through the work of Hughlings Jackson by the 1870s.

[134] Greenblatt (2022:174–182).

[135] Specifically, Ferrier (1873a), but not III:30–96. Ditto III:317n1 where conclusions 4 and 5 from Ferrier (1873a) are reproduced. Greenblatt (2022:174) stated that Jackson "made no reference to Ferrier's paper", meaning Ferrier's first *WRLAMR* paper, in his own two contributions to *WRLAMR* volume III.

Jackson elsewhere.[136] Jackson's evolutionary view of the nervous system, of the dissolution in disease states which permitted the positive symptoms of lower centres to emerge as a consequence of the negative effects of inaction of higher centres, and which was derived from Herbert Spencer rather than from Darwin, was still being developed during the years of Crichton-Browne's superintendency at WRA.[137]

Despite the unequivocal significance of these contributions to *WRLAMR*, establishing Jackson's physical presence at WRA, rather than simply his intellectual influence, is to enter uncertain territory, notwithstanding the confident statements made by some authors in the secondary literature, here presented chronologically.

Dewhurst, writing in 1982, stated that "Jackson kept in touch with psychiatry through his regular visits to the West Riding Asylum" and that he was "Undoubtedly ... fascinated by his visits to Wakefield".[138] Furthermore, Dewhurst also claimed that Jackson gave a lecture "at the Wakefield Asylum 'On temporary mental disorders after epileptic paroxysms' (1875)".[139] Certainly, this was the title of one of Jackson's papers in *WRLAMR* (V:105–129). However, in his classification of all the papers published in *WRLAMR*, Viets noted only two "Papers read at West Riding", those by William Turner (III:1–29) and William Carpenter (IV:1–23).[140] Moreover, none of the published accounts of the 1875 *conversazione* (see Chap. 8 for details) mentioned Jackson amongst "between 300 and 400 medical men" present.[141] The main address on that occasion was given by William Broadbent on the "Theory of construction of the nervous system".[142]

Noting that "Doctors often did autopsies on deceased patients from mental asylums for the poor", Star included Jackson among "Several prominent

---

[136] III:317 and n1, 325; VI:268.

[137] For example, VI:271n1: "a duplex condition ... —negative (loss of control) and positive (over-activity of lower centres)". Dr. Jonathan Miller noted the influence of Francis Anstie (see Chap. 9) on Jackson's hierarchical conception (V:111–112:n1), and also his use of a social model as a metaphor for describing the double symptoms of central nervous system dysfunction (e.g. VI:271, "a duplex condition"), noting that this was written within a few years of the social disorder of the Hyde Park Riots of 1866 (Greaves 2017:160–161, 165).

[138] Dewhurst (1982:16, 18).

[139] Ibid., 80.

[140] Viets (1938:486).

[141] *BMJ* 1875;2:680 (27th November; The West Riding Asylum) from which the quotation is taken; *Medical Times and Gazette* 1875;2:603 (27th November; Conversazione at the West Riding Asylum); *Medical Press and Circular* 1875;20:457 (1st December; Medical Conversazione).

[142] Broadbent (1876). Had Hughlings Jackson lectured, one might have anticipated that it would be covered in the medical press, as so many of his lectures were, although against this supposition the limited reporting of the WRA *conversazione* in the medical press (see Chap. 8) should be noted.

localizationists" who "spent years working in the postmortem rooms and laboratories of these asylums" and furthermore that "Crichton-Browne made it possible for Ferrier and Jackson to do research at West Riding".[143] No documentary evidence to support this statement was offered.

The Critchleys, writing in 1998, stated that Jackson "was able to pay visits to the West Riding Asylum" but specified no dates and cited no references.[144] Michael Trimble stated that Jackson "visited the Wakefield Lunatic Asylum, where he conducted experiments with Crichton-Browne and David Ferrier" and that "together with Ferrier … he went to Wakefield to use the laboratory that Crichton-Browne had established there, in part to conduct vivisection investigations."[145] The syntax here is ambiguous, but the possible reading that Hughlings Jackson conducted animal experimentation can be firmly rejected; according to Henry Head "He never performed an experiment".[146] Millett stated that "Ferrier and Jackson were frequent participants" at the WRA *conversaziones*[147] but offered no evidence, and certainly I am not aware of any evidence for Jackson's attendance (see Chap. 8).

Simon Shorvon and Alastair Compston, perhaps wishing to buttress their assertion that "Jackson was … a visitor to Wakefield", cited the anecdote of

---

[143] Star (1989:31, 32). The references offered in support of the latter statement are: Ferrier's first paper in *WRLAMR* (III:30–96); Jackson's two part *Lancet* publication (1873a) "On the anatomical and physiological localisation of movements in the brain" but with incorrect details (viz. "no. 4 (April): 197–201 [Part 1]; no. 5 (May); 245–48 [Part 2]"); two of Jackson's papers in *WRLAMR* (III:175–195 and VI:266–309); and "Spillane (1981:389)". The latter page mentioned Jackson only in the context of Ferrier's work at WRA to confirm his ideas. None of these references places Jackson at WRA.

[144] Critchley and Critchley (1998:28).

[145] Trimble (2016:122, 123). A similar, erroneous implication was made by Quick (2014:67): "Laycock played a key role in the training of such now-lauded experimentalists as the founders of *Brain*, John Hughlings Jackson and James Crichton-Brown [*sic*], as well as David Ferrier".

[146] Head (1911) (cited by Critchley and Critchley (1998:189)). Similarly, "Jackson cannot strictly be called a physiologist since he did no experimental work" yet he was elected to the Physiological Society (O'Connor 1988:62; also 1991:484). Sharpey-Schafer (1927:82) dated his election to 13th November 1886; O'Connor (1988:62) stated 1885, whereas Star (1989:55) erred in listing "Jackson" amongst the original members of the Physiological Society in 1876 (cf. Sharpey-Schafer 1927:8). According to O'Connor (1988:62), Jackson "took no part in the activities of the Society". He was nevertheless sympathetic to the application of physiological principles to clinical medicine: "The physiological part of our clinical work is not sufficiently methodical; we have medical knowledge, and we have separately physiological knowledge, but our medical knowledge is not sufficiently physiological" (III:181). Likewise, Jackson advocated "what the physiologist does in experimenting on animals; to ascertain the exact distribution of a nerve, he destroys it, and also stimulates it. Indeed, this double kind of study is essential in the investigation of cases of nervous disease for physiological purposes. For limited *destroying lesions* of *some* parts of the cerebral hemisphere produce no obvious symptoms; whilst discharging lesions of those parts produce very striking symptoms" (Jackson 1873a:84 [italics in original]). A blueprint, if one were needed, for Ferrier's studies in the WRA laboratory.

[147] Millett (1998:287). Lazar (2013:96) appears to have followed Millett's formulation.

Sir Wemyss Reid, recounted by Crichton-Browne in 1926,[148] which tells of Reid's encounter with Jackson at a hotel in Clapham, Yorkshire, the latter's attendance reportedly prompted by the desire to escape the stress and anxiety of professional life in London and also to stir up dormant emotions as he had spent his honeymoon at the hotel (he married Elizabeth Dade, his first cousin, in July 1865).[149] This hardly seems compelling evidence for a visit to Wakefield, which is located almost 60 miles away from Clapham.[150] Moreover, Elizabeth Dade Jackson died in May 1876, postdating the hey-day of WRA activity, since by this time Crichton-Browne had left, the *conversazione* were no more, and the final *WRLAMR* was in process of production. Although undated, the earliest possible date of the Reid-Jackson meeting is 1887.[151] Furthermore, would such a (professional) visit to WRA be calculated to assuage the stress and anxiety of professional life? Much as Jackson may have enjoyed visiting Yorkshire, attending a local asylum may not have featured as part of his itinerary.[152] Other biographical materials do not mention Jackson's association with WRA.[153]

An intriguing contemporary comment, perhaps pertinent to this issue, comes from Thomas Clouston. Responding to Crichton-Browne's paper in the *Journal of Mental Science* critiquing the late David Skae's (1814–1873) classification of mental disease,[154] Clouston wrote:

> Surely, Dr. Hughlings Jackson has not been to the West Riding Asylum lately, or we should have had some clinical facts about these convulsive seizures, where they arose, what muscles they affected, whether they were bilateral or unilateral, how long they lasted, whether they were followed by paralysis, or increased

---

[148] Crichton-Browne (1926:84–85). Critchley and Critchley (1998:172) repeated the story, their reference suggesting that it originated from the neurologist Wilfred Harris (1869–1960).

[149] Shorvon and Compston (2019:140 and n28). These authors also stated that "Neurology continued at the West Riding Lunatic Asylum after the departure of Ferrier and Hughlings Jackson" (2019:305) and described Crichton-Browne as "patron of Hughlings Jackson and Ferrier's work in Wakefield" (at 342). Whilst unequivocally true for Ferrier, the latter statement would be difficult to credit even if Hughlings Jackson had visited and worked at WRA, since Jackson was the older man, born 5 years before Crichton-Browne, and well-established in London medical practice some years before Crichton-Browne was appointed at WRA, indeed whilst the latter was still a medical student.

[150] RAC Route Planner (accessed 13/02/2024) suggested a drive time from Clapham, Yorkshire, to Wakefield of 1 h 42 min, so it was hardly on the doorstep.

[151] Greenblatt (2022:408–409 and n265).

[152] Greenblatt (2022:326n108) noted Jackson's refusal "to go to some lunatic asylum and show how the cases of patients there could be classified" (Jackson 1881:329) under his "Hypothesis of Dissolution". See also Chap. 10.

[153] For example, Swash (1986).

[154] Crichton Browne (1875–1876b).

temperature, or cephalalgia, or double vision, or hallucinations of the senses, or the epileptic irritability.[155]

At the risk of overinterpretation, one might read this either as an acknowledgement that Jackson had previously but not recently been to WRA, or possibly as a (slightly sarcastic?) dig that Jackson had not (ever?) been to WRA to assess patients with seizures. (Whichever, the passage certainly attests to Jackson's powers of clinical observation.) In his final *WRLAMR* paper, Jackson, discussing epileptic seizures in asylum patients, reported that "On this matter I again quote Crichton-Browne. In a letter to me in reply to enquiries …" (VI:303), information that surely could have been delivered in person had he (recently) visited WRA.

Hence, I submit that, although absence of evidence does not equate to evidence of absence, "the evidence for his absence is more compelling than for his presence".[156] But wherever the truth may lie concerning Jackson's attendance or otherwise at WRA he was probably known of by all the clinicians who worked there and it is incontrovertible that he profoundly influenced at least two of the key individuals who did work there: Clifford Allbutt and David Ferrier. Moreover, his influence was not only national but also international, including neurologists working in Europe such as Jean-Martin Charcot and Arnold Pick.[157]

T. Lauder Brunton (1844–1916)[158]

Thomas Lauder Brunton qualified (MB, CM) in Edinburgh in 1866 and MD in 1868, the same year that David Ferrier gained his medical qualification.[159] That they were at least acquainted and possibly friends is suggested by several lines of evidence. For example, Sherrington's obituary of Ferrier reported that

---

[155] Clouston (1875–1876:541).

[156] The quotation is from Greenblatt (2022:99) in the context of the meeting of the British Association for the Advancement of Science in 1868 and the non-event of Jackson's debate with Broca (but *cf.* Swash 2024:192). Greenblatt also stated here that Jackson "disliked ceremonial occasions and large meetings" (see also Critchley and Critchley (1998:162): "Formal meetings, committees and assemblies bored him"). If so, this might explain his non-attendance at the WRA medical *conversazione*.

[157] Iniesta and Larner (2011), Larner (2024f).

[158] Biographical material on Lauder Brunton may be found in Fye (1989) reprinted 2003, Waddington (2007), and Hunting (2016). None of these sources mentioned his connection to WRA. Also, Gunn, revised Earles, https://doi.org/10.1093/ref:odnb/32139. Lazar (2013:102n7) erred with "(1844–1914)".

[159] *Edinb Med J* 1868;14(3):266 (Graduation in Medicine at the University of Edinburgh. Candidates who received the Degree of Doctor of Medicine under the New Statutes). *Alphabetical list of graduates of the University of Edinburgh* …, 1889:25. Also D.Sc. (Physiol.), 1870.

when he first moved to London in the early 1870s he shared a house with Lauder Brunton.[160] In the *Medical Directory* for 1871 their addresses are identical (28 Davies St., Grosvenor Sq., W) and also from 1872 to 1874 (23 Somerset St., Portman Sq., W) but by 1875 Ferrier had moved (16 Upper Berkeley St., Portman Sq., W), presumably following his marriage in September 1874.

Both Lauder Brunton and Ferrier were employed by Burdon Sanderson at the Brown Animal Sanatory Institution in the 1870s,[161] and Lauder Brunton was a contributor to Burdon Sanderson's *Handbook for the Physiological Laboratory* of 1873. He was lecturer in materia medica and pharmacology at the Middlesex Hospital in 1870–71, the same years that Ferrier was at the Middlesex (as Lecturer in Physiology), and they were joint authors on four publications on the progress of physiology which appeared in the *Journal of Anatomy and Physiology* in 1871 and 1872.[162] Lauder Brunton's association with WRA may therefore be a consequence of his association with Ferrier, which was not only professional but also domestic.

Very early in his career, whilst still in Edinburgh (1867), Lauder Brunton had found that nitrite of amyl reliably relieved the pain of angina pectoris,[163] a finding which, along with his gold-medal winning thesis on digitalis (1868), was to establish his reputation and presage his career in therapeutics. These studies had included sphygmographic recordings from patients, and self-experimentation with digitalis. Prompted by Lauder Brunton's findings, nitrite of amyl was later used as a medication at WRA for purposes other than the treatment of angina, for example it was the subject of one of Crichton-Browne's papers in *WRLAMR* (III:153–174) in patients with epilepsy.

Lauder Brunton contributed one (long) paper to *WRLAMR* (IV:179–222) entitled "On inhibition, peripheral and central" on the by-line of which he was listed as "Casualty Physician and Lecturer on Materia Medica and Therapeutics at St Bartholomew's Hospital" with an impressive list of degrees

---

[160] Sherrington (1928:ix). Sherrington stated that Milner Fothergill was also with them, but this cannot be correct since he did not arrive in London until 1872, 2 years after Ferrier's move to the capital. Furthermore, as mentioned above, their addresses in the *Medical Directory* do not align.

[161] Romano (2002:73, 182).

[162] Fraser et al. (1871), Brunton and Ferrier (1871, 1872), Rutherford et al. (1872).

[163] Lauder Brunton (1867, 1870a). The latter paper, giving details of a patient admitted to the Royal Infirmary Edinburgh in December 1866, was communicated to the Clinical Society of London by Burdon Sanderson. It included tracings of the sphygmographic recordings of the pulse. Lauder Brunton (1870b), examined the effect of nitrite of amyl on the circulation in dogs and rabbits. See also Fye (1986) (whose reference 28 gave the wrong year for Lauder Brunton (1870b) [as 1871]).

("MD DSc Edin FRS MRCP").[164] His *WRLAMR* paper was much concerned with reflex actions and reflex centres, perhaps betraying the influence of Laycock.[165] It also indicated that Lauder Brunton had undertaken some experimental work at WRA in which he "irritated the brain both by constant and induced currents" in kittens (IV:198–199) but failed to detect inhibitory action by stimulating the brain. This paper was commented on in the editorial pages of the *Lancet* in February 1875[166] and was mentioned by Lawson and Bevan-Lewis (VI:134). Lauder Brunton's work was also cited in other *WRLAMR* papers (e.g. by Mitchell, II:80), and he was also credited with the sphygmograph tracings appearing in one of Milner Fothergill's *WRLAMR* papers (IV:117–118). Lauder Brunton also loaned material exhibited at the 1874 medical *conversazione* at WRA.[167]

Lauder Brunton became the editor of *The Practitioner* in 1874 after the untimely death of Francis Anstie (for whom, see Chap. 9). Occasional papers emanating from WRA were subsequently published therein,[168] as was Lauder Brunton's description of "my friend Professor Ferrier".[169] He witnessed some of Ferrier's monkey experiments in London in 1875,[170] and they collaborated in some experiments to examine the "influence of electrical irritation of the brain and its ganglia on the circulation and respiration" and on muscular discrimination.[171] Although their paths subsequently diverged, it is evident that Ferrier and Lauder Brunton remained in contact, as the latter presented Ferrier's experimental work on monkeys at the Annual Meeting of the British Medical Association in Edinburgh in August 1875.[172]

Although principally known as a pharmacologist, Lauder Brunton evidently maintained some contact with the evolving discipline of neurology, for

---

[164] Lauder Brunton was elected FRS in 1874, hence before Ferrier in 1876, Hughlings Jackson in 1878, and Crichton-Browne in 1883. He was also Gulstonian Lecturer at the Royal College of Physicians in 1877, the year before Ferrier.

[165] James (1996:374) recorded Lauder Brunton as "another [Edinburgh] student of the Laycock era", although Laycock was not specifically mentioned in Lauder Brunton's *WRLAMR* paper.

[166] *Lancet* 1875;1:312–313 (27th February). The fourth volume of *WRLAMR*, containing Lauder Brunton's paper, was reviewed in the *BMJ* of the same date (Table 6.2).

[167] *Medical Times and Gazette* 1874;2:609 (28th November; Annual Conversazione at the West Riding Asylum).

[168] Crichton Browne (1874b), Lawson (1874, 1875a).

[169] Lauder Brunton (1876:133). Also *WRLAMR* IV:199. Ferrier (1876:278) reciprocated when speaking of "my friend Dr. Lauder Brunton".

[170] Ferrier (1875a:447) ("April 7th, 1875"), 460 ("March 9th, 1873"). I take the latter date to be a typographical error for 1875 since this date would fit better with the sequence of experiments reported; furthermore, Ferrier may have been in WRA on March 9th, 1873 (see Larner (2025j) for discussion).

[171] Ferrier (1876:83, 228), respectively.

[172] Ferrier (1875c:277). This may have been because Ferrier's daughter was born on 3rd August 1875, 3 days before the presentation in Edinburgh (*BMJ* 1875;2:186).

example adjudicating in the Ferrier-Schäfer dispute at the Neurological Society of London in 1887 regarding the cortical localisation of the auditory centres in lesioned monkeys.[173] He was President of the Medical Society of London in 1905–1906. Ferrier contributed to Lauder Brunton's obituary notices in 1916:

> many both in the profession and out of it have lost a dear and valued friend. Among these I have the privilege of counting myself; for our friendship dates from our student days in Edinburgh, and continued unimpaired, without even a passing cloud, to the day of his death.[174]

Lennox Browne (1841–1902)

Lennox Browne (no relation to Crichton-Browne or William Browne, to my knowledge) was a noted early practitioner in the discipline of otorhinolaryngology who founded the Central London Throat and Ear Hospital in 1874.[175] His account of his route to WRA (V:271) suggested that, after reading a paper in the *BMJ* issue of "July 19, 1875" on difficulties in speech expression in general paralysis,[176] the only such publication to his knowledge:

> It was with the greatest pleasure, therefore, that early in the spring of this year I accepted the invitation of Dr. Crichton Browne to make some investigations under his guidance of this interesting subject, and the abundant wealth of material at his command offered a rich field for observation.

No doubt, based on the time discrepancy ("July 19, 1875"; "early in the spring of this year") this was a retrospective construction of events.

Lennox Browne's otolaryngological examination of patients at WRA resulted in two papers in *WRLAMR* in 1875, on "Othaematoma, or the insane ear"[177] (V:149–159) and "Laryngoscopic observations in general paralysis"

---

[173] Schäfer (1888:164–165). Discussed in Larner and Griffiths (2025).

[174] *Lancet,* 1916;2:575 (23rd September). Another obituary of Lauder Brunton was written by Allbutt (*Proc R Soc Lond* 1917;89:xliv–xlviii).

[175] Anon (1986a).

[176] Voisin (1875), which in fact appeared in the 19th June issue of the *BMJ*. There was no *BMJ* issue on 19th July 1875 (the nearest was 17th July).

[177] For information on the clinical features and pathogenetic theories of insane ear, see Hare (1990:86–88). Cases of othaematoma or asylum ear encountered at WRA had previously been reported by Nicol (1870b), a paper referred to by Lennox Browne and its conclusions disputed. One of George Thompson's patients with general paralysis of the insane was reported to have developed "slight haematoma auris" (I:65) and the condition was also briefly mentioned by Milner Fothergill (III:124–125) and by Lawson

(V:271–283). Both studies were probably undertaken on the same visit as the reported total number of inpatients at WRA (1424) and their gender distribution (F:M = 717:707) was identical in both reports.

Lennox Browne later loaned "numerous paintings executed by himself, and representing various views at Lemnos and Aix-les-Bains", to the 1875 WRA medical *conversazione*.[178]

H. R. Octavius Sankey (1850–1894)

Herbert Richard Octavius Sankey was the son of William Heney Octavius Sankey (1813–1889), the latter a significant name in medico-psychological circles. W.H.O. had worked at Hanwell Asylum and then Sandywell Park, a private asylum near Cheltenham, published *Lectures on Mental Diseases*, and was appointed Lecturer on Mental Diseases at University College London in 1866,[179] presenting on this subject "in the summer". He was President of the MPA in 1868 (the year before Thomas Laycock).[180] One of the issues he emphasized in his presidential lecture was that medical students should attend compulsory lectures on medico-psychology and that these should be given by asylum doctors.[181]

H.R. Octavius Sankey's single contribution to *WRLAMR*, entitled "A new process for examining the structure of the brain. With a review of some points in the histology of the cerebellum" (V:188–197), gave his affiliation as "Undergraduate in Medicine of the University of London". He does not

---

and Bevan-Lewis ("Recovery from insanity in cases where Haematoma Auris has occurred", VI:127–129). The latter authors noted that "the insane ear, is commonly looked upon as indicative of incurability in insanity". A "Dr. SUTHERLAND" exhibited a sane patient with "insane ear" (*Haematoma auris*), as a consequence of trauma, at the Clinical Society of London on 22nd May 1874 (*BMJ* 1874;1:838 [capitals in original]). This may be Henry Sutherland who was AMO at WRA in the early 1870s before moving to London (see Chap. 5) since he commented that the lesion "resembled in appearance and feeling a haematoma in an old insane patient", perhaps suggesting that he had clinical knowledge of the afflictions of the insane.

[178] *Medical Times and Gazette* 1875;2:603 (27th November; Conversazione at the West Riding Asylum).

[179] *BMJ* 1866;1:162 (Appointments; 10th February).

[180] Obituary: *J Mental Sci* 1889;35:145. Sloffer confused H.R.O. Sankey with W.H.O. Sankey, listing the latter as an author in *WRLAMR* (Sloffer 2023:72n128, 73, 75) which is not the case (see Table 6.1). To my knowledge, W.H.O., unlike H.R.O., had no connection or direct dealings with WRA (although it may be his work which Major alludes to at II:48, 51). Finn stated (2012:73n249) that Crichton-Browne recruited junior clinicians from Sankey's London course but provided no specific evidence. As mentioned (see Chap. 5), the only example I am aware of is John Wilcocks Watson.

[181] Sankey (1868). Renvoize (1991:68). It was not until 1885 that the GMC made a course of instruction a requirement for the final MB and that the examination should embrace insanity.

appear to have worked at WRA.[182] However, a report on the 1875 medical *conversazione* mentions that "Mr. R. H. [*sic*] Octavius Sankey exhibited some beautiful specimens of cerebellar sections prepared by a new and effective method", although it is not entirely clear from the report whether or not he did this in person.[183] His work was mentioned in the *BMJ* ("whose paper in the last number of the *West Riding Reports* [*sic*] well shows the values of his methods of section and preparation"[184]).

At a meeting of the Royal Medical and Chirurgical Society on the 13th March 1877 "A paper was read on 'The pathological anatomy of canine chorea' by Dr. W.R. GOWERS and Mr. H.R.O. SANKEY".[185] This paper was subsequently published in the *Medical Chirurgical Transactions*, wherein Sankey's affiliation was given as "Resident Medical Officer to the National Hospital for the Paralysed and Epileptic", the hospital in London's Queen Square where William Gowers (1845–1915) was an eminent physician.[186] Sankey's appointment as "Resident Medical Officer and Registrar to the National Hospital for the Paralysed and Epileptic" was noted in January 1877.[187] It is not clear whether or not Sankey ever contemplated a career as a physician with an interest in neurology, but 2 years later, in 1879, "H.R. Sankey, Senior AMO Prestwich Asylum" was elected to the membership of the MPA.[188]

A. H. Rabagliati (Andrea Carlo Francesco Rabagliati, 1843–1930)

Andrea Carlo Francesco Rabagliati (*sic*, despite the initials in his *WRLAMR* publication[189]) was the son of an Italian army officer who had emigrated to Scotland after a failed insurrection. Andrea was educated in Edinburgh and attended the University there for his medical education, graduating MB in

---

[182] Finn (2012:181–184) did not include Sankey in his list of those working as either medical officers or clinical clerks at WRA between 1866 and 1876.

[183] *Medical Times and Gazette* 1875;2:603 (27th November; Conversazione at the West Riding Asylum).

[184] *BMJ* 1876;1:51 (8th January; A new histological dye).

[185] *Lancet* 1877;1:388 (17th March; Royal Medical and Chirurgical Society) [capitals in original].

[186] Gowers and Sankey (1877). Although Scott et al. (2012:254) listed Gowers and Sankey's joint presentation and publication in their biography of Gowers, I find no other mention of Sankey. Canine chorea was mentioned by Hughlings Jackson (III:332n1).

[187] *Medical Press and Circular* 1877;23:98 (31st January; Appointments). See also Anon (1960:86).

[188] *J Mental Sci* 1879–1880;25(October 1879):435. R.H. Heurtley Sankey became a member of the MPA in 1894.

[189] But these initials, "A.H.", appear in at least one other publication, *viz.* Rabagliati (1877). This also denotes him as "M.A., M.D.".

1869 and MD in 1872 with a gold medal thesis on relapsing fever.[190] After graduation he became Assistant Medical Officer to the Bradford workhouse in 1870, began private practice in 1872, and was later appointed Assistant Surgeon to the Bradford Eye and Ear Hospital in 1874,[191] surgeon to the Bradford Infirmary in 1877, and Honorary Gynaecologist in 1892.[192] He was to spend the whole of his professional career in Bradford,[193] and was admitted FRCSEd in 1890.[194]

Although Rabagliati did not work at WRA,[195] he was among those reported to be invited to the medical *conversazione* in 1872 and 1873, and accepted an invitation in 1875,[196] which latter meeting he certainly attended.[197] It may be that he had met Crichton-Browne at medical functions held in the West Riding; they were both present at a meeting in late 1872 which decided upon the foundation of the Leeds and West Riding Medico-Chirurgical Society.[198] Moreover, they shared a common background in their Edinburgh medical education although they did not overlap there.

In his single paper in *WRLAMR*, "On classification and nomenclature in nervous disorders" (VI:27–42),[199] Rabagliati's affiliation is given simply as "Bradford". Certainly, he was working there and published from there later in the same decade.[200] Rabagliati may therefore have known Patrick Nicol (see Chap. 5), a former WRA AMO who, according to his three publications in *WRLAMR*, was Physician to the Bradford Infirmary by time of their publication in 1871 and 1872 (Nicol was also invited to the 1872 *conversazione*). In his *WRLAMR* paper, Rabagliati favoured an aetiological classification, as per David Skae, a formulation which had been rejected by Crichton-Browne in

---

[190] *Alphabetical list of graduates of the University of Edinburgh …*, 1879:71, 128.

[191] *Medical Press and Circular* 1874;18:301 (30th September; Appointments).

[192] *Medical Press and Circular* 1892;53:282 (16th March; Appointments).

[193] Obituary: *BMJ* 1930;2:1067 (20th December).

[194] https://archiveandlibrary.rcsed.ac.uk/surgeon/3770984 (accessed 12/11/2023). The *BMJ* obituary gives "F.R.C.S." in error.

[195] Finn (2012:181–184) did not include Rabagliati in his list of those working as either medical officers or clinical clerks at WRA between 1866 and 1876.

[196] For 1872: *Leeds Mercury* 17th October 1872, p.8 (Medical Conversazione at the West Riding Asylum). For 1873: *Yorkshire Post and Leeds Intelligencer* 27th November 1873, p.3 (West Riding Asylum. Medical Conversazione). For 1875: *Leeds Mercury* 20th November 1875, p.3 (Medical Conversazione at Wakefield Asylum).

[197] *BMJ* 1875;2:680 (27th November; The West Riding Asylum).

[198] *BMJ* 1872;2:640 (7th December; Formation of a Medical Society for the West Riding).

[199] Rabagliati returned to this subject matter a few years later, including a presentation to the British Medical Association meeting in Cambridge in August 1880 (Rabagliati 1880, 1881).

[200] Rabagliati (1873). See also Finn and Stark (2015:19).

preference for a symptomatic classification,[201] an irony not lost on a reviewer of the volume.[202]

Rabagliati must have been well thought of by Crichton-Browne since he was amongst the non-WRA individuals reported to be lined up to contribute to the mooted "Monographs on Mental Diseases" on the subject of general paralysis,[203] although he does not appear to have published anything on this subject (unlike a number of individuals working as resident staff at WRA, e.g. Burman, Aldridge, Merson, Bevan-Lewis, Newcombe).

Rabagliati was present as a guest at Crichton-Browne's leaving banquet in Wakefield in April 1876.[204] He subsequently made a number of contributions to the "Critical Digests and Notices of Books" section of *Brain* (Table 6.4) and later to the Reviews and Notices of Books section,[205] as well as publishing elsewhere.[206] In later life he became known for his views on diet, as a convinced vegetarian, on which subject he published a number of books. He does not appear to have pursued any subsequent interest in diseases of the brain.

Henry Clarke[207]

The position of Resident Surgeon at the West Riding Prison, Wakefield, was advertised as vacant in October 1875: "Salary, £400 per annum, with house, coals, gas, and water".[208] Henry Clarke's appointment as "Resident Medical Officer to the West Riding of Yorkshire Prison, Wakefield, vice Wood,

---

[201] Crichton Browne (1875–1876b).

[202] *J Ment Sci* 1877;23(October 1877):380.

[203] *BMJ* 1874;1:210 (14th February; Monographs on Mental Diseases).

[204] *BMJ* 1876;1:516 (22nd April; Dr. Crichton Browne).

[205] Rabagliati (1888).

[206] Rabagliati (1877, 1880, 1881). In the former his affiliation was given as "Surgeon to the Bradford Infirmary". It is possible that he may have become acquainted with Herbert Major (Chap. 5) who moved to Bradford following his departure from the WRA superintendency in 1884. Major had read a paper on behalf of Rabagliati at the Annual Meeting of the British Medical Association held in Cork in 1879 (*J Ment Sci* 1879–1880;25(October 1879):447–449). See Chap. 5 for details.

[207] Triarhou (2021:60) gave his dates as (1845–1909) but I think these refer to Henry Edward Clark [*sic*], author of *An elementary text-book of anatomy* published in 1903. Certainly, Henry Clarke's name disappeared from the list of corresponding members of the MPA between volumes 55 (1909) and 56 (1910) of the *Journal of Mental Science* but I have found no obituary therein, nor in other general medical journals (*Lancet, BMJ*) for 1909. The Wellcome Collection entry for Clarke's *Drawings of Wakefield* gives a date of death of 1921, but again I find no obituary in the *Lancet, BMJ*, or *Journal of Mental Science* for 1921 or 1922.

[208] *BMJ* 1875;2:572 (30th October). Ditto *BMJ* 1875;2:628 (13th November). Compare this salary with that of the Assistant Medical Officers at WRA (Chap. 4).

resigned" in late 1875,[209] having previously been House-Surgeon to Guy's Hospital,[210] might seem to have little to do with the history of the Asylum, as it is unlikely that he ever worked at WRA.[211] However, he seems to have collaborated with the medical staff there from an early stage of his appointment. One may surmise that many individuals labelled as criminal and hence finding their way to the prison in fact had mental health problems, such that there may have been traffic between the Prison and the Asylum, some inmates of the former institution perhaps proving more appropriately managed as patients at the latter.[212]

Clarke was co-author, with Crochley Clapham, on one *WRLAMR* paper "The cranial outline of the insane and criminal" (VI:150–169), indicating a collaboration; Clapham's interest in brain size and weight was already well-established (see Chap. 5). In 1878, Clarke was co-author on one of Bevan-Lewis's seminal papers on cerebral cytoarchitectonics which favoured a five-layer classification of cortical lamination in the motor area and illustrated, for the first time, the large pyramidal ("ganglionic") cells previously described by Betz. The paper was communicated to the Royal Society by Ferrier.[213] Since most of Bevan-Lewis's publications were solo efforts, one wonders exactly what role Clarke played in the genesis of this work; possibly he supplied brain tissue, although there can have been no shortage at the Asylum based on the number of post-mortem examinations undertaken. Another possibility is that he helped with drawing the illustrations. Presumably it was these two collaborative works which contributed to Clarke's election to the membership of the MPA in 1879, at the same time as Bevan-Lewis.[214] Clarke remained as surgeon at the prison until 1908.

In addition to his clinical work, Clarke was a "weekend photographer and serious amateur artist".[215] He illustrated his copy of Henry Clarkson's *Memories*

---

[209] *Lancet* 1875;2:896 (18th December; Medical Appointments). Also *BMJ* 1876;1:30 (1st January; Medical Appointments). For the surgeons William Wood and William Dyson Wood, father and son, who worked at Wakefield Prison, see Chap. 5.

[210] *Lancet* 1876;1:334 (26th February; Medical Appointments).

[211] As was the case for Sankey and for Rabagliati, Finn (2012:181–184) did not include Clarke in his list of junior clinicians at WRA in the Crichton-Browne years.

[212] See for example Burman (1874-1875b:248-250) (Cases II and III). Also pertinent to patients received by the Asylum from the prison is Crichton-Browne (1926:97). Cox and Marland (2022) discussed the distinction between "Criminal or lunatic, prisoner or patient?" (their Chap. 4) with specific examples related to Wakefield Prison and Asylum (at 65, 110), but none was related to the time period covered here.

[213] Lewis and Clarke (1878). For discussion, see Triarhou (2021:59–63).

[214] *J Mental Sci* 1879–1880;25(October 1879):433. Based on a comment in Bevan Lewis (1889:537), Clarke may have undertaken pathological studies in "criminals".

[215] aba.org.uk/book/448146560 (accessed 25/12/2023), drawings of Tivy Side, Cardigan, Wales, 1881; 22 engravings.

of Merry Wakefield (in the reprinted 1889 edition) with drawings of Wakefield scenes, probably done in the 1890s. This volume was later donated by Clarke's daughter, Gladys Taverner Clarke, to Wakefield Corporation in 1960, and hence to the care of the City Librarian. These drawings, 97 in total, were published in 1977 in the *Journal of the Wakefield Historical Society* (volume 4). Although two drawings were views of the prison,[216] the Asylum was not among Clarke's drawings.

Summary: *WRLAMR* Contributors at WRA

Of those non-resident faculty who contributed to *WRLAMR*, several can be shown with certainty to have attended WRA, either for the purposes of assessing patients (Allbutt, Milner Fothergill, Lennox Browne) or undertaking experimental work (Ferrier, Lauder Brunton). It is possible, but not confirmed, that William Browne and Lauder Brunton also saw patients at WRA. Others' attendance at WRA seems to have been confined to the medical *conversazione* (Rabagliati definitely; Sankey possibly). Because of his geographical proximity I think it very likely that Henry Clarke visited WRA (maybe to collaborate with Clapham and/or Bevan-Lewis), but the available evidence suggests that it is decidedly doubtful if not highly unlikely that Hughlings Jackson ever went to WRA despite the affirmative statements to the contrary of previous authors.

Many of these non-resident contributors to *WRLAMR* were distinguished clinicians, holding or later gaining Fellowships of the medical Royal Colleges and of the Royal Society (Lauder Brunton; later Ferrier, Hughlings Jackson, Allbutt). Their contributions to *WRLAMR* undoubtedly enhanced the profile of the journal. Moreover, unlike the resident staff, whose publications in *WRLAMR* have been suggested to have contributed no significant or enduring advance to neurology (Chap. 5), some of the contributions of the non-residents have become recognised as seminal papers in the field of clinical neurology (Jackson) and experimental physiology (Ferrier). As such, they played a role in the establishment of neurology as a clinical discipline in Britain.

---

[216] Clarke (1977:57, 78). Taylor (2005:111).

Part IV

Meetings

…the most fundamental function of a specialist research society: … to provide a forum for presentation and discussion of original investigations by members.[1]

---

[1] French (1975:203).

8

Conversazione at the West Riding Asylum 1871–1875

In addition to a dedicated institution (as discussed in Part I), faculty (Part II) and a house journal (Part III), a series of annual meetings termed medical *conversazione* were staged at the West Riding Asylum at Wakefield (WRA) between 1871 and 1875. This Part firstly examines the nature of these gatherings, the lectures, demonstrations, exhibitions, and entertainments, using reportage from the local popular press to supplement the relatively limited accounts published in contemporary medical journals. In addition, a prosopography is provided encompassing the invited speakers and some of the notable guests.

The *conversazione* evidently provided educational opportunity for invited local practitioners by showcasing the clinical and experimental research work of the Asylum, presented in a manner more immediate than in the house journal. After the fifth and final meeting, many of the personnel involved with the WRA *conversazione* were eventually instrumental in the foundation of another society for the presentation and dissemination of knowledge about diseases of the brain and hence the development of neurology of British neurology, the Neurological Society of London (later the Neurological Society of the United Kingdom).

© The Author(s), under exclusive license to Springer Nature Switzerland AG 2026
A. J. Larner, *The West Riding Asylum and the Origins of British Neurology 1866-1876*,
https://doi.org/10.1007/978-3-032-12591-0_8

Meetings: *Conversazione*[1]

Whilst most clinicians are now familiar with gatherings for educational purposes, designated as conferences and congresses, and even symposia, colloquia, and conclaves, the idea of the conversazione, let alone the experience, may now be unfamiliar, if not entirely alien.

However, the conversazione was a staple of nineteenth-century societies, not only literary and philosophical, but also medical and scientific. Broadly defined, a conversazione was a social gathering held by a learned or art society which commonly included an informal meeting, an exhibition and one or more lectures, in a public or semi-public space. Hence, in addition to its educational purpose, the conversazione provided the opportunity for social encounter, interaction, dialogue, spectacle and entertainment.[2] Certainly the term was in common usage by the end of the nineteenth century:

> … the scientific society opens its museums, its gardens, its library, its laboratories, and its annual *conversaziones* to each of its members, whether he be a Darwin, or a simple amateur.[3]

Origins and Aims of *Conversazione* at the West Riding Asylum

Between 1871 and 1875, James Crichton-Browne organised annual medical *conversazione* at WRA. Although mentioned in passing in historical scholarship relating to WRA,[4] to Crichton-Browne,[5] and to the conversazione as a nineteenth-century cultural phenomenon,[6] no sustained analysis of the medical *conversazione* held at Wakefield has been presented hitherto to my knowledge.[7]

---

[1] Henceforward I use the italicised form solely to describe the WRA meetings, and in direct quotations which used this form.

[2] Alberti (2003), Wood (2006).

[3] Kropotkin (1892:31) [italics in original]. I thank Dr. Guleed Adan for bringing this book to my attention, September 2023.

[4] Todd and Ashworth (n.d.:128–130, 1991:401–402).

[5] Neve and Turner (1995:408).

[6] Wood (2006:88–90).

[7] The WRA *conversazione* were mentioned in passing by Leyland (1888:II:29), Ashworth (1975:69), Todd and Ashworth (1991:401–402), Jellinek (2005:429), Finn (2012:83,145), and Sloffer (2023:56–62). This chapter is based in part on, but much extended from, Larner (2025s).

The conversazione (plural conversaziones or conversazioni)[8] was "a regular event in the calendar of an array of Victorian institutions",[9] not least the pinnacles of London medicine and science, the Royal College of Physicians and the Royal Society. This may have been one of the reasons why Crichton-Browne opted for this nomenclature and format, but there are other possibilities. One of these relates to Crichton-Browne's period of medical training in Edinburgh in the 1850s and 1860s. Conversaziones had been held at the Royal College of Surgeons of Edinburgh at least from the mid-1850s,[10] and the idea was adopted by the Royal Medical Society, the Edinburgh medical students' society, around the same time:

> It having been resolved by this Society, instead of the annual dinner of its members at this season [27th February 1856], to follow the example of the Royal College of Surgeons in its recent and successful conversazione, …[11]

Certainly the Royal Medical Society held a conversazione in 1858 (18th March)[12] and in 1860 (27th March),[13] dates which coincide with Crichton-Browne's time in Edinburgh whilst pursuing his initial medical studies (1857–1862).[14] The Royal College of Physicians of Edinburgh held a conversazione in 1859 (31st January)[15] and in 1860 (21st June),[16] and the Royal College of Surgeons held a series of conversazione in 1861 (25th January; 1st March; 5th April).[17] Hence, this was not a novel or unfamiliar event in the Edinburgh medical calendar of Crichton-Browne's youth.

---

[8] But not "Converzasiones" [*sic*], as in Reynolds and Broussolle (2022:293). I use "conversaziones" henceforth.

[9] Alberti (2003:210).

[10] *Edinb Med J* 1856;1(9):865 (Conversazione of the Royal College of Surgeons).

[11] *Edinb Med J* 1856;1(10):966–967 (Royal Medical Society—Conversazione).

[12] *Edinb Med J* 1858;3(10):955–956 (Royal Medical Society—Conversazione).

[13] *Edinb Med J* 1860;5(11):1051 (Royal Medical Society—Conversazione).

[14] Crichton-Browne's own, retrospective dating (Crichton-Browne 1937:31). Interestingly, and of possible significance, William Browne, Crichton-Browne's father, spoke (his "address occupied close upon two hours in delivery") to the Royal College of Surgeons conversazione held on 30th March 1860, hence just 3 days after the Royal Medical Society conversazione. In this talk "Dr Browne detailed at some length the results of a personal visit to the Bicètre [*sic*] in Paris" (*Edinb Med J* 1860;5(11):1050–1051 (Royal College of Surgeons—Conversazione).).

[15] *Edinb Med J* 1859;4(9):857–859 (Royal College of Physicians—Conversazione).

[16] *Edinb Med J* 1860;6(1):81–82 (Conversazione by the Royal College of Physicians to the Officers of the Channel Fleet).

[17] *Edinb Med J* 1861;6(9):846 (Royal College of Surgeons Conversazione); *Edinb Med J* 1861;6(10):957 (Royal College of Surgeons—Conversazione); *Edinb Med J* 1861;6(11):1047–1049 (Royal College of Surgeons Conversazione).

Other examples, more proximate to the date of inauguration of the WRA *conversazione*, and which might have influenced Crichton-Browne, may also be noted. One such source may have been the 37th Annual Meeting of the British Medical Association (BMA) held in Leeds between 27th and 30th July 1869, where "Dr. Heaton, who is President of the Leeds Literary and Philosophical Society, gives a *conversazione* in the rooms of that institution". The same BMA meeting included a visit to WRA (see Chap. 3).[18] Another conversazione of similar date, and perhaps of greater significance, was held by the Medico-Psychological Association (MPA) at its meeting in York on Monday 2nd August 1869.[19] Thomas Laycock was the MPA President,[20] and Crichton-Browne was in attendance and "proposed a vote of thanks to Dr. Laycock for his address".[21] In the evening a conversazione was held, the description of which[22] bears many resemblances to the subsequent events at WRA.

Funding

How were the WRA *conversazione* funded? As for the Asylum's house journal, no specific information on this point has been found, but a number of possibilities may be considered. One is that Crichton-Browne was able to persuade the WRA Committee of Visitors that, in supporting the public profile of the Asylum, funding of these meetings was a legitimate use of ratepayers' money, and the provision of "liberal refreshment" to the guests was money well spent.

However, the report of the 1873 *conversazione* appearing in the *Wakefield Express* stated that "so much appreciated was the meeting [of 1871] that Dr. Browne (*at whose sole cost they are held*) decided to make the conversazione an

---

[18] *Lancet* 1869;2:175. "Dr. Brown [*sic*], at the West Riding Lunatic Asylum, has issued invitations for an evening party". The visit was described in the *Lancet* 1869;2:312 (28th August; The West Riding Pauper Lunatic Asylum (Wakefield)) and also, in passing, in the *Lancet* 1870;1:17.

[19] Bewley (2008:14–15) suggested that a conversazione had been part of the meetings of AMOAHI, the forerunner of the MPA, at least from 1843.

[20] Laycock's Presidential address was published in the *Journal of Mental Science* in October 1869 (Laycock 1869–1870).

[21] *J Ment Sci* 1869–1870;15(October 1869):470 (Psychological News). Hughlings Jackson was also present at the meeting according to James (1996:64), presumably "Dr. H. Jackson" in the list of attendees, which also included Lawson Tait. At this meeting, Thompson, Mitchell, and Aldridge, all of West Riding Asylum, were elected new members of the MPA, as was Burman (his affiliation at this time was at Devon Asylum).

[22] *J Ment Sci* 1869–1870;15(October 1869):476–477 (Psychological News). James (1996:64) suggested that Laycock did not attend the MPA conversazione of 1869.

annual one".[23] Considering that the refreshments provided included "sand-wiches, cake, fruit, and a choice supply of wine", I am doubtful that Crichton-Browne could have borne the whole cost of entertaining several hundred visitors. Another possibility, not mutually exclusive, is that some form of sponsorship by the commercial enterprises that displayed their products on the *conversazione* stalls (*vide infra*) may have helped to defray costs.

Structure and Content of WRA *Conversazione*

Sources of information relating to the WRA *conversazione* are limited. Printed programmes are available for some of the meetings.[24] Only occasional reports of the meetings appeared in the contemporary medical press such as the *British Medical Journal, Lancet* (perfunctory at best), *Medical Press and Circular*, and *Medical Times and Gazette* (Table 8.1), as well as in the statutory annual *Report of the Medical Superintendent*. As for specialist journals, no account of the WRA *conversazione* has been found in the issues of the *Journal of Mental Science* covering the years 1871–1875, nor in the single issue of the new series of the *Journal of Psychological Medicine and Mental Pathology* pub-lished in this time period (1875), although these journals did carry reviews of *WRLAMR* (Table 6.2). No dedicated neurological journal which might have commented on the WRA *conversazione* existed at this time, since *Brain: a journal of neurology*, the effective successor to *WRLAMR*, did not appear until 1878.

Another source, sometimes more detailed, was reportage in the local press. This finding is concordant with the observation that it was often the case that "the local press were meticulous in detailing who was present at such occasions",[25] perhaps indicative of the social as well as the academic function of these meetings. Local reports were sometimes more widely syndicated, and in places appear to have been the source (or certainly predated) material appearing, almost verbatim, in the general medical journals. I am not aware of any first-hand account of any of the WRA *conversazione* by an attendee.

---

[23] *The Wakefield Express, and Barnsley, Normanton, Pontefract, Ossett, Horbury & Dewsbury Advertiser* Volume 22, No, 1126, 29th November 1873, p.2, cols. 4–7 (Medical conversazione at the West Riding Asylum. Speech by Lord Houghton. Lecture by Dr. Carpenter) [my italics].

[24] WRA archives (WYAS C85/1362) only has programmes for 1872 and 1875 as far as I could find (accessed 23/02/2024) but not for 1871, 1873, or 1874. Title pages of the 1873 and 1874 programmes are illustrated elsewhere without their source(s) being stated: for 1873, Spillane (1974a:704, 1981:389), Todd and Ashworth (n.d.:129), Wood (2006:89), Finn (2012:147), Sloffer (2023:61), for 1874, Ashworth (1975:70).

[25] Alberti (2003:219).

Table 8.1 Summary of medical *conversazione* at WRA 1871–1875

Date of *conversazione*	Published reports of *conversazione*	Keynote speaker and title of lecture	Publication of lecture
1871: 13th October (Friday)	*Lancet* 1871;2:588.	Dr Francis E. Anstie: On the Hereditary Connexions of Nervous Diseases with each other	*J Ment Sci* 1872; 17: 471–484.
1872: 15th October (Tuesday)	*Lancet* 1872;2:615. *BMJ* 1872;2:474–5. *Med Press Circ* 1872;14:360. *Med Times Gaz* 1872;2:466.	Dr William Turner: The convolutions of the human brain considered in relation to the intelligence	*WRLAMR* 1873; III: 1–29.
1873: 25th November (Tuesday)	*Lancet* 1873;2:788. *Med Times Gaz* 1873;2:625.	Dr William Carpenter: Recent advances in the physiology of the brain	*WRLAMR* 1874; IV: 1–23.
1874: 20th November (Friday)	*Med Times Gaz* 1874;2:609–610.	Dr John Charles Bucknill: Responsibility for Homicide	*BMJ* 1874; 2: 667–672.
1875: 19th November (Friday)	*BMJ* 1875;2:680. *Med Press Circ* 1875;20:457. *Med Times Gaz* 1875;2:603.	Dr William Broadbent: Theory of construction of the nervous system	*BMJ* 1876; 1: 371–373, 401–403, 433–436.

These various sources indicate that the format of the WRA *conversazione* changed relatively little across the course of the five meetings. Chairmanship fell to the chair of the Asylum Committee of Visitors or one of the Visiting Justices who, once the invited guests were assembled, made some apposite remarks, often reported in detail in the local press accounts, before the main action of the evening began.

All the *conversazione* featured a high-profile external speaker, professional men of medicine and science at the apex of their particular disciplines which were either directly relevant to and/or interacted with the work of asylum medicine (Table 8.1).

After the speaker, instructive and possibly interactive demonstrations of clinical or experimental methods featured in some of the meetings. The visitors were then able to view the stalls or tables, usually five in number, each manned by members of the Asylum junior staff and displaying work or items from WRA (Table 8.2), as well as from elsewhere.

The guests, invited personally by Crichton-Browne, were generally medical men from around the West Riding area, the largest contingents coming from Wakefield and the nearby conurbations of Leeds and Bradford. In addition to the intellectual fare, they could also enjoy refreshments provided for the

Table 8.2 Stalls at WRA medical *conversazione* 1871–1875

Stall	1871	1872	1873	1874	1875
A: Pathological specimens (and physiological experiments in 1872)	–	Burman	Burman and McDowall	Lawson	Lawson
B: Photographs, stereoscopes	–	Aldridge	Merson	Wallis	Merson
C: Scientific and surgical instruments	–	Woods	Lowe	Benham	Seymour
D: Microscopical preparations	–	Major	Major and Tyler Smith	Major[a]	Major and Bevan-Lewis (and Sankey?)
E: Drugs and medicinal preparations	–	Wood	Watson	Watson (and Bracey)[a]	Arbuckle (and Bracey)

[a]Watson and Bracey were said to have manned the fourth stall, and Major the fifth, in the account of the 1874 *conversazione* published in the *Medical Times and Gazette* 1874;2:609–610 (28th November; Annual Conversazione at the West Riding Asylum)

occasion and enjoy music played by the Asylum band. All the *conversaziones* took place in the Asylum dining hall which was suitably decorated for the occasion.

The West Riding Asylum *Conversazione* 1871–1875

A sequential presentation of each of the five WRA *conversazione* is now given, highlighting the various activities encompassed in each programme.

I: 1871, 13th October

In the *British Medical Journal* (henceforward *BMJ*) dated 14th October 1871, the following note appeared:

> DR. J. CRICHTON BROWNE has issued cards for a medical *conversazione*, to be held in the hall of the West Riding Asylum, Wakefield, on the evening of Friday, Oct. 13th, at eight o'clock.[26]

---

[26] *BMJ* 1871;2:443 (14th October) [capitals and italics in original]. Finn was therefore in error when he stated that "Crichton-Browne … showcased Wakefield through annual conversazione between 1872 [*sic*] and 1875" (Finn 2012:83). He was perhaps misled by the fact that the first of the *conversazione* to be

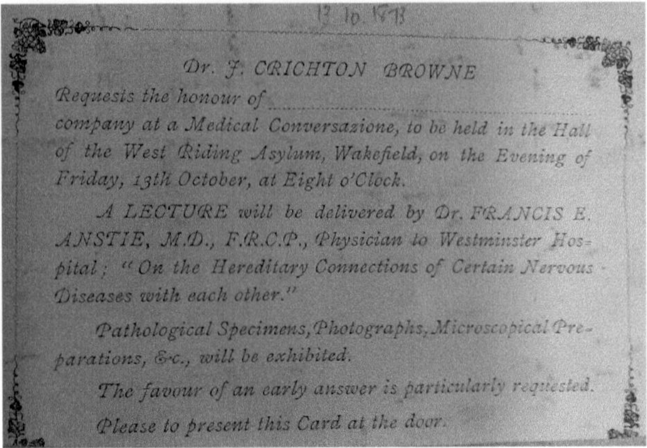

Fig. 8.1 Card for the medical *conversazione*, October 1871

A copy of the said card (Fig. 8.1) reads:

Dr. J. CRICHTON BROWNE
Requests the honour of …
company at a Medical Conversazione to be held in the Hall of the West Riding
Asylum, Wakefield, on the Evening of Friday, 13th October, at Eight o'Clock

A LECTURE will be delivered by Dr. FRANCIS E. ANSTIE, M.D.,
F.R.C.P., Physician to Westminster Hospital; "On the Hereditary Connections
of Certain Nervous Diseases with each other."

Pathological Specimens, Photographs, Microscopical Preparations, &c., will
be exhibited.

The favour of an early answer is particularly requested. Please to present this
Card at the door.[27]

---

reported on (rather than merely announced) in the *BMJ* was that of October 1872 (see below; *BMJ*
1872;2:474–475 (26th October; Medical Conversazione at the West Riding Asylum)), although elsewhere he spoke of "annual conversazioni [*sic*], held yearly between 1871 and 1876 [*sic*]" (Finn 2012:3)
and stated that Crichton-Browne "made the Asylum a profitable place, which gave him the freedom,
starting in 1871, to begin work on … hosting annual conversazione" (Finn 2012:85 [my italics]). It
would be difficult to explain away both dating mistakes as simply typographical errors.

[27] WYAS C85/1382 [capitals in original]. Written in pencil, above the printed words, is "13.10.1873
[*sic*]". If there was a printed programme for 1871 I could find no copy of it in WYAS C85/1382 (accessed
23/02/2024).

The posthoc announcement in the *BMJ*, evidently of no use to any interested party who might wish to travel to Wakefield for the occasion, had no follow up in the pages of the journal. However, in the *Lancet* issue dated 21st October 1871 more information on the event was forthcoming, the report *in toto* reading:

> The West Riding Asylum witnessed on the 13th inst. the first of a series of medical *conversazioni* [*sic*], instituted by Dr. Crichton Browne, with a view to promoting among the profession in Yorkshire the interchange of ideas on scientific medicine in general, and on the treatment of nervous diseases in particular. To an audience of more than one hundred and fifty practitioners Dr. Anstie delivered an address "On the Hereditary Connexions of Nervous Diseases with each other," and received a hearty vote of thanks, proposed by Dr. Chadwick, of Leeds, at the close. In the course of the evening Mr. Brudenell Carter gave an interesting demonstration of the reflecting ophthalmoscope. We congratulate Dr. Browne on the successful initiation of a praiseworthy enterprise.[28]

Thus, a series of annual meetings[29] at the Wakefield asylum was initiated which ran until 1875.

No other report of this first *conversazione* has been found in contemporary medical journals. However, a clear exposition of the purpose of the meeting was forthcoming in the local popular press, specifically the *Wakefield Journal and Examiner* for Friday 20th October 1871 which carried two reports, in adjacent columns of the same page, the second of which explained that Crichton-Browne's inauguration of these meetings was:

> as a means of bringing together the representatives of every branch of the profession in Yorkshire with a view to promote the interchange of experience and ideas on the scientific aspects of medicine, and to afford to those engaged in professional practice facilities for acquainting themselves with the newest and

---

[28] *Lancet* 1871;2:588 (21st October) [italics in original].

[29] Oppenheim (1991:67) stated that "Wakefield Asylum was the centre of neurological interest, and many eminent men congregated there and made their contributions at the monthly [*sic*] medical conversaziones which were organized at that institution by its director". This error concerning the frequency of the meetings presumably originated from Crichton-Browne's obituary in the *British Medical Journal* in 1938 (*BMJ* 1938;1:311). The logistics of organizing monthly, as opposed to annual, meetings would, I suggest, have proved too much even for the administrative talents of Crichton-Browne! The same error is found in Spillane (1974a:702) who wrote of "monthly medical conversaziones" (repeated in Spillane 1981:387–388), and in Finger (2000:163) who noted "special monthly gatherings". Golding (2021:146) erred when stating that "Two medical *conversaziones*, taking place in 1872 and 1875, were held ...", presumably because her source (WYAS C85/1362) only has programmes for these years.

most enlightened methods of dealing with the complex problems of mental disease.[30]

These facilities were listed:

Microscopes, oppthalmoscopes [*sic*], and other scientific instruments were there in abundance and Mr. Manton was in attendance to administer laughing gas to anyone who wished to inhale it.[31]

The *Wakefield Express* stated that "About 100 gallons of 'laughing gas' were in readiness to be administered to any of the guests who might require it, but there was 'only a poor demand'".[32]

Also available for inspection was a table which:

contained the patients' work, [which] seemed to attract considerable attention. Upon it were displayed specimens of book-binding, wood carving, male and female apparel, boots and shoes, tin, iron, and stone work, woollen cloth, dressmaking, Berlin wool work, and, in fact, such a variety of articles as to lead some of the guests to believe that they were at a bazaar. Some of the specimens were remarkably clever and ingenious productions. For instance, we observed an improved axle, to ensure safe travelling in turning sharp curves, which we understand has been patented, …[33]

In his *Report* to the Committee of Visitors for 1871, dated 25th January 1872, Crichton-Browne stated:

By your kind permission I was enabled to introduce to the Hall of the Asylum a large party of visitors of a special class, on 13th of October last. I allude to the

---

[30] *Wakefield Journal and Examiner* 20th October 1871, p.2, col.7 (Medical Conversazione at the West Riding Asylum).

[31] *Wakefield Journal and Examiner* 20th October 1871, p.2, col.6 (Medical Conversazione at the Asylum). I presume "Mr. Manton" was Mr. J.N. Manton, L.D.S., of Wakefield who exhibited dental specimens on Stall A at the 1872 *conversazione* (*Wakefield and West Riding Herald with which is incorporated the Wakefield Journal & Examiner* 19th October 1872, p.6, cols.1,2 (Medical Conversazione at the West Riding Asylum)), rather than Samuel Mitchell who was investigating the physiological and possible therapeutic effects of nitrous oxide at WRA at this time (See Chaps. 5 and 6).

[32] *The Wakefield Express, and Barnsley, Pontefract, & Dewsbury Advertiser* Volume 20, No. 1015, Saturday 14th October 1871, p.8, col.1 (Great gathering of medical gentlemen at the West Riding Asylum. Grand conversazione last night. Lecture by Dr. Ainstie [*sic*]). Also cited in Neve and Turner (1995:408). These authors also stated that the visitors "braved rain and muddy roads"; I have not found this information in the accounts I have seen in the contemporary medical or local press.

[33] *The Wakefield Express, and Barnsley, Pontefract, & Dewsbury Advertiser* Volume 20, No. 1015, Saturday 14th October 1871, p.8, col.1 (Great gathering of medical gentlemen at the West Riding Asylum. Grand conversazione last night. Lecture by Dr. Ainstie [*sic*]).

medical practitioners of the Riding, who then assembled here to the number of 150, and listened to an eloquent and thoughtful address by DR. FRANCIS E. ANSTIE, Assistant Physician to Westminster Hospital, on "The Hereditary Connexion of certain Nervous Diseases with each other." The gathering, which was in all respects eminently successful, besides its social attractions afforded an opportunity for the exchange of experience and views upon medical topics, and for the exhibition of the results of some of the scientific work which is executed by your Medical Officers.[34]

II: 1872, 15th October

The second WRA *conversazione* took place almost exactly 1 year after the first, but this time on a Tuesday rather than a Friday evening. This meeting attracted more coverage in the medical (Table 8.1) and popular press, the former including both the *Lancet* and the *BMJ*, although the account in the *Lancet* was perfunctory:

> On the 15th inst. a medical *conversazione* was held in the West Riding Asylum at Wakefield. Professor Turner of Edinburgh, delivered a lecture to a large and influential audience of local practitioners and men of science on the cerebral convolutions.[35]

No names of those attending, other than the speaker, were given in this notice, nor mention of the purpose of the meeting or any other activities occurring in it. However, a "List of the gentlemen invited" was published in the *Wakefield and West Riding Herald*, a list which included some individuals previously or subsequently involved with WRA and/or *WRLAMR*, including Nicol and "Rabagliata" [*sic*] from Bradford (see Chap. 5 for discussion of Nicol, and Chap. 7 for Rabagliati); Dr. Wright from Wakefield and Mr. W.J. Lancaster from Barnsley (see Chap. 2); Courtenay from Derby, Lawrence from Chester, Lowe from Sedgefield, and Lawson Tait from Birmingham (all discussed in Chap. 5).[36] In all, "Upwards of 250 invitations had been issued, and all with few exceptions, were accepted", not only from the West Riding but also

---

[34] *Report*, 1872:31 [capitals in original]. Note there was no use here of the word "conversazione," which may explain why Sloffer (2023:58) reported that "that term was not used in 1871", perhaps unaware of the notes on the meeting published in the *BMJ* and the *Lancet* both of which used the term, as did the notices in the local press.

[35] *Lancet* 1872;2:615 (26th October).

[36] *Wakefield and West Riding Herald with which is incorporated the Wakefield Journal & Examiner* 19th October 1872, p.6, cols.1,2 (Medical Conversazione at the West Riding Asylum); also *Leeds Mercury* 17th October 1872, p.8 (Medical Conversazione at the West Riding Asylum).

London (Dr J.S. Sabben [*sic*], Mr. J.H. Balfour Browne), Manchester (Dr W.G. Mould), and Edinburgh (Dr J.B. Pettigrew). The *Wakefield Express* specified 210 acceptances from 250 invitations.[37]

According to the report of the meeting appearing in the *Medical Press and Circular*:

> The object of the gathering—which was the second of what we believe is to be a series of annual meetings—was to give an opportunity to the Medical [*sic*] practitioners of the various towns in the West Riding and other districts to see the mode of treatment adopted at this most admirable institution, to discuss and exchange views upon professional topics …

Comment was also made on the décor:

> Stalls were fixed on each side, and at the top of the hall, in the centre of which, and placed here and there, were a number of small stands containing rare plants, ferns, &c.[38]

According to the *Leeds Mercury*:

> The hall had been arranged with great care and taste. Around the walls were displayed a number of pretty coloured banners and paintings. At various points there were choice plants effectively grouped, and ranging round the room were a series of stalls, on which were placed a large variety of objects of interest, while the monotony of the centre of the room was relieved by a number of stands, on which were placed a few plants or some other object of interest.[39]

Likewise, the *Wakefield Express* noted that:

> The arrangements were … perfect, the hall looked beautiful, it felt very comfortable, and the guests thoroughly enjoyed themselves.

However, there was a hitch in that:

---

[37] *The Wakefield Express, and Barnsley, Normanton, Pontefract, Ossett, Horbury & Dewsbury Advertiser* Volume 21, No. 1068, 19th October 1872, p.2, cols.3–4 (Great gathering of medical gentlemen at the West Riding Asylum. Conversazione and lecture by Professor Turner). Here "Dr. Rapagliats" [*sic*] was listed as one of those invited.

[38] *Medical Press and Circular* 1872;14:360 (23rd October; Conversazione and lecture by Professor Turner).

[39] *Leeds Mercury* 17th October 1872, p.8, col. 1 (Medical Conversazione at the West Riding Asylum).

The proceedings were announced to commence at eight o'clock but in consequence of many of the visitors having to travel considerable distances by rail and by road, and the weather being very foggy, it was a quarter to nine before the whole of the guests made their appearance.[40]

The Chairman, Spencer Stanhope, then made some remarks:

there had been a very great increase of knowledge in the treatment of mental diseases, and he had no doubt whatever that that would be materially promoted by such meetings as the present, at which members of the medical profession met together and exchanged their ideas, and enquired into the modes adopted for the treatment of different phases of mental maladies.[41]

Professor Turner then gave his presentation, after which:

The remainder of the evening was spent in examining various objects of medical and scientific interest which had been collected together in the Asylum hall, and arranged in a series of stalls. These included a large assortment of surgical instruments, and pathological specimens from the asylum museum, microscopic preparations, photographs, and drawings by the insane. The stalls were presided over by the medical officers of the asylum, Dr. Mitchell, Dr. Aldridge, Dr. Burman, Dr. Major, Dr. Oscar Woods, and Mr. Bryan Wood. The splendid band of the asylum performed a selection of music at intervals during the evening.[42]

More details of the stalls or tables may be found in the account of the *conversazione* published in the *Medical Press and Circular* of 23rd October, which is quoted here in full:

The first stall, which was described as Stall A, was presided over by Dr. J. Wilkie Burman, and it was covered with pathological specimens and physiological experiments, most of which were from the Pathological Museum of the Asylum. There were also on the stall some interesting contributions from the Leeds School of Medicine, a most extraordinary malformed foetus, exhibited by Dr. Morris, of Barnsley, and a dried ovarian cyst, shown by Dr. Lee, of Bradford. Mr. J.N. Manton, dentist, of Wakefield, exhibited a number of models of jaws,

[40] *The Wakefield Express, and Barnsley, Normanton, Pontefract, Ossett, Horbury & Dewsbury Advertiser* Volume 21, No. 1068, 19 October 1872, p.2, cols.3–4 (Great gathering of medical gentlemen at the West Riding Asylum. Conversazione and lecture by Professor Turner).

[41] *Leeds Mercury* 17th October 1872, p.8, col. 1 (Medical Conversazione at the West Riding Asylum).

[42] *BMJ* 1872;2:474–475 (26th October; Medical Conversazione at the West Riding Asylum). See Chap. 5 for details of these "medical officers of the asylum".

showing many forms of irregularities of the permanent teeth, another series of models containing supernumerary teeth, and a collection of dental specimens. Stall B was presided over by Dr. Charles Aldridge, and it contained a large, valuable, and interesting collection of photographs and stereoscopes from the Asylum collection, together with many others exhibited by Dr. J.B. Pettigrew, Dr. W.A.F. Browne, and Messrs. Harvey and Reynolds, of Leeds. The last named firm again lent a series of oleographs, which were much admired. There was on this stall a very large collection of photographs representing both males and females suffering from almost every variety of insanity. Stall C was presided over by Dr. Oscar Woods, and upon it were arranged a large number of scientific and surgical instruments belonging to the Asylum, together with others lent by Messrs. Harvey and Reynolds, and Messrs. Maw and Son, of London. The next stall, lettered D, was presided over by Dr. Herbert C. Major, and it was filled with a large number of microscopical preparations from the Asylum collection, and others lent by Messrs. J. Fowler, Wakefield; J. Walker, Leeds; E. Yendall, and Dr. James Gilchrist. Stall E was presided over by Mr. W. Bryan Wood, and it contained drugs and Medical [*sic*] preparations, exhibited by Messrs, J. and H. Smith, of Edinburgh and London, Harvey and Reynolds, and McDougall Brothers, Manchester. Another stall,[43] in a corner of the hall, was filled with specimens of the work of the patients, and they were inspected and examined with great interest by many of the visitors. During the evening Dr. Burman performed some experiments on rabbits, rats, and frogs, illustrating the inhibitory power of the vagus nerve over the action of the heart, reflex and galvanic action, and the physiological action of conia, picrotoxine, strychnia, and hydrate of chloral when subcutaneously injected. The curious experiments were witnessed by several gentlemen, who seemed to take the greatest interest in watching the "slaughtering of the innocents".[44] The gathering, which was originated last year by Dr. Crichton Brown [*sic*], is looked upon with great interest by the Profession, and great credit is due to that gentleman and his coadjutors for the manner in which everything connected with it is carried out.[45]

---

[43] In their account of the stalls at the 1872 *conversazione*, Todd and Ashworth (n.d.:128, 130) reported "five stalls were available for the further instruction of the guests" but nevertheless included a "Stall 'F'" where "refreshments were available for the guests attending the conversazione". They did not mention a stall with "specimens of the work of the patients".

[44] Burman's paper on conia in *WRLAMR* (II:1–40) gave some evidence of his readiness to sacrifice experimental animals.

[45] *Medical Press and Circular* 1872;14:360 (23rd October; Conversazione and lecture by Professor Turner). The same report appears verbatim in the *Wakefield Express* (19th October 1872, p.2) which may thus be the source of the *Medical Press and Circular* report. The account of the *conversazione* published in the *Leeds Mercury* (17th October 1872, p.8 (Medical Conversazione at the West Riding Asylum)) confirmed the stall presiders to be Burman, Aldridge, Woods, Major, and W.B. Wood. Hence, contrary to the *BMJ* report (*BMJ* 1872;2:474–475 (26th October; Medical Conversazione at the West Riding Asylum)), there is no mention here of "Dr. Mitchell" as presiding over a stall. I presume that the *BMJ* report was referring to Dr. Samuel Mitchell, but he was no longer one of the "medical officers of the asylum" by this time, having left WRA to become Medical Superintendent at the South Yorkshire Asylum

Evidently then, the stalls featured more than simply material from WRA, but also items from elsewhere, including from commercial outlets.[46]

The programme for this *conversazione* bears out this account, but also drew attention to a "Stall F" for refreshments and also informed attendees that "During the Evening the Band of the West Riding Asylum, conducted by Mr. E. BERRY, will perform the following SELECTION OF MUSIC" including J. Strauss, Verdi, and Rossini. It also gave more details of the specimens from the Pathological Museum (e.g. Arachnoid cyst *in situ*, Syphilitic brain, Brain of epileptic idiot, Brains of monkey, ox, sheep, rabbit, &c."), the Photographs (e.g. the normal and some abnormal arrangements of the cerebral convolutions, changes in the optic disc in cases of general paralysis), and of the microscopical preparations (e.g. sections of the grey matter of the cerebral convolutions in health, in general paralysis of the insane, and in chronic brain wasting).[47]

Crichton-Browne's own account, in his Medical Superintendent's *Report* for 1872 (dated 30th January 1873), was as follows:

> The second Annual Medical Conversazione was held in the Hall of the Asylum, on October 15th. Mr. SPENCER STANHOPE, the Chairman of your Committee, presided upon the occasion, and PROFESSOR TURNER of the University of Edinburgh, delivered a most able and original lecture on the Convolutions of the Cerebrum. Upwards of two hundred medical men were present, some having come from a great distance to take part in a gathering which combines social with scientific attractions, and which is, I believe, powerfully conducive to the successful administration of the Asylum.[48]

---

around March 1872 (e.g. *BMJ* 1872;1:303; see Chap. 5 for further details), although this does not of course exclude the possibility that he attended this *conversazione*. The "List of the gentlemen invited" published in the report of the *conversazione* which appeared in the *Leeds Mercury* (17th October 1872, p.8) did not include Mitchell's name. He was invited to the 1873 *conversazione* according to *Yorkshire Post and Leeds Intelligencer* 27th November 1873, p.3 (West Riding Asylum. Medical Conversazione).

[46] Jones (2013:116) has noted, in her study of Medical Trade Catalogues, that "In the 1870s, both Maw and Reynolds & Branson [*sic*] set up stalls at the West Riding Asylum, Wakefield for its annual medical conversazione with the hope of selling products to the country's leading mental health practitioners", with a reference to 15th October 1872. The programme for this meeting notes exhibits by "Messrs. HARVEY & REYNOLDS, Leeds" and "Messrs. MAW & SON, London" but there is no "Branson" mentioned, likewise in the quoted *Medical Press and Circular* report (ditto the programme for the 1875 *conversazione*); also by Lawson (VI:82). Harvey and Reynolds of Briggate, Leeds, also retailed the clinical thermometer designed by Allbutt (*BMJ* 1868;2:447). From our (early twenty-first century) perspective on medical meetings, we might perhaps wonder whether or not these commercial interests sponsored the *conversazione* in any way or paid a premium to the Asylum in order to attend.

[47] WYAS C85/1382, "West Riding Asylum, Wakefield. Medical Conversazione, 15th October, 1872".

[48] *Report*, 1873:25–26 [capitals in original].

Also of possible relevance to this *conversazione* is the account given by Finn, that:

> Late in 1872, when Crichton-Browne's good friend and fellow Scotsman Ferrier visited Wakefield for the annual conversazione, the two talked about many things, and Fritsch and Hitzig's results were chief among them.[49]

The absence of Ferrier's name in the contemporary accounts of the *conversazione* appearing in the medical press does not absolutely exclude his presence at this meeting, since absence of evidence does not necessarily equate to evidence of absence. Certainly, at this stage of his career Ferrier was not a highly notable name so might have gone unremarked in the throng, perhaps as one of the gentlemen "having come from a great distance". However, the "List of the gentlemen invited" published in the local press reports does not include Ferrier's name.

III: 1873, 25th November

The programme for the 1873 *conversazione* advertised William Carpenter to give a lecture on "RECENT ADVANCES IN THE PHYSIOLOGY OF THE BRAIN", David Ferrier to give a demonstration of "THE LOCALISATION OF FUNCTION IN THE BRAIN", and Richard Norris "Will exhibit some New Experiments in Cohesion, Attraction, &c., designed to explain the nature of certain leading phenomena of Inflammation, Stasis of the Blood, and Transudation of its Corpuscles through the walls of vessels, without interference with structural continuity, as observed by Addison, Wallis, Williams, Cohnheim, and others".[50]

This meeting was noted in the *Lancet*, of Saturday 29th November 1873, the report *in toto* reading:

> The medical conversazione held at the West Riding Asylum on Tuesday evening last [25th November] was a brilliant success. An admirable address was delivered by Dr. Carpenter on the Functions of the Brain. Among those present were

---

[49] Finn (2012:139). Finn cited no source(s). I have previously cast doubt on Ferrier's attendance at the 1872 *conversazione*, for want of any definitive evidence to the contrary (Larner 2023c, 2025j; also Chap. 7), although he was certainly present at the 1873 meeting.

[50] The title page of the 1873 programme was reproduced by Spillane (1974a:704, 1981:389), Todd and Ashworth (n.d.:129), Wood (2006:89, who misdated the meeting as 28th November [at 88]), Finn (2012:147), and Sloffer (2023:61) [capitals in original]. I found no copy of this programme in WYAS C85/1382 (accessed 23/02/2024).

Lord Houghton, Dr. Harrington Tuke,[51] Dr. Ferrier, Dr. Crichton Browne, Dr. Paley of Melbourne,[52] &c.[53]

Not the most in-depth reportage, but it is perhaps of note that Ferrier's name preceded that of Crichton-Browne, perhaps understandably in this, his *annus mirabilis*.[54]

The account in the *Medical Times and Gazette* was similarly perfunctory, not even using the word *conversazione*:

> Lord Houghton presided, and delivered an address, at an important meeting of medical practitioners at the West Riding Asylum, Wakefield, on Tuesday. Dr. Carpenter afterwards gave a lecture on the recent experiments by Professor Ferrier on the localisation of the functions of the brain.[55]

No account of the 1873 *conversazione* has been found in the *BMJ*, but an article titled "Brain-force and blood-supply" in the issue of 29th November (i.e. 4 days after the Wakefield meeting) alluded to two lectures recently given by Carpenter on the functions of the brain,[56] one of which must surely have been that given at WRA.

More detail was available in the local popular press,[57] although the focus was generally more on the chairman's address rather than on Carpenter or Ferrier. The account in the *Yorkshire Post and Leeds Intelligencer* of Thursday 27th November 1873 gave details of the those invited, the stalls, the talks and Ferrier's demonstration. Amongst those invited were several with prior involvement with WRA or who were to have later contact with it or publish in *WRLAMR*, including Clifford Allbutt from Leeds (Chap. 7), Mitchell from Sheffield (Chap. 5), Lancaster from Barnsley (Chap. 2), Rabagliati from Bradford (Chap. 7), and Wright from Wakefield (Chap. 2).

---

[51] Thomas Harrington Tuke (1826–1888) was MPA President in 1873.

[52] I presume "Dr. Paley of Melbourne" to have been Dr. Edward Paley (1827–1886), Inspector of Asylums in Victoria, Australia, between 1863 and 1883, who had worked at Chapeltown in Yorkshire from 1860 to 1863 (Crowther 2003). He appears to have been the only international visitor to any of the WRA *conversazione*.

[53] *Lancet* 1873;2:788 (29th November).

[54] As detailed in Larner (2023c) and more extensively (2025j).

[55] *Medical Times and Gazette* 1873;2:625 (29th November).

[56] *BMJ* 1873;2:641 (29th November).

[57] For example, *Yorkshire Post and Leeds Intelligencer* 27th November 1873, p.3 (West Riding Asylum. Medical Conversazione); *Leeds Mercury* 27th November 1873, p.7 (Medical Conversazione at the West Riding Asylum); *The Wakefield Express, and Barnsley, Normanton, Pontefract, Ossett, Horbury & Dewsbury Advertiser* Volume 22, No, 1126, 29th November 1873, p.2, cols. 4–7 (Medical conversazione at the West Riding Asylum. Speech by Lord Houghton. Lecture by Dr. Carpenter).

This year, the stalls were presided over by Burman and McDowall (pathological specimens),[58] Merson (photographs, stereoscopes),[59] Lowe (scientific and surgical instruments), Major assisted by Mr. E. Tyler Smith (microscopical preparations), and "Mr Watson" (drugs and medicinal preparations).

According to the *Leeds Mercury*, following Carpenter's talk, "A series of experiments were afterwards made by Dr. Ferrier upon a cat under chloroform in demonstration of the localisation of function in the brain."[60] A more detailed account appeared in the *Yorkshire Post and Leeds Intelligencer*. After Carpenter's talk:

> a most interesting part of the business of the evening took place. In a small room off the hall, Professor Ferrier gave to parties of 12 or 14 gentlemen at a time, demonstrations of "The Localisation of Function in the Brain." The experiments were made upon a cat, which having been placed under chloroform, the covering of the brain was removed. The interest and importance of the experiments consisted in the definiteness and certainty with which certain muscular movements were produced, on the application of the electrode to certain portions of the brain. … The interest evinced in the experiments was very great, there being quite a rush of gentlemen to witness them. … The company did not separate until a late hour.[61]

A further, technical experimental point was mentioned in the *Wakefield Express,* specifically that Ferrier:

> applied the electrodes of a galvanic battery … first testing the strength of the current … by applying them to his own tongue, and predicting the movements which would ensue.

Furthermore, "When the experiments were completed the animal was destroyed…".[62]

Crichton-Browne's account of this *conversazione*, in his Medical Superintendent's *Report* for 1873 (dated 29th January 1874), was as follows:

---

[58] *Leeds Mercury* gives "T.W. McDavall" [*sic*].

[59] *Leeds Mercury* gives "John Moxon" [*sic*].

[60] Cited by Crowther (2013:13, n13). Other papers reported that Ferrier demonstrated "the localisation of friction [*sic*] in the brain", e.g. *Morpeth Herald* 29th November 1873, p.6 (Medical Conversazione at the West Riding Asylum).

[61] *Yorkshire Post and Leeds Intelligencer* 27th November 1873, p.3 (West Riding Asylum. Medical Conversazione)

[62] *The Wakefield Express, and Barnsley, Normanton, Pontefract, Ossett, Horbury & Dewsbury Advertiser* Volume 22, No, 1126, 29th November 1873, p.2, cols. 4–7 (Medical conversazione at the West Riding Asylum. Speech by Lord Houghton. Lecture by Dr. Carpenter).

The Medical Conversazione of 1873 was held on the 25th of November. The Right Honourable Lord HOUGHTON occupied the Chair, and that veteran physiologist, Dr. W.B. CARPENTER, who has done so much for science in this Country, addressed an audience of nearly 300 medical men on "Recent Advances in the Physiology of the Brain." The address had special reference to the discoveries of PROFESSOR FERRIER, as to the Localization of Function in the Brain, and had special interest as being delivered in the place where those discoveries were achieved. I know it will not be a matter of indifference to the inhabitants of the West Riding that their County Asylum was the scene of PROFESSOR FERRIER'S labours, and of the new revelation in which these labours resulted—a revelation which must ultimately vastly augment our knowledge of human nature and of the ills to which it is subject, and our power of curtailing and alleviating those ills.[63]

IV: 1874, 20th November

The programme for the 1874 WRA *conversazione* advertised John Bucknill's lecture on "Responsibility for Homicide" on the front page and gave details of the stalls on another.[64]

No report of this meeting has been found in either the *Lancet* or the *BMJ*, although Bucknill's address, "Read to an audience of medical men assembled at the West Riding Asylum, November 20th, 1874", was published in the latter.[65] However, the *Medical Times and Gazette* for 28th November carried a report,[66] in which the social importance of the meeting was emphasized:

For those living in large towns, and enjoying many opportunities of meeting personally, it is almost impossible to judge of the importance of an annual gathering of medical men who have almost no other chance of meeting in a body or of watching the practical progress of medical science than that afforded by the courtesy of the director of a large public provincial institution.

---

[63] *Report*, 1874:24–25 [capitals in original]. I would imagine that Crichton-Browne's rhetorical flourish "I know it will not be a matter of indifference to the inhabitants of the West Riding that their County Asylum was the scene of PROFESSOR FERRIER'S labours" was counterfactual.

[64] The programme is reproduced by Ashworth (1975:70). I found no copy of this programme in WYAS C85/1382 (accessed 23/02/2024).

[65] Bucknill (1874). This address was also noted in *BMJ* 1874;2:685 (28th November; Dr. Bucknill's address at the West Riding Asylum) which promised that "Of the address, the place, and the occasion, we shall have more to say next week". My search of the *BMJ* issue for 5th December 1874 has found nothing which corresponds to the item promised.

[66] *Medical Times and Gazette* 1874;2:609–610 (28th November; Annual Conversazione at the West Riding Asylum).

Between 200 and 300 medical practitioners had been invited. In the "large and well-proportioned hall of the Asylum … decorated and arranged for the purpose of conducing to the comfort and edification of the professional visitors" the following stalls were noted:

A well-filled table of pathological specimens, supplied mainly from the museum of the West Riding Asylum, was furnished, in addition, with preparations of great illustrative value from the collection of the Leeds School of Medicine and from the private museum of Dr. John Duncan, of Edinburgh. An excellent table of photographs, illustrative of cases at present or formerly in the Asylum, was superintended by Dr. John Wallis. A stall for scientific and surgical instruments was presided over by Dr. T. W. Benham [*sic*], who, in the course of the evening, demonstrated Ludwig's Strom-uhr as a method of determining the amount of blood passing through any vessel in a given time. At this stall the instruments in the possession of the Asylum were supplemented by others lent by Dr. Lauder Brunton and Messrs. Maw, Son, and Thompson. The fourth stall, superintended by Mr. C. E. Watson, of King's College, assisted by Mr. Bracey, the Apothecary of the Asylum, was fitted with numerous specimens of new drugs, and many magnificent samples of crystallised alkaloids, etc., lent by Messrs. Smith, of Edinburgh. At the fifth table Dr. Herbert Major exhibited some of the results of his microscopic researches into cerebral histo-pathology, which have done so much to identify the West Riding Asylum with the progress of brain-histology. At the same time, Dr. Major showed some brain-sections by Dr. Tempest Anderson, which could not possibly fail to elicit expressions of enthusiastic admiration from anyone who had ever attempted to prepare microscopic slides. At the same stall, brain-slides by Dr. Clifford Gill and Dr. Batty Tuke, and lucid micro-photographs from the collection of Dr. Gray, of the New York Asylum, Utica, were exhibited, to the satisfaction of all professional visitors.

Hence, as previously, there was a commercial input to the proceedings, and also an international flavour with exhibition of materials from as far afield as the USA.

The meeting was also reported in the local press,[67] confirming the stalls and their superintendents and also mentioning a sixth stall providing refreshments. In addition, some of these reports noted that Lawson was at the

---

[67] For example, *Wakefield and West Riding Herald with which is incorporated the Wakefield Journal & Examiner* 21st November 1874, p.5, col.6 (Medical Conversazione at the Asylum); *Leeds Mercury* 21st November 1874, p.7 (Medical Conversazione at Wakefield Asylum); *Yorkshire Post and Leeds Intelligencer* 21st November 1874, p.5 (Medical Conversazione at Wakefield Asylum); *The Wakefield Express, and Barnsley, Normanton, Pontefract, Ossett, Horbury & Dewsbury Advertiser* Volume 23, No. 1178, 28th November 1874, p.2, cols 6–7 (West Riding Asylum. Fourth annual conversazione. Address by Dr. Bucknill).

pathological specimens table, and that at Major's table "Mr Clifford Gill, of York, exhibited on the same stall preparations of brain and other organs, showing injection of the vessels combined with logwood staining" .

> During the supplementary transactions of the conversazione, Dr. Heaton, Mr. Wheelhouse, Dr. Bucknill, Mr. Ernest Hart, and Dr. Clifford Allbutt expressed incidentally their high appreciation of the West Riding Asylum as an institution for the treatment of the insane and a school of original scientific observation; and subsequently many of the visitors from a distance had an opportunity of inspecting the Asylum and of judging for themselves of the high and progressive character of the retreat as an institution comfortable to all who reside in it, and gratifying to all who may visit it.[68]

Although there does not appear to have been any experimental demonstration at this *conversazione*, other than Benham's display of Ludwig's Strom-uhr, as in previous meetings entertainment was on hand:

> During the course of the evening, the band of the Asylum, containing about thirty attendants, played classical selections from Auber, Strauss, Verdi, Bellini, etc.[69]

Ernest Hart "in an able speech, proposed a vote of thanks to the Chairman which was seconded by Dr. Clifford Allbutt".[70]

V: 1875, 19th November

> DR. CRICHTON BROWNE has issued cards for his annual medical *conversazione* in the hall of the West Riding Asylum, for Friday, Nov. 19th. Dr. Broadbent will deliver an address on the Theory of Construction of the Nervous System.[71]

The programme for this meeting (Fig. 8.2), covering four pages in total, gave details of the lecture "On the theory of construction of the nervous system" to be delivered by Dr. W.H. Broadbent, Physician to St Mary's Hospital, London,

---

[68] *Medical Times and Gazette* 1874;2:609–610 (28th November; Annual Conversazione at the West Riding Asylum).

[69] Idem.

[70] *Wakefield and West Riding Herald with which is incorporated the Wakefield Journal & Examiner* 21st November 1874, p.5, col.6 (Medical Conversazione at the Asylum).

[71] *BMJ* 1875;2:618 (13th November) [capitals and italics in original].

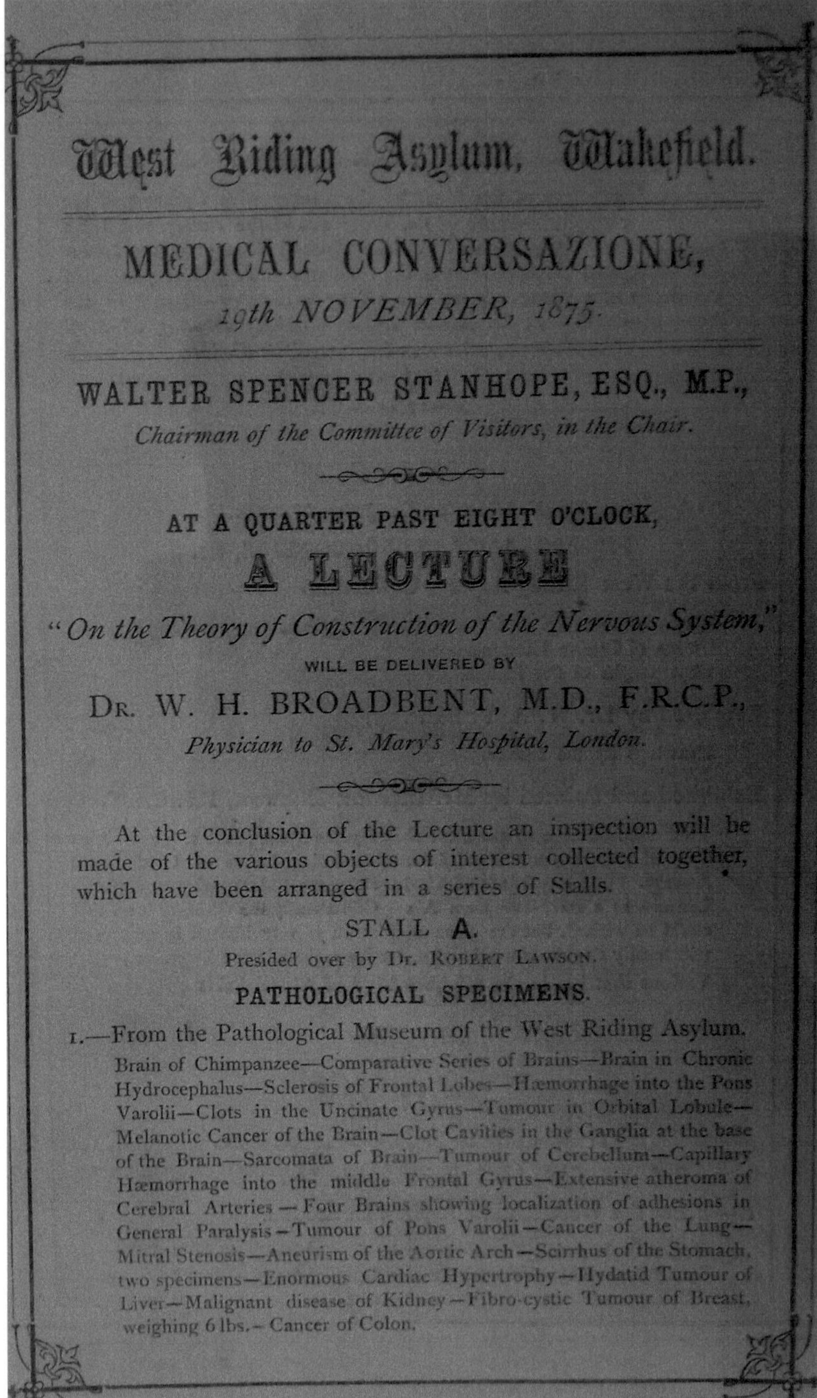

Fig. 8.2 Programme for the medical *conversazione*, November 1875

as well as the various stalls, and the selection of music to be played by the Asylum Band, including Verdi, "Waldtenfel" (presumably Waldteufel), and Meyerbeer.[72] Stalls A-E were respectively presided over by Robert Lawson (pathological specimens), John Merson (photographs, stereoscopes, &c.), Charles Seymour (scientific and surgical instruments), Herbert Major and "Bevan Lewis" (histology), J.H. Arbuckle and Mr. G Bracey (drugs and medicinal preparations).

The account of the 1875 *conversazione* published in the *BMJ* issue of 27th November stated that the meeting "came off last week with great success".[73] It reported that "There were present … between 300 and 400 medical men of the locality", hence a significant increase from the number of "more than 150 practitioners" reported at the inaugural meeting of 1871.[74] Amongst those attending, the names of Clifford Allbutt of Leeds and Dr. Rabagliati of Bradford were mentioned, and from London Dr. Harrington Tuke (as in 1873), who proposed the vote of thanks to the Chairman, but there was no mention of either Hughlings Jackson or Ferrier, unlikely omissions if either had indeed been present. Ernest Hart was also present (as in 1874), and he:

> moved a vote of thanks to the orator, observing that English medical science boasted in the last generation a Bell and a Marshall Hall, who laid the foundations of progress in the anatomy and physiology of the nervous system, and the treatment of diseases of the mind and nervous system. We might add now to the list Lockhart Clarke, Ferrier, Hughlings Jackson, and Broadbent, as no unworthy followers in the footsteps of those benefactors of mankind. The West Riding Asylum, under the initiative of its present most able director, was affording facilities for the furtherance of the studies of these men, and for the application of their work to the treatment of mental disease; and in doing so, with the hearty concurrence of the visiting magistrates, Dr. Browne was setting a high example, which could not but be fruitful in great results, and might well be widely imitated.[75]

The *BMJ* report concluded:

> The good results of the infusion of the spirit of scientific research into a great curative establishment are nowhere more apparent than at the West Riding

---

[72] WYAS C85/1382, "West Riding Asylum, Wakefield. Medical Conversazione, 19th November, 1875".

[73] *BMJ* 1875;2:680 (27th November; The West Riding Asylum).

[74] *Lancet* 1871;2:588.

[75] *BMJ* 1875;2:680 (27th November; The West Riding Asylum).

Asylum, which, under the singularly able direction of Dr. Crichton Browne, is in every respect a credit to the county and an honour to this country.[76]

The meeting was also noted in the *Medical Press and Circular*, just a few lines which failed to mention anything or anyone,[77] and no account has been found in the pages of the *Lancet*. However, the *Medical Times and Gazette* devoted the best part of a column to a description of the proceedings.[78]

As previously, in addition to the guest lecturer, Dr. William Broadbent, there were stalls or tables to view. The *BMJ* reported that:

Among the objects displayed from the West Riding Asylum were many pathological specimens of value shown at a table presided over by Dr. Robert Lawson, one of the medical officers of the asylum. They included a very instructive preparation of the brain of a chimpanzee, and a comparative series of brains, most useful for the study of function. Four brains, showing localisation of adhesions in general paralysis, were prepared by a new method (steeping in a nitric acid solution). This method is obviously very superior to the ordinary modes of removing the membranes, and promises to yield useful results. The table presided over by Dr. Herbert Major and Dr. Bevan Lewis was crowded with a quite unique collection of microscopic preparations from the collection belonging to the asylum, illustrating the histological condition of the convolutions of the human brain in the healthy adult, in the foetus, and in various forms of insanity; and similar series of the medulla oblongata, spinal cord, sciatic nerve, and sympathetic ganglia. Among these preparations were the series illustrating Dr. Major's thesis for the M.D. degree of Edinburgh, which received the gold medal, and his own and Dr. Lewis's papers in the West Riding Reports.[79]

More details were found in the *Medical Times and Gazette* report:

Around the handsome hall of the Asylum were ranged several stalls for the exhibition of objects of interest to the medical profession. The first, presided over by Dr. Robert Lawson, was for the display of selected specimens from the large pathological museum of the West Riding Asylum. Amongst the most interesting of these objects were specimen [*sic*] of brains from which the membranes had been removed, after submersion in dilute nitric acid, so as to show the precise localisation of the adhesions of the membranes to the grey matter in general paralysis of the insane. Several interesting specimens were contributed

---

[76] Idem.

[77] *Medical Press and Circular* 1875;20:457 (1st December; Medical Conversazione).

[78] *Medical Times and Gazette* 1875;2:603 (27th November; Conversazione at the West Riding Asylum).

[79] *BMJ* 1875;2:680 (27th November; The West Riding Asylum).

to this table by the Leeds School of Medicine. At the second stall, which was under the charge of Dr. John Merson, was a selection from the magnificent collection of photographs of insane patients now or formerly resident in the Asylum. This table was also enriched by a number of drawings by insane patients, lent by ex-Commissioner W. A. F. Browne. Mr. Lennox Browne also supplied the stall with numerous paintings executed by himself, and representing various views at Lemnos and Aix-les-Bains. The table for surgical and other instruments, presided over by Mr. Charles Seymour, M.R.C.S., held instruments in use at the Asylum, and a fine collection lent by Messrs. Salt and Son (Birmingham), Harvey, Reynolds, and Co. (Leeds), Maw and Son (London), and J. C. Elliott and Son (Leeds). The histological table, under the charge of Dr. Herbert C. Major and Dr. Bevan Lewis, was one of great interest as affording good evidence of the special original work done at the West Riding Asylum. Slides illustrative of the minute structure of the brain in health and disease, in foetal and adult life, were objects of great interest, as also were preparations showing the comparative histology of the cerebrum and cerebellum in man, birds, and batrachia [a clade of amphibians including frogs and salamanders]; and sections showing health-structure and pathological changes in the medulla oblongata, spinal cord, and sciatic nerves. Dr. Tempest Anderson and Mr. Clifford Gill contributed valuable material to this stall; and Mr. R. H. [*sic*] Octavius Sankey exhibited some beautiful specimens of cerebellar sections prepared by a new and effective method. The drug-stall was under the charge of Dr. J. H. Arbuckle, and was rich in new medicinal agents.[80]

In conclusion:

The meeting, which was an exceedingly happy and successful one, was enlivened by the performance by the large and admirable band of the Asylum of a long programme of classical and general music. The whole of the arrangements were perfectly carried out, and in both their conception and execution reflected great credit on Dr. Crichton Browne and his subordinate officers.[81]

Consistent with its social, as well as intellectual, rationale, this meeting was, like some of its predecessors, reported in the local popular press.[82] The *Leeds Mercury* noted the stalls presided over by Lawson, Merson, Seymour, Major and Lewis, and Arbuckle and Bracey. It also listed the "accepted invitations" which included a number of clinicians previously associated with WRA, such

---

[80] *Medical Times and Gazette* 1875;2:603 (27th November; Conversazione at the West Riding Asylum).

[81] Idem.

[82] *Leeds Mercury* 20th November 1875, p.3 (Medical Conversazione at Wakefield Asylum); *Sheffield Daily Telegraph* 20th November 1875, p.2 (West Riding Asylum, Wakefield. Medical Conversazione).

as "Mr W.J. Lancaster" of Barnsley, "Dr. Rabagliati" of Bradford, "Dr. Wright" of Wakefield, and "Mr. C. Clapham" of York. The meeting was even mentioned in the London *Times* of 23rd November which described it as "an important annual convention of medical scientists".[83]

Also of possible relevance to this *conversazione* is Dewhurst's statement that Jackson gave a lecture "at the Wakefield Asylum 'On temporary mental disorders after epileptic paroxysms' (1875)",[84] which was subsequently published in *WRLAMR*, specifically "On temporary mental disorders after epileptic paroxysms" (V:105–129). If this was indeed the case, it was not delivered in the context of the annual medical *conversazione*. The evidence accrued here is in agreement with Viets's finding of only two papers read at WRA which subsequently appeared in *WRLAMR*,[85] namely those by Turner and Carpenter given at the second and third *conversazione* respectively. At time of writing, any evidence for Hughlings Jackson ever attending WRA, let alone lecturing there, has yet to be found (see Chap. 7).

The End of the WRA *Conversazione*

At the 1875 *conversazione*, the Chairman, W.S. Stanhope, M.P., declared that "It was exceedingly desirable that meetings such as this should be continued, and at all events he hoped they would be continued".[86] At the close "The meeting … after doing honour to the liberal refreshment provided by Dr. Browne for his guests, dispersed well pleased with an evening of rare professional interest".[87] Yet despite the hopes expressed and the positive assessment delivered, echoing the responses to the earlier meetings, this was to prove the last of the WRA *conversazione*.[88] Like the house journal, *WRLAMR*, the *conversazione* did not survive after Crichton-Browne left Wakefield to become Lord Chancellor's Visitor in Lunacy in 1876. If it was indeed the case that "the West Riding's scientific spirit did not fade with the departure of

---

[83] *Times* (London), 23rd November 1875, p.7, as cited by Finn (2012:3n10).

[84] Dewhurst (1982:80).

[85] Viets (1938:486).

[86] *Leeds Mercury* 20th November 1875, p.3 (Medical Conversazione at Wakefield Asylum). Although not officially announced until December 1875, Stanhope's comment suggests that there were at least inklings that Crichton-Browne was going to depart, perhaps occasioned by his temporary appointment to the Visitorship in the absence of Bucknill through ill health (*Lancet* 1875;2:896 (18th December; Medical Appointments); see Chap. 5 for details) and hence concern that the *conversazione* would not continue in his absence.

[87] *BMJ* 1875;2:680 (27th November; The West Riding Asylum).

[88] Wood (2006:82) erred in stating the meetings were held "between 1866 and 1876".

Crichton-Browne, but was continued by successive superintendents",[89] why were there no further *conversazione?*

As for *WRLAMR*, it may be that Herbert Major, Crichton-Browne's immediate successor as Superintendent, was not willing to continue with the *conversazione*, even though he had been a consistent contributor to the meetings between 1872 and 1875. Similar reasons for such a decision might be advanced, principally a lack of time and energy, perhaps abetted by a disinclination to undertake yet more administrative work. Enthusiasm may have ebbed as the optimism for scientific breakthroughs in understanding the brain diseases underpinning insanity and developing effective treatments increasingly appeared misplaced. Moreover, Major, being a less prominent figure on the local and national stage than Crichton-Browne, may have lacked the pull to attract top quality speakers to meetings at WRA. Additionally, if it was indeed the case that Crichton-Browne had bankrolled the *conversazione* out of his own pocket (see Funding), money may also have been an issue, if not the critical issue.

WRA *Conversazione*: Precursor of the Neurological Society of London?

Were the WRA *conversazione* the forerunners of clinical meetings held by neurologists in later years, in a manner analogous to that in which *WRLAMR* was the forerunner of the neurological journal *Brain* (Chap. 6)? As with *WRLAMR* and *Brain*, some continuities may be traced between the WRA *conversazione* and the meetings of the Neurological Society of London (NSL), inaugurated in 1886 as "Britain's first society of neurology",[90] at least in terms of the personnel involved. (As from 1903, it became the Neurological Society of the United Kingdom.[91]).

---

[89] The claim of Wallis (2017a:9).

[90] Critchley and Critchley (1998:157–158), Casper (2014:30).

[91] For example: *Brain* 1903;26(1):141–152; *BMJ* 1903;2:41 (4th July; Edinburgh meeting of the Neurological Society): "The Neurological Society of the United Kingdom met in Edinburgh …". It is thus peculiar that Schurr (1985:147), Casper (2014:37), and Reynolds and Broussolle (2022:292) all dated the change of name to 1905. Schurr cited no sources, but as the then President of the Section of Neurology of the Royal Society of Medicine (RSM) he presumably had access to the same RSM Archives used by Casper. Reynolds and Broussolle's only reference is to Schurr. However, there is no doubt that the first usage of "Proceedings of the Neurological Society of the United Kingdom" published in *Brain* occurred in 1903, and indeed this date also appeared in Casper (2014:40). Penelope Hunting (2002:264) correctly dated the name change to 1903.

As previously shown (Chap. 6), all the key players in the inception of *Brain* had some link, major or minor, to WRA, and these individuals were also present at the beginnings of the NSL: Hughlings Jackson was the first President of the Society, Crichton-Browne was one of the two inaugural Vice-presidents, and Ferrier and Bucknill were on the Council. It has been suggested that Hughlings Jackson, along with William Broadbent, took the lead in founding the Neurological Society, or that it was largely Jackson's initiative,[92] whilst a retrospective account claimed that "Sir James Crichton-Brown [*sic*] had a good deal to do with the inception of the Society".[93] However, a case can also be made in favour of Armand de Watteville (1845–1926) being the prime mover in initiating the NSL; he was at this time the sole editor of *Brain*, in place of the original quadrumvirate.[94]

There was, moreover, a notable difference in timing: whilst the first issue of *Brain* (April 1878) followed the last issue of *WRLAMR* (dated 1876, but published no earlier than January 1877; see Chap. 6) by just over a year, almost a full decade separated the final WRA *conversazione* (19th November 1875) from the first meeting to discuss the possibility of the NSL (14th November 1885, at de Watteville's house). The subsequent, inaugural NSL meeting took place in January 1886.

In terms of the shape of the NSL meetings, these also had some overlap with the WRA *conversazione*. For example, distinguished speakers gave talks on topical issues, usually at the invitation of the Council, and there were also dedicated meetings to show pathological specimens. However, there appears to have been more discussion following the didactic presentations at NSL than was the case at WRA. Moreover, the NSL featured dedicated clinical meetings at which patients ("clinical cases") were demonstrated before the crowd of onlookers. NSL meetings were more frequent than WRA, six times per year as stipulated by the Rules of the Society.[95] The provision of refreshments does not appear to have been a feature of NSL meetings, far less the opportunity to listen to classical music or inhale laughing gas if required. The opportunity for social encounter, interaction, and dialogue was common to both the WRA *conversaziones* and NSL meetings, but spectacle and entertainment seem to have been confined to WRA, as might be anticipated since these

---

[92] Bailey (1895:102–103), Hunting (2002:263), Shorvon and Compston (2019:131).

[93] Hunting (2002:263), citing Thomas Buzzard. Buzzard's letter, dated 1st February 1908, survives in the archives of the Neurological Society held at the Royal Society of Medicine (NS/A/2, unpaginated).

[94] *BMJ* 1886;1:219 (30th January; The Neurological Society of London); *Lancet* 1886;1:218 (30th January; The Neurological Society of London); *Medical Press and Circular* 1886;41:104 (3rd February; Another Medical Society). For de Watteville, see Larner and Triarhou (2025b).

[95] Larner (2026a).

were features typical of the genre of the conversazione,[96] a terminology not used by the NSL.

Discussion

The proposition of an evening meeting taking place in late autumn, beginning at 8 p.m. or later and not finishing until around 11 p.m., located in a West Yorkshire lunatic asylum at some distance from the nearest urban centre, may not seem the most inviting of prospects in retrospect. Yet the WRA medical *conversazione* regularly achieved an audience of between 150 and 400 attendees, if published sources are to be believed, some of whom had travelled considerable distances by road and rail to attend, sometimes in spite of adverse weather conditions. What was it that attracted these practitioners to WRA? More than simply the "liberal refreshment" one presumes, but what exactly was to be gained from attending these annual meetings? Examining the stated purposes of the *conversazione* may give some explanation for their traction.

In 1872 Crichton-Browne reported that the great object he had in view was:

> in the first place to contribute in every possible way to the relief of the suffering and the cure of the inmates committed to his care; and, in the second place, to advance by every possible means the cause of medical science, by making the Asylum as much as possible what did not exist in the country—a medical school for physiological study.[97]

The benefits which might accrue from the WRA *conversazione* undoubtedly differed according to perspective: institutional or individual.

For WRA, the attendance of metropolitan professional men of medicine and science at the *conversazione* gave a gloss of scientific respectability to the institution (as did the nomenclatura publishing in *WRLAMR*, such as Hughlings Jackson, Ferrier, and Allbutt). In addition, it allowed the Asylum to advertise its work locally and, to a lesser extent, nationally. As Clifford Allbutt remarked "these meetings were but part of a very great intellectual movement which was going on in the asylum".[98]

---

[96] Alberti (2003), Wood (2006).

[97] *The Wakefield Express, and Barnsley, Normanton, Pontefract, Ossett, Horbury & Dewsbury Advertiser* Volume 21, No. 1068, 19 October 1872, p.2, cols.3–4 (Great gathering of medical gentlemen at the West Riding Asylum. Conversazione and lecture by Professor Turner.).

[98] Idem; also, verbatim, in *BMJ* 1872;2:475.

The physical isolation which had been deemed desirable in planning the siting of county asylums, as recommended by Samuel Tuke and as enacted at Wakefield, might also occasion an intellectual isolation, particularly injurious for the junior staff, the Assistant Medical Officers. The *conversazione* presented an opportunity for the resident medical staff to see and be seen as part of an institution devoted not merely to the custodial and therapeutic functions of a county asylum but also integrated into broader networks, social, medical and scientific.

As shown by the published invitation lists, most of those invited to the WRA *conversazione* were local practitioners.[99] By inviting practitioners not directly involved in asylum medicine into the Asylum, by allowing them to transcend both the physical and the figurative walls of the institution, the *conversazione* helped to mediate WRA and its work to outsiders, to demystify its procedures, and to emphasize its adherence to a science-oriented philosophy. In an era when public asylums were perceived as grim and forbidding places, closed to the external gaze (aside from the obligatory visits of the Commissioners in Lunacy), the *conversazione* provided good publicity and reputational enhancement for WRA.

As previously mentioned, for those invited to attend the *conversazione*:

> The object of the gathering—…—was to give an opportunity to the Medical [*sic*] practitioners of the various towns in the West Riding and other districts to see the mode of treatment adopted at this most admirable institution, to discuss and exchange views upon professional topics …[100]

As implied in the term "conversazione", the meeting was not simply a one-way transmission of expert knowledge,[101] as might occur with an erudite lecture delivered by an expert in the field. Even if "illustrated by diagrams", this could prove largely an exercise in (more or less) passive listening. But the WRA *conversazione* also provided a chance for those attending to interact with those who were demonstrating techniques and experiments and manning the stalls, to ask questions, to share experience with the staff and with other delegates, and possibly even to have an opportunity to use the

---

[99] Perhaps comprising "the medical talent and enterprise that abound more or less in the neighbourhood of every asylum" (Crichton-Browne 1878–1879:367).

[100] *Medical Press and Circular* 1872;14:360 (23rd October; Conversazione and lecture by Professor Turner). The phrase "to discuss and exchange views upon professional topics" also appeared in *The Wakefield Express, and Barnsley, Pontefract, & Dewsbury Advertiser* Volume 20, No. 1015, Saturday 14th October 1871, p.8, col.1 (Great gathering of medical gentlemen at the West Riding Asylum. Grand conversazione last night. Lecture by Dr. Ainstie [*sic*]).

[101] Alberti (2003:223).

ophthalmoscopes, stereoscopes, and microscopes on display. Ensuring greater immediacy of effect and proximity of encounter, Brudenell Carter's ophthalmoscopic demonstration in 1871 was reported to have taken place "in a room adjoining the great hall",[102] as was the case with Ferrier's experimental demonstration in 1873.

Beyond these practical outcomes, "Participating in a conversazione had symbolic significance, a collective affirmation of identity".[103] The account of the 1872 meeting in the *Medical Times and Gazette*, whilst noting Professor Turner's lecture and the many objects of interest, held that:

> These are all very excellent, no doubt, as incentives to conversation and an easy means of introducing subjects of conversation a little less hackneyed than the weather and the price of coals, but we do not conceive the value of such meetings to rest so much on the acquisition of information or even of new ideas, but rather as affording the means of social intercourse so sadly lacking among the members of our Profession. Isolation is always dangerous; supreme rule in a limited sphere is most disastrous to mental improvement—in short, it is only by finding out that there are many men quite as clever as ourselves in the world that we learn to estimate others at their true value, and escape for our own part the intolerance of an overweening self-conceit. But such escape is only possible by contact with our fellows, and it is for this reason that meetings such as those inaugurated by Dr. Crichton Browne are so much to be commended.[104]

This was of particular significance for those practitioners living in regional, as opposed to metropolitan, settings, as was recognised in the report appearing in the *Medical Times and Gazette*. This allowed those attending a meeting based in "a large public provincial institution":

> to engage in the profitable converse which busy practitioners widely separated have rarely the opportunity of enjoying.[105]

Hence these meetings might be understood as part of a process of the socialisation of knowledge.

Another perspective may also be detected in the WRA *conversazione*, beyond the educational, self-improving one. Each of the *conversazione* was

---

[102] *The Wakefield Express, and Barnsley, Pontefract, & Dewsbury Advertiser* Volume 20, No. 1016, Saturday 21st October 1871, p.2, col.5 (The medical conversazione at the West Riding Asylum).

[103] Alberti (2003:224).

[104] *Medical Times and Gazette* 1872;2:466.

[105] *Medical Times and Gazette* 1874;2:609–610 (28th November; Annual Conversazione at the West Riding Asylum).

held in the dining hall of the Asylum, a space which served multiple purposes for the benefit of the patients beyond simple refectory, including the production of dances, concerts and theatrical entertainments.[106] The overlap between these theatrical performances and the *conversazione* was not merely spatial. The hall "presented the appearance of a philosophical saloon in which science and pleasure were blended".[107] That the *conversazione* had a theatrical element was partially recognised even at the time. In 1872, the Chairman of the meeting, Spencer Stanhope, was briefly indisposed, requiring to be helped from the platform; returning later he "remarked that as that was his first performance on a theatrical platform he felt the effects of the footlights, though Professor Turner and Dr. Browne did not seem much the worse".[108] At the *conversazione* the following year, the Chairman, Lord Houghton, noted that "if the only peculiarity [?] of the institution was that it had become the theatre of such meetings as the present, it would deserve some special remark".[109] This theatricality is notable, even perhaps palpable, in the sense of engagement and excitement afforded to the local practitioners when viewing the drama of Ferrier's experimental demonstration in 1873, perhaps as close as these practitioners would ever get not only to the "cutting edge" of modern physiological science but also to a scientist who was currently something of a celebrity. At the same time, one may feel abhorrence at reading of this needless vivisection, perpetrated essentially for entertainment rather than scientific advance (ditto Burman's experimental demonstration in 1872 characterised as the "slaughtering of the innocents"). This was a spectacle, and the audience had come to see it. Such public exhibition of experiments was soon to be rightly prohibited under the terms of the Cruelty to Animals Act of 1876.[110]

The WRA *conversazione* thus differed from the annual meetings of the MPA which seem, from the accounts of their transactions as published in the *Journal of Mental Science*, rather procedural, with little intellectual material aside from certain of the Presidential addresses. Indeed, the MPA conversazione was held separate from the main meeting. At the WRA *conversazione*,

---

[106] Golding (2021).

[107] *The Wakefield Express, and Barnsley, Normanton, Pontefract, Ossett, Horbury & Dewsbury Advertiser* Volume 22, No, 1126, 29th November 1873, p.2, cols. 4–7 (Medical conversazione at the West Riding Asylum. Speech by Lord Houghton. Lecture by Dr. Carpenter).

[108] *The Wakefield Express, and Barnsley, Normanton, Pontefract, Ossett, Horbury & Dewsbury Advertiser* Volume 21, No. 1068, 19 October 1872, p.2, cols.3–4 (Great gathering of medical gentlemen at the West Riding Asylum. Conversazione and lecture by Professor Turner.).

[109] *The Wakefield Express, and Barnsley, Normanton, Pontefract, Ossett, Horbury & Dewsbury Advertiser* Volume 22, No, 1126, 29th November 1873, p.2, cols. 4–7 (Medical conversazione at the West Riding Asylum. Speech by Lord Houghton. Lecture by Dr. Carpenter) [my transcription; uncertain].

[110] Ryan (1963), Ozer (1966), French (1975), Bone and Larner (2024).

according to one judgment of posterity, it would appear that "Knowledge and skill were being disseminated to other professionals, rather in the manner of the modern academic conference".[111] However, these were not dedicated meetings for the presentation of research findings, which may be deemed one of the defining features of a separate clinical discipline.[112]

The winter of 1875–6 marked the end of an era in the life of WRA. A different dispensation was beginning, even though Herbert Major might have been seen as a "continuity candidate" when appointed as Superintendent to succeed Crichton-Browne. Hence, this is the logical time point at which to examine the question of what role WRA may have played in the origins of British neurology, the subject to be addressed in the final chapter.

---

[111] Wood (2006:90). The same may be said of the meetings of the Neurological Society of London.
[112] French (1975:203).

9

Prosopography: Contributors to WRA *conversazione*

The purpose of this chapter is to present a prosopography of the invited speakers at the WRA *conversazione* (listed in Table 8.1), but this is relatively brief since these individuals were generally well-known, unlike the resident staff (Chap. 5). Moreover, the visiting lecturers probably contributed nothing to the work at WRA beyond their single presentations, other than possibly inspiring new or ongoing local work, unlike the visiting staff and those who contributed papers to *WRLAMR* (Chap. 7) and may have collaborated with or inspired the resident staff.

In addition to the *conversazione* speakers, information on some of the guests attending and/or contributing materials to be exhibited at the various stalls, and not hitherto mentioned (Chap. 7), is included.

Francis E. Anstie (1833–1874)[1]

Francis Edmund Anstie was the invited lecturer at the inaugural WRA *conversazione* held on 13th October 1871.

At this time, as Crichton-Browne noted, Anstie was an assistant physician at the Westminster Hospital in London, as of 1860, and from 1868 the

---

[1] Biographical material on Anstie may be found in Buzzard (1876), Earles, https://doi.org/10.1093/ref:odnb/583. Obituaries: *BMJ* 1874;2:392 (19th September); *Medical Times and Gazette* 1874;2:352 (19th September); *Le Progrès Médical* 1874;2(39):585 (26th September).

A. J. Larner, *The West Riding Asylum and the Origins of British Neurology 1866-1876*,
https://doi.org/10.1007/978-3-032-12591-0_9

founding editor of *The Practitioner: a monthly journal of therapeutics*[2] wherein Crichton-Browne had already published.[3]

Possible reasons for Anstie's selection as lecturer at WRA may have included his known interests in diseases of the nervous system. A graduate of King's College Hospital, London, he was said to have had great affection for his teacher Robert Bentley Todd (1809–1860) who had described post-ictal paralysis, known as Todd's palsy, in 1849,[4] a subject later discussed by Hughlings Jackson (VI:266–309). Anstie had written on neuralgia, then understood in broader terms than current neurological usage, including a monograph published in 1871 and a chapter in Russell Reynolds' *System of Medicine* (1872, as well as chapters on hypochondriasis and alcoholism). Of possible interest to some clinicians at WRA, he had also given two lectures on the sphygmograph (see Chap. 6) at the Royal College of Physicians in 1867.[5] His 1864 work on *Stimulants and narcotics* had proved influential on Hughlings Jackson's thoughts about over-action in lower brain centres, consequent upon inaction in higher centres.[6] He had published in the *Journal of Mental Science*,[7] and later published "Lectures on Diseases of the Nervous System" in the *Lancet*. In 1873 he was appointed full physician to the Westminster Hospital.[8]

Anstie's lecture at the medical *conversazione* was later published, in the January 1872 issue of the *Journal of Mental Science*.[9] In a footnote, it records

---

[2] Later, from 1873, volume 10, it became "*The Practitioner: a journal of therapeutics and public health*". *The Practitioner* continued in print until 2022. At time of writing, a limited archival website persists (www.thepractitioner.co.uk)

[3] Crichton Browne (1871e). A number of other WRA clinicians and/or *WRLAMR* contributors also subsequently published in *The Practitioner*, e.g. Burman (1872b), McDowall (1873), Crichton Browne (1874b), Lawson (1874, 1875a, 1876b), Rabagliati (1877), as well as Allbutt, Milner Fothergill, and Lauder Brunton, although several of these publications postdate Anstie's untimely death at the age of 41 in 1874. He was succeeded as editor of *The Practitioner* by Lauder Brunton (for whom, see Chap. 7).

[4] Reynolds (2005).

[5] Anstie (1867).

[6] For example, see *WRLAMR* V:111-112n1. The influence of Anstie on Jackson was mentioned by Temkin (1971:343n229). Anstie's work on *Stimulants and narcotics* was also quoted or mentioned by Samuel Mitchell in *WRLAMR* (I:52–54 and II:80, 85, 87–88, 89, 95). Anstie was also named in *WRLAMR* by Hughlings Jackson (III:326) and by Merson (IV:92).

[7] Anstie (1865–1866).

[8] *Medical Press and Circular* 1873;15:502 (4th June; Appointments).

[9] Anstie (1871–1872:471–484) (January 1872). The index to this volume of the *Journal of Mental Science* (1871–1872:629) gives the first page of Anstie's paper as 472, in error, and also lists the author as "Anstie, Dr. E. Francis". There is a spelling difference between the title of the published paper ("connections") and both the report in the *Lancet* (1871;2:588) and Crichton-Browne's note (*Report*, 1872:31) of the presentation given at the *conversazione* ("connexions" and "Connexion" respectively). Some of Anstie's lecture was also printed in *The Wakefield Express, and Barnsley, Pontefract, & Dewsbury Advertiser* Volume 20, No. 1016, Saturday 21st October 1871, p.2, cols.4–5 (The medical conversazione at the West Riding Asylum).

that "The substance of this paper was delivered as an address at a Conversazione of medical men of the West Riding, at the West Riding Ayslum [*sic*], Wakefield.".[10] Drawing particularly on the work of Henry Maudsley, Anstie, "in addressing you gentlemen, who are biologists", made a distinction between "active hereditary neurosis" and "dormant hereditary neurosis". None of the clinicians at WRA seems to have made a particular study of hereditary factors in brain disease, although both Crichton-Browne and Henry Clarke later published on the topic in *Brain* (see Table 6.4; "Heredity in epilepsy" and "Heredity and crime in epileptic criminals" respectively).[11]

Robert Brudenell Carter (1828–1918)[12]

As reported in the *Lancet*, "Mr. Brudenell Carter gave an interesting demonstration of the reflecting ophthalmoscope" at the inaugural WRA *conversazione* on 13th October 1871.[13]

Robert Brudenell Carter was one of the pioneers of ophthalmology as an independent clinical discipline. At the time of the WRA *conversazione*, he was Lecturer in Ophthalmic Surgery at St. George's Hospital Medical School in London and Ophthalmic Surgeon to the hospital. His credentials as a clinician with an interest not only in the eyes but also in the nervous system were established early in his career, with a book on *The pathology and treatment of hysteria* (1853) and, 2 years later, on *The influence of education and training in preventing diseases of the nervous system* (1855).[14] He translated Adolf Zander's book on the ophthalmoscope from the German (1864),[15] and later included a chapter on ophthalmoscopy in his book *A practical treatise on diseases of the eye* (1875). At the Medical Society of London in 1871, he "showed his ophthalmological instruments at the conversazione" (not dated),[16] so perhaps this presentation may have prompted his invitation to Wakefield to deliver a similar demonstration.

---

[10] Anstie (1871–1872:471).

[11] On the subject of heredity, Ferrier (IV:57) later noted that "The leading action of the left hemisphere may, however, be merely an accident of education or heredity, and there is no reason why articulate speech should not be the function of the right side."

[12] Biographical material on Brudenell Carter may be found in James (1941), Shorvon and Compston (2019:367n72); *Plarr's Lives of the Fellows online*, Carter, Robert Brudenell (1828–1918) (rcseng.ac.uk).

[13] *Lancet* 1871;2:588.

[14] Crammer (1996:216) reported that "*On the Pathology & Treatment of Hysteria* [*sic*] ... sold 135 copies in its first year, (the author gave away another 54 copies, apart from review copies)."

[15] Carter (1864).

[16] Hunting (2003:222).

The *Wakefield Express* noted that Brudenell Carter's demonstration "greatly attracted the attention of the medical men present".[17] Although undoubtedly of general interest, the demonstration would probably have been of particular interest to the two clinicians who had practiced ophthalmoscopy extensively at WRA: Clifford Allbutt and Charles Aldridge (if they were present[18]). Allbutt had previously published ophthalmological findings in patients seen at WRA from 1867.[19] Charles Aldridge, who was Assistant Medical Officer at WRA from late 1868 to 1872, pursued a particular interest in ophthalmoscopy during his time at Wakefield, eventually publishing three papers on the subject in *WRLAMR* (I:71–128; II:223–253; IV:291–304). Later, Hughlings Jackson also published an ophthalmological case with illustration in *WRLAMR* (IV:24–29).[20]

By strange coincidence, Brudenell Carter was called in by Francis Anstie in the latter's fatal illness in 1874.[21] In later years, Carter was President of the Medical Society of London in 1886, the year before Hughlings Jackson held this honour, and he became the first Ophthalmic Surgeon appointed to the National Hospital, Queen Square (1886–1899). In 1889 he was elected an Ordinary Member of the Neurological Society of London. During this period (1889–90) he led an attempt "to establish a hospital for the treatment of early cases of mental disorder" which also involved Allbutt, Ferrier, and Crichton-Browne, but eventually came to naught.[22] As a member of the London County Council he moved "That a Committee be appointed to inquire and report on the advantages which might be expected from the establishment, as a complement to the asylum system, of a hospital with a visiting medical staff for the study and curative treatment of insanity". This was one of the early steps along

---

[17] *The Wakefield Express, and Barnsley, Pontefract, & Dewsbury Advertiser* Volume 20, No. 1016, Saturday 21st October 1871, p.2, col.5 (The medical conversazione at the West Riding Asylum), where he is referred to as "Bendenell Carter".

[18] At time of writing, no list of those attending the first medical *conversazione* has been located. Allbutt was certainly present at the 1872 *conversazione*: *BMJ* 1872;2:474–475 (26th October; Medical Conversazione at the West Riding Asylum). As a local, and one already associated with WRA, I think it is reasonable to suppose it likely that he was present. Rolleston's biography of Allbutt says nothing about attendance at the WRA *conversazione* in this, or any other, year.

[19] See Chap. 7 for details. Brudenell Carter had previously commented on some of Allbutt's material from WRA, e.g. *BMJ* 1868;1:257. One might speculate that Allbutt may have suggested to Crichton-Browne that Brudenell Carter be invited as a speaker at the WRA *conversazione*.

[20] It might be mentioned here that Jellinek (2005:429) stated that Allbutt published on ophthalmoscopy in *WRLAMR*, but I do not find this to be the case; neither of Allbutt's *WRLAMR* contributions relate to ophthalmoscopy (Table 6.1), his ophthalmological material from WRA having been published elsewhere, *viz*. Allbutt (1868a, b, c, d, 1871a) (see Chap. 7 for details).

[21] *BMJ* 1874;2:392 (19th September).

[22] Shorvon and Compston (2019:342–344). The "Report of the Committee of the London County Council on a Hospital for the Insane" was published in Burdett (1891:159–247).

the tortuous path leading eventually to the founding of the Maudsley Hospital in London, opened as a psychiatric hospital in 1923.[23] Whether Brudenell Carter's experience of attending WRA, some 18 years earlier, played any part in the genesis of his proposal remains unknown, but the subsequent Committee report ignored the asylums.[24] Brudenell Carter later, in 1899, published a chapter on medical ophthalmology in Allbutt's *A System of Medicine*.[25]

William Turner (1832–1916)[26]

William Turner who gave the address at the second annual *conversazione* held on 15th October 1872 was Professor of Anatomy in the University of Edinburgh. He had been appointed to this post in 1867, some 10 years after he came to prominence with his *Atlas of human anatomy and physiology*. He was also one of the co-founders and editors of the *Journal of Anatomy and Physiology*[27] and a correspondent of Charles Darwin. The *Wakefield Express* considered him "perhaps the most eminent teacher of anatomy now living".[28]

From Crichton-Browne's recollections, published over 50 years later (1926), some insights into Turner's reception as a visiting guest may be obtained:

> Professor Turner (afterwards Sir William Turner) was spending three days with us in October 1872, and delivered a very important and suggestive address at

---

[23] Walk (1976, 1990:23).

[24] According to Walk (1990:26), the subsequent Committee report "pointedly ignored" the asylums, presumably because "only two psychiatrists of standing, Batty Tuke and Crichton-Browne" were called as witnesses and "Maudsley was not called" (1990:23). This view does not coincide with my reading of Burdett (1891:159–247).

[25] Carter (1899).

[26] Biographical material on William Turner may be found in Sturdy, https://doi.org/10.1093/ref:odnb/36590; Wessels et al. (2016); *Plarr's Lives of the Fellows online*, Turner, Sir William (1832–1916) (rcseng.ac.uk).

[27] For the early years of the *Journal of Anatomy and Physiology*, founded 1866–1867 (it subsequently became the *Journal of Anatomy*), see Morriss-Kay (2016). It was sometimes referred to as 'Humphry and Turner's Journal' because of the founding roles of George Murray Humphry of Cambridge and William Turner of Edinburgh. Ferrier had co-authored a number of review articles published in the journal in 1871 and 1872 (Brunton and Ferrier 1871, 1872; Fraser et al. 1871; Rutherford et al. 1872). Other WRA related papers published in this journal include Ferrier (1873b), Galton (1872, 1874), and Major (1879).

[28] *The Wakefield Express, and Barnsley, Normanton, Pontefract, Ossett, Horbury & Dewsbury Advertiser* Volume 21, No. 1068, 19 October 1872, p.2, cols.3–4 (Great gathering of medical gentlemen at the West Riding Asylum. Conversazione and lecture by Professor Turner.).

our medical conversazione on "The Convolutions of the Human Brain in relation to the Intelligence".[29]

It was presumably during this visit that Crichton-Browne "proposed to show him [Turner] round the hospital, and we entered first the ward for female mental defectives, where some 30 idiots and imbeciles were seated in chairs surrounded by toys, flowers and pictures and every comfort, and attended by nurses".[30]

Turner's anatomical work had been instrumental in establishing the delimitation of the frontal, temporal, parietal and occipital lobes of the brain,[31] hence the subject of his WRA lecture on "The convolutions of the human brain considered in relation to the intelligence", which was reported to be "illustrated by diagrams".[32] The lecture was subsequently printed as the first item in the third volume of *WRLAMR* (III:1–29), published in 1873, immediately preceding Ferrier's substantive article (III:30–96).[33] In a footnote, Turner stated that "I have added various numerical and other details, which for want of time could not conveniently be introduced into an oral discourse" (III:1n). In addition, the printed text mentioned an abstract of Ferrier's results and made clear that Turner was aware of, although had not seen, Ferrier's substantive *WRLAMR* paper.[34]

---

[29] Crichton-Browne (1926:111).

[30] Ibid., 47. A review of Crichton-Browne's reminiscences in this volume entitled *Victorian jottings* stated that he "made the West Riding Asylum famous for the men who worked there for a time, such as Sir Clifford Allbutt, Sir William Turner, and Sir David Ferrier" (*BMJ* 1926;2:1190 (18th December; Sir James Crichton-Browne)). Rolleston (1929:56) also listed William Turner amongst the "young men keen on research" attracted to WRA by Crichton-Browne "to work, write for his *Reports*, and attend the annual meeting there", an ambiguous statement but possibly suggestive that Turner worked at WRA. However, I have found no evidence that Turner attended WRA at any time aside from his lecture at the medical *conversazione* in October 1872. Incidentally, his son, William Aldren Turner (1864–1945) became a neurologist and worked with Ferrier at King's College Hospital, London, undertaking experimental research related to cerebral localization and publishing several papers with him, as well as contributing an obituary piece on him (Aldren Turner 1928). Aldren was the maiden name of William Turner's mother, Margaret (Larner 2024g).

[31] For example, Turner (1866).

[32] *Medical Press and Circular* 1872;14:360 (23rd October; Conversazione and lecture by Professor Turner).

[33] I have suggested (Larner 2025j:59) that the proximity of these two papers in *WRLAMR* may have occasioned Crichton-Browne's later lapse (1926:111) to the effect that, when visiting WRA in October 1872, "Reviewing Ferrier's recent observations in my laboratory on the localisation of function in the brain, he [Turner] said ...", an impossibility since Turner's lecture (October 1872) preceded Ferrier's work in the WRA laboratory (Spring 1873) although Turner's *WRLAMR* publication (probably early August 1873) postdated Ferrier's time at WRA. I now also wonder whether this misdating by Crichton-Browne might be the source for the claim that Ferrier attended the 1872 *conversazione* (Finn 2012:139), as discussed in Chap. 7) for which attendance I have identified no evidence.

[34] III:25 and n2. The "abstract" was Ferrier (1873a). The substantive paper was III:30–96. Turner, as co-editor of the *Journal of Anatomy and Physiology*, was perhaps instrumental in Ferrier's subsequent publication in that journal: Ferrier (1873b) (as suggested in Larner 2025j:59).

Turner's paper discussed the mass and weight, external configuration, internal structure, and vascular supply of the brain. Some of his comments on the relation between brain weight and sex were informed by the findings of Crochley Clapham at WRA (III:4 and n1), whose statistics on the weight of the brain were reportedly compiled "at the instigation of Professor Turner" (III:285). On the internal structure of the brain, Turner noted that "the grey matter is observed to be laminated" and that its characteristic cells were "the structures in which the molecular changes occur, which occasion the evolution or disengagement of the special form of energy named nerve-energy or nerve-force" (III:16–17). Accordingly, it was "an important object of enquiry to determine the extent and thickness of the grey cortex in the different parts of the same brain, as well as in different brains", to which Turner added a footnote referring to an "ingenious little instrument named a Tephrylometer … recently … invented for this purpose by Dr. H. C. Major" (III:17 and n1). The study of the minute structure of the grey matter Turner judged to be:

> comparatively untrodden ground. With the improved methods of observation which have of late years been introduced, and with the still further improvements which may reasonably be looked for, any competent observer who will devote his time to working at this subject will find a rich reward for his labour in the new facts which he will acquire. (III:18)[35]

In the final section of his lecture, Turner addressed the question of the functional differences of the convolutions, noting pathological, physiological and anatomical evidence in support of this possibility. The pathological material included Broca's observations on "lesion of the posterior third of the inferior left frontal convolution, with loss of the cerebral faculty of speech" (III:25). The physiological material included the experimental work of Fritsch and Hitzig as well as Ferrier.

Turner later contributed to Herbert Major's 1879 paper on the anatomy of the brain of the white whale, published in the *Journal of Anatomy and Physiology*: "For the following note of the general plan of the convolutions I am indebted to the kindness of Professor Turner, who has drawn it up from the examination of a photograph of the left hemisphere which I sent to

---

[35] I speculate that Turner's observation here may have acted as a stimulus to the work of Herbert Major, as he later investigated the laminar structure of human and non-human primate brains, particularly in his MD thesis (Major 1875; also Major 1877a). This work has been described in Larner and Triarhou (2024a, b). Bevan-Lewis also addressed cortical laminar structure (see Chap. 5).

him.".[36] The brain structure of Cetacea was a subject on which Turner himself had previously published (III:22).

J.H. Balfour Browne (1845–1921)

John Hutton Balfour Browne (1845–1921) was Crichton-Browne's younger brother, the son of William Browne, but family connection was not the sole reason for his presence as an invited guest at the *conversazione* of 1872.

A barrister, Balfour Browne was the author of *The medical jurisprudence of insanity* wherein he acknowledged "the kindness and assistance which he had received" from his brother. Some case material from WRA was included in the work.[37] He had also published in the *Journal of Mental Science* and had written a paper on kleptomania which appeared in the *British and Foreign Medico-Chirurgical Review*.[38] With Dr. J.T. Sabben [*sic*], he had more recently written *Handbook of law and lunacy; or, the medical practitioners complete guide in all matters relating to lunacy practice*.[39] The publishers, J. & A. Churchill, took the opportunity to advertise a number of their other publications in the end papers of this book, including Volume 1 of the *West Riding Lunatic Asylum Medical Reports*. Further publications by Balfour Browne on issues related to mental health and law were to follow.[40]

James Bell Pettigrew (1832–1908)[41]

James Bell Pettigrew was at this time best known for his work on the anatomy of the cardiac musculature, undertaken in Edinburgh in the late 1850s whilst still a medical student and which earned him not only the Edinburgh gold

---

[36] Major (1879:127–128). I presume this refers to Plate X, between pages 136 and 137. Also Wallis (2017a:165).

[37] Balfour Browne (1871a:viii; 173–175). The book was reviewed in *J Ment Sci* 1871;17(October 1871):399–407, and *BMJ* 1872;1:369 (6th April).

[38] Balfour Browne (1870–1871, 1871b).

[39] Sabben and Balfour Browne (1872). The book was reviewed in *Br Foreign Med Chir Rev* 1873;51(101):41–46. J.T. Sabben [*sic*] had also published in the *Journal of Mental Science* (Sabben 1870–1871).

[40] For example, Balfour Browne (1872–1873, 1873, 1873-1874) (the 1873 essay was reviewed in *J Ment Sci* 1872–1873;18(January 1873):587–590).

[41] Biographical details on James Bell Pettigrew may be found in Todd and Ashworth (n.d.:130–131); D'A Power rev. Bevan, https://doi.org/10.1093/ref:odnb/35498; and Gardner (2017) (Wikipedia gives Pettigrew's date of birth as 1834).

medal for his thesis but also the Croonian Lectures of both the Royal Society and the Royal College of Physicians of London. He was elected FRS in 1868.

He attended the *conversazione* of 1872,[42] contributing photographs to Stall B.[43] It may have been on the same visit to WRA that he examined the hearts of patients with general paralysis along with Crichton-Browne and Milner Fothergill (III:113).[44]

Crichton-Browne later wrote a letter supporting Pettigrew's application for the chair of physiology in the University of Edinburgh,[45] a position which he did not obtain. Later he became Professor of Medicine and Anatomy at St Andrews University.[46]

William B. Carpenter (1813–1885)[47]

William Benjamin Carpenter was a distinguished physician, physiologist, and zoologist, Registrar of the University of London, who had longstanding interests in brain function and dysfunction and had championed the idea of unconscious cerebration. He was mentioned and/or his work was cited by various authors in *WRLAMR*, including Thompson (I:63–64), Mitchell (II:88, 94), Crichton-Browne (II:110; V:230), Milner Fothergill (IV:96–97), Lauder Brunton (IV:189, 216), Lawson (IV:250–251), and Clapham and Clarke (VI:160). The presence of this "big hitter" at the WRA *conversazione* held on 25th November 1873 was undoubtedly called forth by the dramatic experimental findings of Ferrier at WRA earlier in the year and their dissemination at meetings of the British Medical Association and British Association for the Advancement of Science, as well as in the medical literature (see Chap. 7).

Carpenter's lecture at the medical *conversazione*, "On the physiological import of Dr. Ferrier's experimental investigations into the functions of the brain", was later published, in the fourth (1874) volume of *WRLAMR*

---

[42] *The Wakefield Express, and Barnsley, Normanton, Pontefract, Ossett, Horbury & Dewsbury Advertiser* Volume 21, No. 1068, 19th October 1872, p.2, cols.3–4 (Great gathering of medical gentlemen at the West Riding Asylum. Conversazione and lecture by Professor Turner).

[43] *Medical Press and Circular* 1872;14:360 (23rd October; Conversazione and lecture by Professor Turner). The same report appears verbatim in the *Wakefield Express* (19th October 1872, p.2).

[44] Todd and Ashworth (n.d.:131) stated that "Pettigrew assisted Fothergill in his researches at the Wakefield Asylum for his paper The Heart Sounds in General Paralysis".

[45] *BMJ* 1874;2:158–-159 (1st August). See also Crichton-Browne (1926:172–174; 1937:31).

[46] The Bell Pettigrew Museum of natural history at the University of St Andrews is named after him.

[47] Biographical material on Carpenter may be found in Leyland (1888:I:20–29); Smith, https://doi.org/10.1093/ref:odnb/4742

(IV:1–23). Carpenter cited verbatim from Ferrier's work on the cat, dog, and rabbit brain from his substantive paper in the third volume of *WRLAMR*,[48] and noted his further work on monkeys "of which the details are as yet unpublished" (IV:15). Based on Ferrier's findings, Carpenter's conclusions as to their import included the reflex nature of cerebral function as well as support for his concept of unconscious cerebration (based on the evidence that "'discharging lesions' of the Cerebrum, take place without any consciousness whatever"; IV:19). Moreover, the experimental evidence indicated to Carpenter that the cerebrum did not act immediately on motor nerves but served to "co-ordinate and direct" muscular contractions by excited primary centres, the crossed action of some of these centres being confirmed.

Carpenter's publication in *WRLAMR* was later criticised by Hitzig. In a German publication, he added an English footnote:

> The fourth Volume of the West Riding Lunatic Asylum Medical Reports, which has just been published, contains (under Nr. 1) a paper by Dr. William B. Carpenter, entitled "On the Physiological Import of Dr. Ferrier's experimental Investigations into the Functions of the Brain." Dr. Carpenter here, as well as on previous occasions, commits the slight mistake to use Dr. Ferrier's name where he should say Fritsch and Hitzig. In order to assist him in avoiding similar errors, which ought to be most unpleasant to himself, I write this remark in his own language, and I shall take the liberty of forwarding him a copy of this paper.[49]

Carpenter's subsequent work entitled *Principles of Mental Physiology* was reportedly "in type" when he became aware of Ferrier's 1873 publication, requiring additions to the text, and including an Appendix the contents of which overlapped with Carpenter's publication in *WRLAMR*.[50]

Richard Norris

Some sources report that Richard Hill Norris was born in 1830, studied medicine at Edinburgh, was the Professor of Physiology at Queen's College,

---

[48] For example, Carpenter's Figs. 1, 2, and 3 correspond to Ferrier's Figs. 3, 6, and 8, but omit the monogram of the illustrator, John Galton (see Chap. 5). Lazar (2013:97) stated that Carpenter "observed his [Ferrier's] experiments and even aided in recording data" but offered no source(s) and I have found no evidence to suggest such a collaboration. Burdon Sanderson and Lauder Brunton witnessed some of Ferrier's later experiments (Ferrier 1875a:447, 460).

[49] Hitzig (1874: 410n1). An interesting insight into Hitzig's character! (see Breathnach 1992).

[50] Carpenter (1874:129, 709–722) (Appendix—left hand pages headed "Appendix—Dr. Ferrier on the brain"). Young (1970:109) reported that Carpenter "held up publication in order to take account of these important findings". Also Young (1970:214–215).

Birmingham, from 1862 until 1891, and died in 1916.[51] An obituary in the *BMJ*,[52] however, stated that "He was for a time assistant demonstrator of physiology in Queen's College, Birmingham, and afterwards settled in practice at Aston [in Birmingham]" and gave his date of death as 30th November 1919 at the age of 66, which is incompatible with a date of birth in the 1830s (hence may be a typographical error). His entry in the "Former Fellows of the Royal Society of Edinburgh, 1783–2002" gives his election as FRSE in 1878, but gives his date of death as 1921![53]

Norris certainly published in the *Proceedings of the Royal Society*, in 1862, 1869, and 1871, including papers entitled "A consideration of causes of various phenomena of attraction and adhesion in solid bodies, films, vesicles, liquids, globules, and blood corpuscles" and "On statis of the blood, and exudation". He had interests in photography and microscopy. However, he does not appear in Sharpey-Schafer's history of the Physiological Society,[54] nor in O'Connor's biographical dictionary of the founders of British physiology, despite discussion of developments in Birmingham.[55]

How Norris came to be invited to the WRA *conversazione* of 25th November 1873, to present alongside Carpenter and Ferrier, is unclear. If he was an Edinburgh graduate, and if he was born in 1830, he would not have overlapped with Crichton-Browne. Presumably his research interests prompted the invitation. Of possible significance, he had given an experimental demonstration at the annual meeting of the BMA on 6th August 1873 "illustrative of his views regarding the formation of rouleaux by the blood corpuscles" which was "brilliantly illustrated and most lucidly explained".[56]

As per the published programme, some press reports of the WRA *conversazione* stated that "Dr. Norris ... exhibited some new experiments".[57]

---

[51] Richard Hill Norris—Wikipedia (accessed 01/02/24).

[52] *BMJ* 1919;2:801 (13th December).

[53] https://www.royalsoced.org.uk/cms/files/fellows/biographical_index/fells_indexp2.pdf   (accessed 01/02/24).

[54] Sharpey-Schafer (1927).

[55] O'Connor (1988:229) reported that "until 1880 all medical teaching was given in Queen's College of Birmingham. Medical training had however become stagnant." As of 1881, John Berry Haycraft was appointed to a newly founded chair of physiology (O'Connor 1988:240–241).

[56] *BMJ* 1873;2:241 (23rd August; Physiological demonstrations). Ferrier presented at the same meeting, 2 days later (Idem). See also *Medical Record* 1873;8:507 ("Experiments on blood-corpuscles" followed by "Experiments upon the brain").

[57] For example, *Morpeth Herald* 29th November 1873, p.6 (Medical Conversazione at the West Riding Asylum) and *Central Glamorgan Gazette* 28th November 1873, p.4 (Medical Conversazione at the West Riding Asylum.). As these are identical, including misnaming "Dr Crighton [*sic*] Browne" and reporting Ferrier's demonstration of "the localisation of friction [*sic*] in the brain", I presume these are by the same author whose work, by hearsay, was syndicated.

However, the *Wakefield Express* reported that Crichton-Browne informed the audience that "Dr. Norris …. had just sent a telegram to say that he was unable to attend",[58] and hence the *Yorkshire Post and Leeds Intelligencer* noted that "owing to that gentleman's absence, from illness, this portion of the proceedings was omitted".[59] The extended build-up for Norris in the advertisement for the *conversazione* thus in the end came to nothing. Nevertheless, his inclusion in the *conversazione* programme gives further indication of the calibre of individuals Crichton-Browne wished to associate with the WRA meetings.

John Charles Bucknill (1817–1897)[60]

When he spoke at the WRA *conversazione* on 20th November 1874, John Charles Bucknill was Lord Chancellor's Visitor in Lunacy, the role Crichton-Browne was later to assume. Bucknill's appointment had come at the culmination of a long and distinguished career in asylum medicine. At age 26 he was appointed superintendent of the newly opened Devon County Lunatic Asylum at Exminster near Exeter. He co-authored with Daniel Hack Tuke (1827–1895) the significant textbook, *A Manual of Psychological Medicine* (first published 1858, four editions to 1879),[61] in which his contribution dealt with the diagnosis, pathology and treatment of insanity. He was the founding editor of the *Asylum Journal* in 1853, the official journal of the Association of Medical Officers of Asylums and Hospitals for the Insane (AMOAHI), and served as editor until 1862, renaming it the *Journal of Mental Science* in 1858.[62] He was later to become one of the four founder editors of *Brain: a journal of neurology* (Chap. 6). He became a Fellow of the Royal College of Physicians of London in 1859, where he was Lumleian

---

[58] *The Wakefield Express, and Barnsley, Normanton, Pontefract, Ossett, Horbury & Dewsbury Advertiser* Volume 22, No, 1126, 29th November 1873, p.2, cols. 4–7 (Medical conversazione at the West Riding Asylum. Speech by Lord Houghton. Lecture by Dr. Carpenter).

[59] *Yorkshire Post and Leeds Intelligencer* 27th November 1873, p.3 (West Riding Asylum. Medical Conversazione).

[60] Biographical material on Bucknill may be found in Langley (1980), Scull et al. (1996:187–225), Beveridge (1998), Scull, https://doi.org/10.1093/ref:odnb/3874, and Larner and Gardner-Thorpe (2023) (reprinted in adapted form, Larner 2025q).

[61] *WRLAMR* authors alluding to or quoting from the authority of "Bucknill and Tuke", various editions, include: Crichton Browne (I:8n1); Bywater Ward (I:162), Nicol (I:201), Major (II:44; IV:231), Sutherland (II:65), Milner Fothergill (IV:108–109, 110), Bevan Lewis (V:95, 97), Hughlings Jackson (V:106), Newcombe (V:207), Merson (VI:107). For Bucknill, Tuke, and the *Manual,* see Beveridge (1998). Bucknill's clinical authority was also appealed to elsewhere in *WRLAMR* (VI:145).

[62] The *Journal of Mental Science* became the *British Journal of Psychiatry* in 1963.

lecturer in 1878 (speaking on "Habitual drunkards and insane drunkards"), and of the Royal Society in 1866. As befitting an erudite gentleman physician, he took an interest in the works of Shakespeare, publishing books on *The Psychology of Shakespeare* (1859) and *The Medical Knowledge of Shakespeare* (1860).

Bucknill's lecture at the medical *conversazione* was later published, in the *BMJ* issue of 28th November 1874, hence only days after it was delivered in Wakefield.[63] It was also the subject of an editorial in the *Medical Times and Gazette* of 28th November.[64]

The same journal's *conversazione* report had noted that "Dr. Bucknill's able address, which we have noticed fully in one of our leading articles, was devoted to the subject of responsibility for homicide, though it in reality rather related to the law of murder".[65] Although this subject was a departure from the previous lectures at the *conversazione*, which had focussed on brain anatomy and physiology, the legal aspects of insanity were not wholly foreign to the meetings. For example, Balfour Browne, a barrister with an interest in the legal ramifications of insanity, had attended in 1872, and it should not be forgotten that Ferrier held the chair of Forensic Medicine at King's College London as of 1872 and was co-author with William Guy, his predecessor in the chair, of a well-respected textbook, *Principles of forensic medicine*, as of its fourth edition, published in 1875.[66]

Bucknill was later not only one of the editors of *Brain* but also an assiduous contributor to the early volumes, publishing in the "Critical Digests and Notices of Books" section of the inaugural issue of April 1878 (as did Ferrier), and continuing to contribute until 1885 (in all, 15 publications). He was also involved with the Neurological Society of London from its inauguration in 1886, a founder member who served on the Council (with Ferrier; Hughlings Jackson was president, Crichton-Browne was one of the two vice-presidents).[67] His obituary in the *Journal of Mental Science* was written by an alumnus of WRA, Crochley Clapham.[68]

---

[63] Bucknill (1874). Curiously, Bucknill's is the only name of the five lecturers at the WRA medical *conversazione* to be omitted by Leyland (1888:II:29).

[64] *Medical Times and Gazette* 1874;2:605–606 (28th November; The law of homicide).

[65] *Medical Times and Gazette* 1874;2:609–610 (28th November; Annual Conversazione at the West Riding Asylum).

[66] Likewise further editions: 5th in 1881; 6th in 1888; 7th in 1895. William Augustus Guy (1810–1885) was professor of forensic medicine at King's College London from 1838 to 1872 and first published his *Principles of forensic medicine* in 1844.

[67] *BMJ* 1886;1:219 (30th January; The Neurological Society of London).

[68] Clapham (1897). Other notices and obituaries: *BMJ* 1897;2:233 and 255 (24th July); *Lancet* 1897;2:228–229 (24th July).

Tempest Anderson (1846–1913)[69]

Tempest Anderson, mentioned in the report of the 1874 *conversazione* appearing in the *Medical Times and Gazette*, was the son of William Charles Anderson, a general practitioner in York who went on to become an ophthalmic surgeon in the city. In 1850 Hughlings Jackson was "apprenticed to Dr William Charles Anderson and his son, Dr Tempest Anderson, who were general practitioners in York",[70] but if, as seems likely, this referred to the same "William Charles Anderson" then it cannot be entirely true since Tempest was Jackson's junior by more than 10 years, hence around 4 years of age at the time Jackson was apprenticed.

Tempest Anderson later became famous for his expeditions and his work in vulcanology. He is said to have taken a great interest in the dissemination of science to the public. At the 1875 *conversazione* he exhibited "Sections of Tumours of the Brain",[71] possibly the same material as in 1874, but it is not clear if he was present in person.[72]

He may have crossed paths with Jackson in October 1904, when at the inauguration of the University of Leeds both were awarded the honorary degree of Doctor of Science.[73]

Clifford Gill (1846–1883)

Henry Clifford Gill graduated at University College London before, by "accident rather than inclination", entering asylum medicine, initially at Bethlem Hospital and Nottingham Asylum before arriving in Yorkshire in 1869, initially at the North Riding Asylum, Clifton, York, and then, as of 1874, the superintendency of the York Lunatic Asylum until his death in 1883. He was President of the York Medical Society in 1882. "The most divers forms of

---

[69] Biographical material on Tempest Anderson may be found in Suthren, https://doi.org/10.1093/ref:odnb/37115

[70] Greenblatt (2022:10–11); see also Reynolds (2020:711). Shorvon and Compston (2019:131) also described Jackson as "apprenticed (20 October 1850) to Dr. William Anderson and his son Tempest" but called them "physicians" rather than general practitioners. Could it be that William Anderson conducted his medical practice as a business, "Anderson & Son", hence the claim that Jackson was also apprenticed to Tempest, age notwithstanding? Taylor, revised Walton of Detchant (https://doi.org/10.1093/ref:odnb/34137) simply stated that William Anderson was the father of Tempest Anderson. The Anderson's home, 23 Stonegate, York, now serves as the home of the York Medical Society.

[71] WYAS C85/1382, "West Riding Asylum, Wakefield. Medical Conversazione, 19th November, 1875".

[72] Commemorations of Tempest Anderson include the Tempest Anderson Room at the York Medical Society and the Tempest Anderson Hall attached to the Yorkshire Museum in York.

[73] Critchley and Critchley (1998:184).

scientific enquiry successively attracted him"[74] according to his *BMJ* obituary. This was reprinted in the *Journal of Mental Science* with a single paragraph addendum which noted that "Ten years ago [i.e. ca. 1873], when a fresh impetus was given to the investigation of the brain in the insane [by Ferrier's findings, perhaps?], Mr. Gill threw himself with ardour into the inquiry, and prepared a large number of microscopic sections, many of which are unsurpassed to the present day".[75] This may explain why his preparations of brain slides were displayed at the WRA *conversazione* of both 1874 and 1875. This latter obituary also noted that "Mr. Gill's communications to the work of his own special department were not numerous".[76]

Ernest Hart (1835–1898)[77]

When he attended the 1874 medical *conversazione* at WRA, Ernest Abraham Hart was the editor of the *British Medical Journal*, a post to which he had been appointed on 11th August 1866, just over a month after Crichton-Browne's appointment to the WRA superintendency. Hart had trained at St George's Hospital in London and held various posts, including in ophthalmic and aural surgery at St Mary's Hospital, London, before turning to medical journalism. Of possible significance, Hart was adviser on medical literature to the publisher Smith, Elder & Co., the publishers of the third to sixth volumes of *WRLAMR* (1873–1876), and also of John Galton's translation of Ecker's *On the convolutions of the human brain* (1873) and Ferrier's monograph on *The functions of the brain* (1876 and 1886).

Crichton-Browne had published a number of times in the *BMJ* during Hart's editorship, including his series of "Clinical lectures on mental and cerebral diseases".[78] Ernest Hart was later Crichton-Browne's guest at the time of

---

[74] Obituary: *BMJ* 1883;1:387 (24th February). In the *Medical Directory* for 1874 he was "Asst. Med. Off. N. Riding Asyl. Clifton, York" (429) but in 1875 "Res. Med. Superintend. Lunat. Hosp. York" (438).

[75] Obituary: *J Ment Sci* 1883;29(April 1883):136–137. I have not encountered Gill's name in any other material relating to WRA.

[76] He did publish (e.g. Gill 1882–1883) including "one on Hyoscyamine in the treatment of the insane" which "was much appreciated" (according to *J Ment Sci* 1883;29(April 1883):137). In this paper, which appeared in 1878, Robert Lawson's work on hyoscyamine was mentioned (Gill 1878:93), although Gill was not referred to in Lawson's two *WRLAMR* papers on this subject.

[77] Biographical material on Ernest Hart may be found in his obituaries: *BMJ* 1898;1:175–186 (15th January), *Lancet* 1898;1;191–193 (15th January); also Bartrip, https://doi.org/10.1093/ref:odnb/12475; Heaman (2003:56–57), Collins (2024).

[78] Crichton-Browne (1871d, f, 1872b, 1873, 1874a). Other *BMJ* publications were 1871a, 1874c, 1875a.

the performance of *Pygmalion and Galatea* at WRA (2nd April 1875)[79] and also attended the 1875 WRA *conversazione*.[80]

William Broadbent (1835–1907)[81]

Born in Huddersfield, West Yorkshire, William Henry Broadbent's initial medical training was in Manchester before he moved to London where he eventually became Physician to St Mary's Hospital, Paddington.

Although perhaps best known to posterity for his interests in cardiology, he also published on neurological subjects which undoubtedly prompted his invitation to lecture at the WRA *conversazione*. These included a paper of 1866 which tried to explain the sparing of axial muscles in hemiplegia,[82] a subject of interest to Hughlings Jackson who was trying to explain these clinical phenomena, and he cited Broadbent in his *WRLAMR* papers (e.g. III:338, 339, 341 and n1)[83] and elsewhere. William Turner cited Broadbent's paper on the cerebral convolutions in a deaf and dumb woman[84] in the publication based on his 1872 *conversazione* lecture (III:15n3), and Broadbent's work was also mentioned by Carpenter in the publication based on his 1873 *conversazione* lecture (IV:21).[85] Broadbent had also published on the cerebral mechanisms of speech[86] and had credited the efforts of Allbutt and Hughlings Jackson with establishing the place of the ophthalmoscope in "English medicine".[87]

One of Broadbent's letters was quoted in the memoir of his life edited by his daughter:

---

[79] Crichton-Browne (1926:150) (see Chap. 3 for details of this performance). The Wellcome Collection holds a letter from Hart "To My Dear Stone from West Riding Asylum, Wakefield, undated but includes a programme for Gilbert's Pygmalion & Galatea, staged at the Theatre Royal Stanley-Cum-Wrenthorpe, 2 April 1875" (MS 8915), on notepaper headed "West Riding Asylum, Wakefield." presumably sent to Thomas Madden Stone, sometime librarian of the Royal College of Surgeons of London. Crichton-Browne also dined at Ernest Hart's, date unspecified (Crichton-Browne 1926:170), and elsewhere recounted one of his experiences as editor of the *BMJ* (Crichton-Browne 1931:74).

[80] *BMJ* 1875;2:680 (27th November; The West Riding Asylum).

[81] Biographical material on Broadbent may be found in Fye, 1990/2003 (cardiology); Brown, https://doi.org/10.1093/ref:odnb/32077, Eadie (2015), Larner (2025t) (neurology).

[82] Broadbent (1866). He also published in the *Journal of Mental Science*: Broadbent (1870–1871).

[83] Also VI:291n2. Major referenced Broadbent at VI:2.

[84] Broadbent (1870).

[85] Despite the notice taken of his work by contemporaries, one of the judgments of posterity has been that "Broadbent didn't perform 'research' so much as he made clinical observations" (Heaman 2003:60–61)

[86] Broadbent (1872a). This work was cited by Ferrier (1876:273n1).

[87] Broadbent (1872b:633).

Then in October [1875] I was invited to give the address at Dr Crichton Browne's Annual Conversazione at the Wakefield Asylum.

It was too great an honour and too good an opportunity to refuse, and, being a great opportunity, demanded adequate preparation.

I took for my subject "The Theory of the Construction of the Nervous System," and for the first time in my life gave a long address without notes. It was a success, except that the reporters were puzzled by the names.[88]

Broadbent's address at the *conversazione* on 19th November 1875 was reported by the *Leeds Mercury*, wherein he was misnamed as "Dr. W.H. Broadhead", to have "embodied the leading points in the papers in which Dr. Broadbent has of late years forcibly enunciated some extremely interesting views as to the construction and functions of the nervous centres, and still further developed their applications to the study of disease. The lecture was full of matter of great interest and value".[89] The lecture was subsequently published in the *BMJ*.[90]

Later in life, Broadbent apparently claimed Jackson as a lifelong friend,[91] and he was apparently the first to propose the foundation of the Neurological Society of London in 1885, seconded by Jackson.[92] He delivered the third Hughlings Jackson Lecture of the Neurological Society of the United Kingdom on 5th November 1903[93] (he had previously, in 1895, been President of the Neurological Society of London, succeeding Ferrier). Hence one might have anticipated that Jackson would have attended Broadbent's lecture at the WRA *conversazione* if it were possible, making his absence from the listings of those invited or attending even more notable.

---

[88] Broadbent (1909:180–181).

[89] *Leeds Mercury* 20th November 1875, p.3 (Medical Conversazione at Wakefield Asylum).

[90] Broadbent (1876).

[91] The story emanated from Harvey Cushing (Greenblatt 2022:40n70) but is plausible in that both men were born in the same year and both were Yorkshiremen living and working in London.

[92] Bailey (1895:102).

[93] Broadbent (1903).

Charles Seymour

Charles Seymour, who presided over Stall C at the 1875 *conversazione*, has not been encountered in any other material relating to WRA. He appears in the *Medical Directory* for 1877 (645) "M.B. Aberd. and C.M. 1876; M.R.C.S. Eng and L.S.A 1876" with an address in Hampshire but no other details. He does not appear in the 1879 *Medical Directory*. Considering the role he played at the *conversazione* of 1875, he may have been a Clinical Clerk or Clinical Assistant, but no evidence to corroborate this supposition has yet been identified.[94]

Summary: Guests at the WRA *conversazione*

This section has covered only a very small number of the hundreds of guests invited to and attending the WRA *conversaziones* held between 1871 and 1875, mostly practitioners from the area of the West Riding. Moreover, with the exception of those who proposed toasts, there is no individualised information about response to the meetings, although the overall tenor seems to have been one of satisfaction and enjoyment. It should not be forgotten that at this time the opportunity to attend such meetings was rare for most clinicians, especially outside London.

Did these individuals contribute anything to the origins of neurology in Britain during this era? Although none were specific to WRA, it may be argued that Turner contributed to neuroanatomy through his nomenclature of the lobes of the brain; Anstie's work influenced Jackson; Bucknill contributed to the foundation of *Brain*; Hart published papers from WRA in the *BMJ*; and Broadbent was one of the inaugural members of the Neurological Society of London. Whilst none of these contributions is epochal, in the way of Ferrier or Hughlings Jackson, they all added to the conducive, permissive environment in which neurology emerged in Britain. To this subject we now turn, in the concluding chapter.

---

[94] His name does not appear in Finn's listing (2012:181–184) of junior clinicians at WRA in the Crichton-Browne years.

10

Synthesis: The Origins of British Neurology, 1866–1876

The story of how the field of neurology emerged in Britain is one that defies easy retrospective reconstruction of the process.
Casper (2014:14).

Introduction: Neurology or Psychiatry?

The preceding chapters have outlined the development of the West Riding Asylum at Wakefield (WRA), in particular focussing on the years when James Crichton-Browne was the medical director and superintendent (1866–1876). They have detailed: the changes in the institutional infrastructure (Part I); the resident medical staff of the Asylum and their activities (Part II); the clinicians visiting and/or associated with the Asylum and its house journal, the *West Riding Lunatic Asylum Medical Reports* (*WRLAMR*; Part III); and the annual meetings, the medical *conversazione*, and those addressing these meetings and some of those contributing in other ways (Part IV).

The purpose of this final chapter is to assess what contribution, if any, these individuals and their activities at WRA had on the origins of British neurology during the years 1866 to 1876. More particularly, it seeks to address E.D. Adrian's (1939) assertion that this was "a classical period in the history of medicine, the period when neurology became a science".[1]

Such an assessment needs first to be contextualised by reference to previous arguments related to the origins of British neurology. That WRA may indeed

---

[1] Adrian (1939:433). Cited in Todd and Ashworth (1991:416).

© The Author(s), under exclusive license to Springer Nature Switzerland AG 2026
A. J. Larner, *The West Riding Asylum and the Origins of British Neurology 1866-1876*,
https://doi.org/10.1007/978-3-032-12591-0_10

be relevant to these origins is perhaps suggested by the brief accounts of the happenings there during this time period which have appeared from time to time in the neurological literature written by medical historians.[2] On the other hand, WRA barely registered a mention in a history of neurology in Britain written by a historian of medicine.[3] To my knowledge, the only full-length study of the relationship of WRA to the "making of the modern brain sciences" is Michael Finn's unpublished thesis.[4] This relative neglect hitherto of the role of WRA in the origins of British neurology also merits examination.

A distinct difference of opinion may be found in the secondary literature between those who have argued for the origin of British neurology within the context of general internal medicine and those who favour an origin within psychiatry (the latter term will be used here, at risk of anachronism, in preference to others, such as asylum medicine, alienism, or medical psychology).

Frank Clifford Rose (1926–2012), a clinical neurologist with an interest in medical history,[5] argued that "In the UK, neurology stemmed from general (internal) medicine rather than psychiatry".[6] Certainly, many neurologists, perhaps in the context of their training, will have imbibed what might playfully or facetiously be termed the "standard creation myth" of British neurology, *viz.* that it all started with the foundation of the National Hospital for the Paralysed and Epileptic which opened in Queen Square, London, in 1860.[7] From the outset, this institution was staffed by physicians, namely Charles Édouard Brown-Séquard (1817–1894) and Jabez Spence Ramskill (1824–1897),[8] followed by Charles Bland Radcliffe (1822–1889)[9] and John Hughlings Jackson (1835–1911). It should be remembered that at this time in the 1860s, neurology both as a clinical interest and as a diagnostic method

---

[2] For the distinction between "medical historians" and "historian of medicine" as used in this text, see comments in the Preface. For examples of works by members of the former group, see Spillane (1974a, 1981:387–389); WFN Research Group on the History of the Neurosciences (1997), Wilkins (1997), Pearce (2003a), Pearce and Lees (2013), Rollin and Reynolds (2018).

[3] Casper (2014):29, 39. At the latter page, speaking of the founding of *Brain*, Caspar includes Bucknill as a member of the "West Riding Asylum cohort". As shown in Chap. 9, Bucknill only attended WRA for the purpose of giving a lecture, in November 1874.

[4] Finn (2012).

[5] For example, see Rose (1999, 2012).

[6] Rose (2010:613).

[7] Shorvon and Compston (2019) have provided the most comprehensive history of the National Hospital at Queen Square.

[8] For biographical material on Brown-Séquard, see Aminoff (1993), Celestin (2014). I am not aware of any dedicated biographical work on Ramskill, but some information may be found in Shorvon and Compston (2019:98n3, 99n5), and Swash (2024:183), who stated that Ramskill "was influential in ensuring Jackson's appointments both at Queen Square and the London".

[9] For biographical material on Radcliffe, see Eadie (2007), Larner and Triarhou (2024c).

was still evolving. Even the basics of the current neurological examination were not established: the knee jerk reflex was not described in the medical literature until 1875,[10] Babinski's sign not until 1896[11]; Gordon Holmes (1876–1965), credited with systematising the neurological examination, was not yet born.

In contrast to Rose, William Bynum, a historian of medicine, argued for the psychiatric origins of British neurology.[12] Whilst acknowledging that "the years between 1870 and 1890 saw the emergence of a critical and mature neurological profession in Britain … located largely in the London hospitals", nevertheless Bynum was of the view that "If the flowering was in London, the roots are usually placed in the West Riding of Yorkshire, in the fruitful interchange between neurologists, psychiatrists, scientifically orientated general physicians, and pathologists in the newly created pathology laboratory of the West Riding Lunatic Asylum, presided over by the genial and long-lived psychiatrist, James Crichton-Browne".[13]

Is this discrepancy anything more than a realisation of the differing perspectives to be anticipated as emanating from, respectively, a trained neurologist who also studied medical history versus a trained historian who chose to study the history of medicine? Of course, such a binary—psychiatry or neurology?—is exclusive, reductive, and simplistic. Moreover, in searching for origins, the risk of projecting back upon earlier times is apparent.

Nevertheless, using liminality analysis, a methodology which may be applied to explain historical transitions from one state to another in a wide range of divergent situations,[14] it is clear that the 1860s to 1870s was a liminal period for neurology as a discipline. From our current historical vantage point, we know that from this threshold neurology went on to become an independent clinical specialty with its own dedicated body of knowledge, clinicians expert in that knowledge, researchers working to further that knowledge base in both clinical and laboratory settings, journals and meetings to disseminate that knowledge, and training programmes to instil that knowledge into the clinicians and researchers of the future. In other words, beyond this threshold neurology became both a clinically-based and a research-oriented discipline. But the outcome might have been different: beyond this

---

[10] Lazar (2022), Adan and Larner (2025).

[11] van Gijn (1996).

[12] Bynum (1985); reprinted Bynum (1990).

[13] Bynum (1985:95, 96).

[14] For a brief discussion of liminality analysis and liminal periods, ideas which originate from the work of the cultural anthropologists Arnold van Gennep and Victor Turner and the African historian Humphrey Fisher, see Larner (2024d).

threshold in the 1860s and 1870s, neurology might have become simply one branch of internal medicine pursued by general physicians,[15] or a branch of psychiatry, perhaps as neuropsychiatry (as occurred in Germany). How was it that matters turned out the way they did in the British context?

As previously argued (see Introduction: Professionalisation and specialisation), one of the defining features of a profession is the possession and development of an exclusive body of specialised knowledge acquired and articulated through specific and dedicated institutions, faculty, journal(s), and meetings. Here, each of these four factors is reconsidered in the context of Adrian's claim that this was "the period when neurology became a science".

Institution

What kind of an institution was WRA in the 1860s and 1870s? In one sense, this is very easily answered: as a county asylum, it was essentially custodial, though avowedly therapeutic, accommodating the many hundreds of poor individuals from around the locality, and sometimes beyond, whose behaviour was disturbed to the point where they could not be more appropriately cared for by relatives or in other custodial institutions such as the workhouse or the prison.[16] In this respect, WRA was no different from every other county asylum in the country.

However, in addition to this function, it has been argued that WRA was a research laboratory[17] or a research school, the activities of which contributed to the "making of the modern brain sciences".[18] These judgments of posterity were in fact rehearsed in contemporary observations: for example, Crichton-Browne aspired to the creation of a "medical school for physiological study",[19] or a "Pathological Institute".[20] According to John Charles Bucknill, writing in 1874, WRA had become a "school of observation and a college of instruction",[21]

---

[15] Medical culture was generally hostile to specialisation at this time, an ethos which persisted in some locations into the 1950s (e.g. Liverpool, where Professor Henry Cohen remained a tenacious opponent despite, ironically, being one of the founding members of the Association of British Neurologists in 1932. Casper 2007 and 2014:121, 126).

[16] In the words of Charles Aldridge: "before their acts necessitate their removal from home" (II:227).

[17] Easterbrook (1938:297), Gatehouse (1981).

[18] Finn (2012:passim). Finn based his argument on the features postulated to characterise a "research school" by Morrell (1972).

[19] *Wakefield and West Riding Herald with which is incorporated the Wakefield Journal & Examiner* 19th October 1872, p.6, cols.1,2 (Medical Conversazione at the West Riding Asylum).

[20] *Report*, 1873:28.

[21] Bucknill (1874:667).

so much so that it had become a paragon for other similar institutions: "It is lamentable to see how little use is made of the vast material in our great asylums, and how imperfectly the example of the West Riding Asylum is followed in other asylums of this country".[22] As President of the Medico-Psychological Association (MPA) in 1878, Crichton-Browne advocated "the conversion of our asylums into clinical schools to a far greater extent than has yet been attempted".[23]

As previously discussed (see Chap. 2), when WRA was first designed the pursuit of scientific research within its walls was not envisaged, nor was this the case for several decades after its opening. Thus, reconfiguration of the existing institution to provide the infrastructure for research was necessary in order to realise any ambition for a dedicated science-oriented profession. It was necessary for Crichton-Browne to effect changes not only in the buildings of WRA to accommodate this approach (Chap. 3) but also in its ethos. The former was addressed principally by the construction of a dedicated laboratory to promote pathological and experimental investigations. Moreover, possession of a laboratory afforded an intellectual credibility necessary to an institution professing scientific values.[24] But in addition to bricks and mortar, Crichton-Browne needed to change the ethos of WRA from one of custodial care to one of clinical and experimental inquiry.[25] In this context, the existing paradigm for the understanding of insanity needs to be examined, specifically the influence of phrenology, and how the institution moved from this pseudoscience to the more exact sciences.[26]

Phrenology at WRA

From the outset, the precepts of phrenology were integral to medical practice at WRA. The first superintendent, William Ellis, was a phrenologist, as was Disney Alexander, one of the earliest appointed visiting physicians. A local newspaper report from 1873 noted that "… when Dr. (afterwards Sir William)

---

[22] *BMJ* 1876;2:722 (2nd December). Ward (1877) subsequently suggested reasons why this neglect might be the case.

[23] Crichton-Browne (1878–1879:368).

[24] Quick (2014).

[25] My analysis here thus differs from that of Finn and Stark (2015:16) who argued that "provincial county asylums … were home to a wealth of scientific and medical research in the nineteenth century". See also Crichton-Browne's Preface (I:iii-v) which noted "a frequent charge that no scientific work is accomplished" in the public lunatic asylums. Of course, there were occasional exceptions, e,g, Alfred Walter Campbell working at Rainhill Asylum in the final decade of the nineteenth century (*vide infra*).

[26] Finn (2012:15) stated that "In Wakefield [Asylum], the ancestral problem was phrenology", taking the "ancestor problem" terminology from Ravetz (1971); also Finn (2012:134).

Ellis was the director, 45 years ago [hence ca. 1828], Dr. Spurzheim, one of the founders of the science of phrenology, made post-mortem examinations at the asylum to demonstrate the possibility of unfolding the convolutions of the brain".[27] A biography published shortly after Spurzheim's death confirmed that he made a visit to Wakefield in 1829 but without specific mention of WRA or Ellis.[28]

Crichton-Browne's father, William, had been a committed phrenologist in his early career, dedicating his celebrated lectures of 1837 to Andrew Combe (1797–1847) "as an acknowledgment of the benefits conferred on society, by his exposition of the application of phrenology in the treatment of insanity and nervous diseases".[29] Indeed, Crichton-Browne was later to describe his father as "a phrenologist of the old school",[30] some evidence for which may be found in William Browne's solitary paper in *WRLAMR*, which begins with Gall and refers to publications in the *Phrenological Journal* which had been founded by Andrew Combe along with his brother George (1788–1858) and others in 1823. Perhaps skating over William Browne's earlier phrenological beliefs, a later incumbent of the Crichton Royal Institution superintendency maintained that Browne had "always upheld mental disease has a bodily or physical basis".[31] Certainly it appears from his paper in *WRLAMR* that he was able to make a seamless transition to the ideas on the cortical localisation of language function initiated by Broca (II:278–301).

It has been argued that phrenology "remained an essential context for the neurological bent"[32] of James Crichton-Browne. The visitor interviewing "Horniblow", alias Crichton-Browne, in 1873 observed that "We certainly owe much to Gall and the phrenologists for drawing attention to the study of the brain, and for trying, however imperfectly, to localise the faculties".[33] However, any enduring support for the tenets of phrenology on the part of Crichton-Browne might be questioned in light of "A Lecture of Phrenology" which featured in the "Grand Astronomical Night" theatrical performances at WRA held on 2nd January 1867: "By the original ORION, 'Great Orion,

---

[27] *The Wakefield Express, and Barnsley, Normanton, Pontefract, Ossett, Horbury & Dewsbury Advertiser* Volume 22, No, 1126, 29th November 1873, p.2, cols. 4–7 (Medical conversazione at the West Riding Asylum. Speech by Lord Houghton. Lecture by Dr. Carpenter).

[28] Spurzheim (1836:95). There is no mention of WRA in Carmichael's (1833) memoir of Spurzheim.

[29] Browne (1837:iii). See also Cooter (1976a:5). William Browne's commitment to phrenology was extensively examined by Finn (2012:21–45).

[30] Crichton-Browne (1924), cited in Walmsley (2003:22).

[31] Easterbrook (1938:295).

[32] Neve and Turner (1995:401). See also Finn (2012:48–54).

[33] Anon. (1873:472). Finn (2012:1) wrongly ascribed this statement to Horniblow rather than his interviewer. Also discussed in Larner (2025e).

sloping slowly to the West!' who, notwithstanding his tendency to slope will certainly appear on this occasion".[34] It seems unlikely that such a performance lampooning phrenology would have happened if Crichton-Browne were a dedicated adherent, especially occurring so soon after he took up his appointment at WRA.

Certainly, by the early 1870s a different mood was beginning to prevail with respect to phrenology, thanks in part to the researches of Fritsch and Hitzig in Germany and Ferrier's work at WRA and then in London. For example, Milner Fothergill, a visitor to WRA for clinical research purposes, observed that "the localization of function in the brain has been established by the brilliant observations of Dr. Ferrier. The empirical guesses of Gall and Spurzheim, and the more accurate pathological observations of Schroeder van der Kolk, are now having direction and precision given to them by the close clinical studies of Hughlings Jackson, and the direct experiments of Fritsch and Hitzig, and still more of our countryman Ferrier" (IV:106). Whilst there were passing references to phrenology in *WRLAMR*,[35] for the most part these were negative. For example, McDowall, writing on colour vision, referred to "the phrenological hypothesis. Gall and his followers place the organ of colour in that part of the brain situate [*sic*] immediately above the eye and beneath the eye-brow. Although most men may agree that there must be such an organ as the phrenologists maintain there is, perhaps few will consider the evidence sufficient to justify the position selected for it by that school of cerebral physiologists" (III:147).

Considering Crichton-Browne's admissions of the influence of Laycock on his training, the latter may have been instrumental in determining his programme for WRA. Laycock presumably had Crichton-Browne (and possibly others) in mind when he stated that "the scientific development of psychological medicine must depend on the qualifications of those who may succeed their teachers in office". Laycock also noted that asylum physicians:

knowing the need for reform in their methods, and that high and true scientific culture can alone give them their rightful position in the profession and in the world of science and letters, will earnestly set to work in the right way. It is matter of congratulation that the work has been begun, at least, by my friend Dr. Crichton Browne of the West Riding Asylum.[36]

---

[34] WYAS C85/1382, programme for "Theatre Royal, Stanley-cum-Wrenthorpe".

[35] For example: II:91 (Mitchell); III:24 (Turner: "Gall and Spurzheim, and the other writers of their school of Phrenology, also claim to have been able to subdivide the convolutionary surface of the hemispheres into areas, or organs, each of which is the seat of a particular faculty."); IV:23 (Carpenter).

[36] Laycock (1874:4, 50).

But Batty Tuke responded vigorously, pointing out that:

No one will seek to gainsay the great value of the work which Dr. Crichton Browne has done at Wakefield … but if we inquire into the nature of his work, it will be found how little it has been influenced by the teachings of his master, Prof. Laycock. The papers which compose the mass of the West Riding Reports [*sic*] are devoted to anatomy, physiology, pathology, general and morbid, and therapeutics, which sciences are applied in a manner diametrically opposed to the theoretical method of Laycock.[37]

As well as contemporary assessments, some retrospective judgments of phrenology at WRA are also available. For example, Crochley Clapham, who devoted much time and energy to measuring skulls, discussed the newer "lobar phrenology" of Ferrier as against the older "lobular phrenology" of Gall and Spurzheim in a presentation to the MPA in Sheffield in February 1898.[38]

In the early 1920s (i.e. around 50 years after the events at WRA considered here) it was suggested by Bernard Hollander (elected to the MPA in 1900) that Crichton-Browne's motive for inviting Ferrier to Wakefield was "to confirm – or possibly to contradict – phrenology".[39] However, to my knowledge there is no documentary evidence to support Hollander's contention that this was Crichton-Browne's intention; he himself certainly wrote of the motor and sensory centres in the brain,[40] no doubt a reflection of Ferrier's findings. Crichton-Browne was intensely proud of the role of WRA in facilitating Ferrier's work.

---

[37] Batty Tuke (1874:109). References to Laycock in *WRLAMR* are indeed few: I:194n2 (Nicol); III:23 (Turner); IV:139–140 (Milner Fothergill); IV:249 (Lawson, re "maximum hours of death"); V:110, 111, 114 (Hughlings Jackson).

[38] Clapham (1898b). Another WRA alumnus, J.A.M. Wallis, was interested in the shape of patients' skulls when superintendent at Hull (Bickford 1981:51).

[39] Cited in Oppenheim (1991:68). Hollander's text (1921:406–407) reads: "Sir James Crichton Browne is a very learned man who was then, as he is now, doing his utmost to promote the progress of medical science. Seeing that Hitzig had proved the most fundamental principle of Gall's doctrine — the multiplicity of centres in the brain — the denial of which had for 50 years obstructed the advance of our knowledge of brain functions, he invited a young friend and former fellow student (of Dr. Laycock, Professor of Medicine of Edinburgh University) — DAVID FERRIER (1843–), who then was engaged in quite a different department, being Lecturer on Toxicology (1872–1889) in succession to Dr. Guy in King's College, London — to come to Wakefield and repeat Hitzig's experiments on the brains of animals and to confirm — or possibly to contradict — phrenology." Rather than "Lecturer on Toxicology", Ferrier was Professor of Forensic Medicine at King's College Hospital from 1872 (see Chap. 7). Hollander had previously tried to suggest that Ferrier's findings supported the old phrenology: *BMJ* 1890;1:86–87 (11th January; The old and new phrenologies). For more on Hollander, see McEniery (2021).

[40] VI:222, 225, 227, 228, 230, Crichton-Browne (1926:101–103). Both Milner Fothergill and Lauder Brunton had adopted the terminology of "motor centre" by 1874 (see their papers in *WRLAMR* IV), perhaps unsurprisingly as both were close colleagues of Ferrier. It was also used by Lawson (V:58), Bevan-Lewis (V:103, 104), and Hughlings Jackson (VI:269, 277, 278, 284, 292, 296, 297, 298, 301).

Although Ferrier has been credited with demonstrating the "scientific basis of phrenology",[41] I find no use of the word or its cognates in Ferrier's publications based on his WRA researches.[42] A brief item which appeared in the *Medical Press and Circular* of 24th September 1873 reporting Ferrier's address entitled "On the Localisation of the functions of the brain" presented on Friday 19th September at the 43rd Annual Meeting of the British Association for the Advancement of Science held in Bradford, West Yorkshire, hailed an "entirely new system of phrenology",[43] and a report of the same meeting appearing in *The Examiner* noted that "we shall have a scientific phrenology, instead of, as at present, an empirical phrenology".[44] William Rutherford's address at the same meeting gave a clear exposition of the matter:

These researches of Jackson, Fritsch and Hitzig, and Ferrier, mark the commencement of a new era in our knowledge of brain-function. Of all the studies in comparative physiology there will be none more interesting, and few so important, as those in which the various centres will be mapped out in the brains throughout the vertebrate series. A new, *but this time a true*, system of phrenology will be founded upon them; by this, however, I do not mean that it will be possible to tell a man's faculties from the configuration of his skull, but merely this, that the various mental faculties will be assigned to definite territories of the brain, as Gall and Spurzheim long ago maintained, although their geography of the brain was absurdly erroneous, and their notions regarding the indications afforded by the configuration of the skull ridiculous.[45]

The published abstract of Ferrier's first Croonian Lecture to the Royal Society (March 1874) credited him with the view that "A scientific phrenology is regarded as possible".[46] Later, in *The functions of the brain*, a title perhaps

---

[41] Casper (2014:29).

[42] Specifically, nothing in III:30–96 or IV:30–62, nor in Ferrier (1873a, b). Likewise, the term does not appear in Ferrier (1878a).

[43] *Medical Press and Circular* 1873;16:275. For the address, see Ferrier (1873c).

[44] "WAH" (1873:966). Also, "In stating that the first fruits of the new line of inquiry will probably be a scientific phrenology, we correctly indicate what is their value with reference to the science of mind. All that phrenology, if true, could have done, is now likely to be achieved".

[45] Rutherford (1873:392) [italics in original]. Slightly different text appeared in Rutherford (1874:122), omitting the words "of Jackson, Fritsch and Hitzig, and Ferrier," and the italicisation of "but this time a true", and ending simply "although their geography of the brain was erroneous".

[46] Ferrier (1874b:232) (cited by Sherrington 1928:xiii, as noted by Young 1968:264; also in Spillane 1981:389). The paper was read to the Royal Society by Burdon Sanderson but the full manuscript was, notoriously, never published because of the objections of the reviewers, principally Foster and Huxley (see Larner 2026b). The handwritten manuscript is held in the archives of the Royal Society (AP/56/2 The localisation of function the brain). This reads (at Sheet 144; page numbered 134 by Ferrier) "The line of research is one which is likely to lead to valuable results, and may form the basis of a scientific phrenology" [my transcription].

knowingly echoing Gall's *Sur les fonctions du cerveau* (1822–5),[47] Ferrier briefly discussed the "phrenological hypothesis as to the functions of the cerebellum".[48] Ferrier's findings had in fact established the principle of cerebral localisation as physiological fact rather than, as previously, phrenological speculation and served to confirm the views of Hughlings Jackson on the pathology of epilepsy as a discharging lesion.[49] It may be, however, that in the final analysis Crichton-Browne could not shake off the old "empirical phrenology" for the new "scientific phrenology".

Nearly 50 years after his departure from WRA Crichton-Browne stated that the phrenologists had "battled for basic principles now unimpeachable".[50] (However, in addition, he considered the "phrenologists were the first eugenicists", citing the actions of Andrew and George Combe, and that "eugenism is really the acme of evolution. It is ethical selection, and like natural selection aims at the elimination of the unfit and the preservation of the fit",[51] views which might suggest that Crichton-Browne had reinterpreted phrenology in Darwinian terms.) One might, then, agree with Cooter's analysis of phrenology as a "provocation to progress",[52] but not as a catalyst, merely something to be improved upon, escaped from, or set on an empirical research-oriented basis.

Hence, even before Crichton-Browne's departure from WRA, it was deemed to be not only an asylum but also a centre for research. It was said that "Great scientific activity pervades the institution"[53] and Crichton-Browne had been responsible for "the infusion of the spirit of scientific research into a great curative establishment".[54] The annual *conversazione* was "an important annual convention of medical scientists"[55] and Crichton-Browne had "raised the character of the Institution to such a point that its name is now known

---

[47] Young (1970:246).

[48] Ferrier (1876:121–125). I presume this is the reference alluded to by Hollander (1921:407) who noted that Ferrier mentioned Gall only once. The phrenologists attributed the sexual function of amativeness to the cerebellum, a position argued against by William Carpenter on the basis of the experimental evidence that it was involved in coordination of movement (Quick 2014:57–58). According to Spillane (1981:240), "Ferrier also felt it necessary to consider Gall's view [of the cerebellum] and although he thought that a few clinico-pathological observations offered some support, he found no evidence from his own experiments and concluded that there was no foundation for the theory".

[49] Young (1970:234–248).

[50] Crichton-Browne (1924), cited in Neve and Turner (1995:401).

[51] Crichton-Browne (1926:72–73).

[52] Cooter (1976b), spoke of the "provocation of progress" whereas Pressman (1998:399), referencing Cooter, spoke of the "provocation to progress".

[53] *BMJ* 1875;1:488–489 (10th April; The West Riding Lunatic Asylum), quotation at 489.

[54] *BMJ* 1875;2:680 (27th November; The West Riding Asylum).)

[55] *Times* (London), 23rd November 1875, p.7, as cited by Finn (2012:3n10).

and respected throughout the scientific world".[56] Although hardly an impartial observer, Shaw Bolton thought the Asylum under Crichton-Browne had attained "not only a national but a European fame both for the treatment of the insane and for the prosecution of scientific research".[57] The judgment of posterity has credited Crichton-Browne with having "integrated neurological research with asylum administration"[58] and of pursuing a "biological psychiatry".[59]

Experimental Science at WRA

> Between 1865 and 1875 medical research began to take a new direction and to look more and more to the causes, rather than to the results of disease.[60]

This was the retrospective assessment of Thomas Lauder Brunton, a physician with links to WRA, albeit briefly (see Chap. 7), who was later described as "a scientific practitioner who wanted to use the laboratory to enhance treatment and diagnosis".[61]

But how did this shift to a more scientific outlook come about at WRA? How did Crichton-Browne go about transforming an administrative, bureaucratic institution, infused with the ideas of phrenology and typical of the profession of asylum medicine at the time, into a research-oriented school infused with a scientific culture? Although the construction and equipping of a pathological laboratory at WRA in the early 1870s was a sure sign of his intent, Crichton-Browne had no personal experience of laboratory work from his time in Scotland, England, or France (admittedly details on his time in Paris are sparse). Did he have any particular model upon which to base these developments?

An obvious candidate might be Charles Darwin, perhaps the most prominent scientist of the day as a result of his evolutionary theory. As a correspondent of Crichton-Browne,[62] and a student friend of William Browne, it might be imagined that Darwin was an influence on the changes wrought at

---

[56] *J Ment Sci* 1875–1876;21(January 1876):633n (Appointments).

[57] Bolton (1928:607). Also 625 re scientific progress.

[58] Neve and Turner (1995:399).

[59] Walmsley (2003).

[60] Lauder Brunton (1909:198). Cited in Fye (1986:228).

[61] Waddington (2007:275). Despite this label, Lauder Brunton was also amongst the contributors to Hack Tuke's (1892) *Dictionary of psychological medicine*.

[62] Other correspondents of Darwin who had some association with WRA were Lawson Tait (Chap. 5) and William Turner (Chap. 9).

WRA. He was, for his own purposes, interested in the work occurring there, citing both Crichton-Browne and Patrick Nicol in *The expression of the emotions in man and animals* (Chap. 3). Darwin was the subject of passing references in *WRLAMR*,[63] but his ideas may not have been entirely understood. Lauder Brunton, for example, wrote that:

> If a stimulus excites to action once it will tend to do so again, and if it affects the vessels, glands, or ideational centres once it will have an increased tendency to affect these structures on a subsequent application. These tendencies are transmitted to posterity, and the son of a man in whom a stimulus leads to action will have more chance of possessing this quality than the progeny of a man whose leanings are towards reflection. (IV:209).

suggesting a Lamarckian rather than Darwinian viewpoint.[64] Although a champion of an evolutionary view of brain function and dysfunction, Hughlings Jackson's principal influence was Herbert Spencer,[65] not Darwin. Moreover, intellectual debts aside, Darwin ran no institutional laboratory or collaborative research programme, being essentially a solitary worker and thinker, so could not have advised Crichton-Browne on these points. His practical influence on WRA may therefore have been minimal.

The change of name of asylum medicine's professional organisation, from the Association of Medical Officers of Asylums and Hospitals for the Insane (AMOAHI) to Medico-Psychological Association (MPA), was welcomed, as "the new name really expresses its essential scientific aim".[66] This name change occurred in 1865, coinciding not only with William Browne's Presidency of the MPA but also with James Crichton-Browne's first appointment as an asylum superintendent, in Newcastle-upon-Tyne.[67] The new name may have expressed the essential scientific aspirations of asylum medicine, but practice may have fallen well short of such aims in the absence of appropriate infrastructure and manpower. The dilemma was this: should scientifically trained medical men be encouraged to work in the asylum; or should asylum men be

---

[63] For example: II:124 (Crichton-Browne); IV:132 (Milner Fothergill); IV:214 (Lauder Brunton); VI:136–137, 146 (Lawson & Bevan Lewis).

[64] Possibly also evident at IV:220.

[65] Jackson's references to Spencer are found at: III:189, 195, 325, 344–346, 348; VI:287, 298. Other references to Spencer were made at I:5 (Crichton-Browne); II:85, 94 (Mitchell); III:22 (Turner); III:73 (Ferrier); IV:193, 212, 213 (Lauder Brunton); VI:136 (Lawson & Bevan Lewis).

[66] Anon. (1865). Reprinted in *J Ment Sci* 1865–1866;11(October 1865):441–442 (The Medico-Psychological Association) [quote at 441]. See also Bewley (2008:23).

[67] *J Ment Sci* 1865–1866;11(July 1865):295 (Appointments).

sent to the scientific centres to be trained?[68] Crichton-Browne opted for the former approach, in part no doubt because of the impracticability of the latter at this time.

In the 1860s and 1870s, the German-language universities were the acknowledged leaders in the field of experimental physiology.[69] Following the example of Johannes Müller (1801–1858), working in Bonn and then Berlin, a number of his students had developed their own research careers and physiological laboratories, for example Emil du Bois-Reymond (1818–1896) and Hermann von Helmholtz (1821–1894).[70] Had these developments influenced Crichton-Browne in any way? Whilst John Galton had worked in Vienna, he did not arrive at WRA until 1873, hence too late to affect Crichton-Browne's plans. One clinician visiting WRA, however, had experience of Germany and a German university: David Ferrier.[71]

Ferrier had visited Germany in 1864, attending the University of Heidelberg where, according to his first biographer writing in 1888, "he prosecuted his psychological studies, and also began the study of Anatomy, Physiology, and Chemistry".[72] However, it is unclear with whom he actually studied; some later commentators have placed him with Hermann von Helmholtz and Wilhelm Wundt (1832–1920).[73] Certainly, Helmholtz was in Heidelberg at this time, having moved there in 1858, not only to the chair but also to the directorship of a new Physiological Institute; by 1864 he was working on the third volume of his *Physiological Optics*.[74] Study with Wundt would also have been logical for Ferrier because of Wundt's shared interests with Alexander Bain, Ferrier's teacher in Aberdeen. However, in his biographical work on Wundt, Diamond placed Ferrier in Heidelberg as a pupil of neither Wundt nor Helmholtz, but of Friedrich Arnold (1803–1890), Wundt's maternal

---

[68] See Chap. 4 (Non-resident faculty: Visiting clinicians and external collaborators) for the differing views of Crichton-Browne and Maudsley on this point.

[69] Geison (1978). Snow (1967:38) judged Germany to have "been the great educating force of the nineteenth century".

[70] See, for example, Otis (2007a), Finkelstein (2013).

[71] Lauder Brunton had also visited German-language universities in the 1860s, specifically Berlin, Vienna, and Leipzig, as well as working in the Netherlands, in between his time at Edinburgh and his move to London (Hunting 2016:433), but as he in all likelihood followed Ferrier to WRA (see Chap. 7) I think it unlikely that he influenced the development of Crichton-Browne's laboratory. Of note in this context, Hughlings Jackson "did not know German" (Critchley and Critchley 1998:146).

[72] Leyland (1888:II:61). Corroboration of Ferrier's attendance at Heidelberg may be found in *BMJ* 1913;1:692 (Obituary. J.J. Kirk Duncanson). Also Ferrier's obituary in the *BMJ* (1928;1:525) stated that "He then studied psychology in Heidelberg in 1864". However, Purves-Stewart (1939:44) said that Ferrier "carried off a philosophical fellowship which entailed working in Germany".

[73] For example, Pearce (2003b), Sandrone and Zanin (2014:1247). These authors did not cite any primary source(s) to support their claims.

[74] Otis (2007a:125).

uncle, the Director of the Anatomical Institute.[75] Hence it is not entirely clear whether or not Ferrier gained any laboratory experience whilst in Germany. However, his ability to pursue independent research for his MD thesis in 1869–70 suggests a familiarity with laboratory practices, as does his employment by the physiologist John Burdon Sanderson following his move to London in 1870, work pursued possibly at the Brown Animal Sanatory Institution in London's Wandsworth Road,[76] possibly elsewhere.[77] Moreover, by 1871 Ferrier was Assistant-Demonstrator of Practical Physiology in the Department of Physiology at King's College Hospital where William Rutherford, another Edinburgh man, was Professor.[78] Ferrier's immediate model for his experimental subject and methodology at the time when he came to WRA derived from the 1870 paper of Fritsch and Hitzig, working in Berlin, a paper of which Ferrier was certainly aware by early 1871.[79]

As previously discussed (Chap. 7), how and when Ferrier became involved with WRA is, to my knowledge, unknown. No evidence as to whether Ferrier had communicated with Crichton-Browne about laboratory requirements before his arrival has been identified, or indeed whether any specific provisions might have been a condition of his attendance at WRA.[80] However, considering the pace at which his animal research work developed at WRA, with his first publication appearing within weeks of his arrival,[81] it seems unlikely that he was starting from scratch.

Another possibility, raised by Finn, is that Crichton-Browne was "well-informed of recent developments in nervous physiology from … scientific stars of Germany's state-sponsored research hospitals" through the agency of

---

[75] Diamond (1980:18). Diamond's source was Fürbringer (1903:71). For Arnold's possible influence on Ferrier, see Larner (2026c).

[76] Romano (2002:182).

[77] Specifically, "a room over a stable in Howland Street" which Burdon Sanderson had converted into a pathological laboratory (according to Wilson 1979:172); or Burdon Sanderson's "own private laboratory [at his house] in Queen Anne Street, collaborating there with the pioneer neurologist David Ferrier" (according to Richards 1987:127). The latter address was the location for the meeting in March 1876 at which the proposal for founding The Physiological Society was adopted, with Ferrier one of those in attendance (Sharpey-Schafer 1927:8).

[78] Rutherford may have been a student of Laycock (Hollander 1921:405). However, he was not mentioned in James, 1996.

[79] Fraser et al. (1871:396).

[80] Luring the best scholars with research facilities was one aspect of the workings of the German-language university system in the nineteenth century (Otis 2007a:12).

[81] Ferrier (1873a). Finn (2012:135) argued that "Ferrier did not conduct his initial experiments in provincial isolation" on the grounds that "he arrived at an institution already committed to investigating brains and the specific changes they underwent in lunatic patients". My argument (*vide infra*, Conclusion/Epilogue: Endings) differs from Finn's, suggesting that the relative, provincial isolation of WRA in fact facilitated the innovative developments which occurred there.

Thomas Laycock, and accordingly sought to incorporate "the German-inspired, laboratory-based microscopical and experimental approach" at WRA.[82]

Faculty

To be fruitful, a research-oriented institution or programme generally needs to involve a community of individuals, both established experts and enthusiastic juniors:

> … it is by pressing forward with scientific endeavour on a wide front and by enlisting the dedicated efforts of bold, gifted and enterprising men at the right time, that disciplines can hope to bring about salutary advances which have so often transformed whole subjects within a short time.

One might easily imagine this quotation to be from Crichton-Browne, circa 1866–1876, but in fact it dates from more than a century later.[83] One of Crichton-Browne's abilities was to persuade established clinicians to work at WRA and/or to publish in *WRLAMR* as well as attracting those at the beginning of their careers to be employed at WRA. He was thereby able to mould a critical mass of like-minded clinicians, a key to the inception of a self-regulating, autonomous profession.

The extended prosopography presented in Chaps. 5, 7, and 9, has shown the distinct differences in terms of career trajectory between the resident WRA staff and those either visiting and/or associated with the Asylum during the period 1866–1876. The former group, the asylum doctors, were essentially either destined for a career in asylum medicine or merely "birds of passage".[84] Although they contributed the majority of papers to *WRLAMR* (Table 6.1) and several were elected to membership of the Medico-Psychological Association (Table 5.1), very few gained qualifications as physicians beyond the basic licentiate (LRCP, LRCP Edin, or LM).

Was it possible to bridge the divide between the practice of asylum medicine and the career of a physician, or were the two mutually incompatible, divergent career trajectories, fundamentally irreconcilable? For the resident WRA clinicians there was at least one possible model of note: Thomas

---

[82] Finn (2012:49, 76). He did not cite any primary source(s) to support these claims.

[83] From Professor Martin Roth's Maudsley Lecture of 1971 after his induction as the inaugural President of the Royal College of Psychiatrists (Roth 1972).

[84] Dodds et al. (1890:44).

Laycock. Although a physician by training, his interests spanned the professional divide, such that he attended MPA meetings and indeed was MPA President in 1869, as well as being a physician (FRCPEd) and a university professor of the principles and practice of physic. He certainly inspired a number of students, mostly through his course in medical psychology at Edinburgh University, to later become either asylum doctors (Crichton-Browne, Major, McDowall, Lawson) or physicians with an interest in the workings of the brain (Hughlings Jackson, Ferrier, Milner Fothergill, and possibly Lauder Brunton).

Despite this model, very few of the resident WRA staff styled themselves as "physician" in their ultimate appointments (Nicol, Major, Clapham), or had contact with clinicians and/or societies devoted to neurology in later years. Their scientific credentials were therefore extremely limited, and aside from their publications in *WRLAMR* few continued to contribute to the medical, let alone the neurological or scientific, literature after departure from WRA. Notable exceptions were Henry Sutherland and Crochley Clapham (see Chap. 5 and below).

There is little evidence to suggest that, as a group, the WRA resident staff made any contribution to the beginnings of British neurology, either as a discipline or as a body of knowledge, despite the fact that several subsequently published in *Brain*, a journal dedicated to neurology (Table 6.4). A possible exception might be claimed for Robert Lawson's description of alcoholic amnesia,[85] although his observations were largely neglected both at the time and by posterity (in favour of those of Korsakoff). George Thompson has been described as a "man of science", but this related to his later career in Bristol.[86]

In contrast to the resident staff, the clinicians invited to visit, and/or otherwise associated with, WRA, for example through *WRLAMR*, were usually physicians and/or academics, heavily involved in clinical and laboratory research as well as pursuing clinical careers, with affiliations to teaching hospitals and universities. Many held fellowships of the Royal College of Physicians, the Royal Society, or both. Evidently, they were at more advanced, established stages of their careers than the resident WRA staff, and hence better positioned to contribute to neurology, either as an emerging discipline or as a body of knowledge.

Despite these differences, interactions between the resident staff and those visiting WRA evidently occurred, some of which may be traced in the pages

---

[85] Lawson (1878–1879). His observations were not made at WRA.
[86] Tobia (2017:250).

of *WRLAMR*. Herbert Major evidently worked with Allbutt (II:203) and provided material to Milner Fothergill (III:214; IV:105). Aldridge made ophthalmoscopic examinations for Milner Fothergill (IV:115, 117). Ferrier thanked both Galton and McDowall (III:96); his contacts with Lawson and Bevan-Lewis probably post-dated his time at WRA as neither had been appointed at the time when Ferrier can be placed at WRA. Galton provided illustrations for Ferrier and also for Milner Fothergill; moreover, his translation of Ecker was likely to have been of assistance to Ferrier. Lennox Browne mentioned both Lawson and Merson (V:153). However, none of these contacts amounted to a scientific collaboration in the sense that this is now understood; there were no mentors and protégés, research assistants who subsequently developed their own independent research laboratories and programmes.

Oppenheim was of the view that "Wakefield Asylum was the centre of *neurological* interest, and many eminent men congregated there and made their contributions at the monthly [*sic*] medical conversaziones which were organized at that institution by its director".[87] To be sure, this was a post hoc judgment, but nevertheless it is worth looking at some of the key faculty members to assess to what extent their interests were essentially neurological, and hence may have contributed to the origins of neurology as an independent discipline at WRA in the period 1866–1876.

James Crichton-Browne

Was James Crichton-Browne a neurologist? The question might seem odd, since his clinical training (discussed in Chap. 5), which might perhaps be deemed to have begun in his childhood home at Crichton Royal Institution, was that of an asylum doctor, one who was "fast-tracked" to asylum superintendency. This might also explain his otherwise puzzling comments on John Conolly (1794–1866), admittedly written many years after his time at WRA:

> There is no member of my profession whom I have ever met, except Lord Lister, who has left as deep and gracious an impression on my mind as Dr. John Conolly. … He was a benefactor of his species, and no member of his profession – except Jenner and Lister – has done a tithe as much as he to ward off and alleviate human suffering. It is to Conolly that we really owe the modern

---

[87] Oppenheim (1991:67) [my italics].

humane treatment of the insane as it exists to-day [*sic*] in all its beneficent ramifications.[88]

Perhaps Crichton-Browne had forgotten the revelations of the Ruck case, and the excoriating judgment of "Dr. Wycherley" in Charles Reade's *Hard Cash* (1863) or perhaps had not realised that Wycherley was a caricature of Conolly.[89]

Nevertheless, by his own admission, Crichton-Browne's most inspiring teacher was Thomas Laycock, a physician with an interest in the workings of the brain (although, as aforementioned, Batty Tuke believed that at Crichton's Browne's WRA the "sciences are applied in a manner diametrically opposed to the theoretical method of Laycock"). Unlike Laycock, however, Crichton-Browne was never appointed to the membership or fellowship of any of the Royal Colleges of Physicians, and indeed despite his eminence in later life, and his appointments as both FRSE and FRS, he never became either FRCP or FRCPEd, not even in an honorary capacity.[90]

Crichton-Browne not only interacted with neurologists during his years at WRA but continued to move in neurological circles thereafter. He played a role, possible a very significant one, in the foundation of *Brain: a journal of neurology* in 1878 (see Chap. 6). He was one of the two inaugural vice-presidents of the Neurological Society of London founded in 1886,[91] with Hughlings Jackson as the first President,[92] and was President himself in 1888.[93] Crichton-Browne's presidential address noted that "the journal *Brain* had passed into their hands",[94] a fortuitous coincidence with his Presidency of the Society. By his own (undated) report, he was once introduced to Gladstone

---

[88] Crichton-Browne (1926:326–329), quote at 326–327.

[89] Scull (1985). Oddly, Scull referred to "Wycherly" rather than "Wycherley", as per Reade.

[90] Walmsley (2003:22) noted that "Sir James Crichton-Browne was not prominently linked with the Colleges of Physicians". In this respect he was unlike Henry Maudsley (FRCP 1869), who had been a physician at the West London Hospital (Henry Maudsley | RCP Museum; cf. Wikipedia which says FRCP 1870, presumably because he gave the Gulstonian Lectures in that year), and W.H.O. Sankey (FRCP 1865) who had charge of a fever hospital in Islington for 5 years before turning to the study of mental disease (William Henry Octavius Sankey | RCP Museum (rcplondon.ac.uk), accessed 29/04/2024).

[91] According to Hunting (2002:264) "Thomas Buzzard retrospectively (1907; shortly after dissolution) claimed that Sir James Crichton-Brown [*sic*] had a good deal to do with the inception of the [Neurological] Society. Buzzard's letter, dated 1st February 1908, survives in the archives of the Neurological Society held at the Royal Society of Medicine (NS/A/2, unpaginated). However, the contemporary evidence suggests that William Broadbent, John Hughlings Jackson, and Armand de Watteville were the more likely instigators.

[92] Casper (2014:37). Reynolds and Broussolle (2022:292).

[93] As noted by Easterbrook (1938:297).

[94] *Lancet* 1888;1:325–326 (18th February; Neurological Society of London); quotation at 326.

as a neurologist,[95] and in an address delivered in 1897 when referring to the history of medicine he noted "*In my own department, neurology*, it is certain that progress has hinged on the genius and labours of a few great men - Charles Bell, Marshall Hall, Claude Bernard, Brown-Séquard, and Hughlings Jackson".[96]

Despite these associations, it has been stated that Crichton-Browne "severed his ties with neurology, although he made no public announcement of the divorce" at sometime between 1891 and 1894, a claim which was apparently based on the disappearance of his name from the membership list of the Neurological Society of London between these two dates.[97] Speculating on possible reasons for this apparent parting of the ways, Oppenheim cited Bynum to the effect that the NSL made the psychiatric members feel less welcome,[98] but this argument carries little credence since asylum-based clinicians continued to be NSL members,[99] made presentations,[100] and some were later appointed to the Presidency (*vide infra*) not only in 1894 but into the first decade of the twentieth century. It was Oppenheim's opinion that the likeliest reason for Crichton-Browne's departure from NSL membership centred on his "recoil from the implications of materialism that he found in the

---

[95] Crichton-Browne (1926:133). Obviously the introduction must have occurred before 19th May 1898.

[96] Crichton-Browne (1897:995) [my italics].

[97] Oppenheim (1991):74. It is certainly true that Crichton-Browne's name is not to be found in the 1894 NSL Members list: *Brain* 1894;17(Table of Contents):13–17. Ditto (1897): *Brain* 1897;20(4):A13–A18 (where A = addendum, after p.549). In my preliminary examination of the Neurological Society Council Minutes 1886–1898 (Royal Society of Medicine, NS/A/1) I have found no mention of his resignation from the Society (*cf.* Bevan Lewis: NS/A/1, p.70); merely a note on his retirement from the Council on 17th December 1889 (NS/A/1, p.41), the statutory end of his tenure on the Council. Following Oppenheim, Finn (2012:163) was undoubtedly in error with his statement that "In 1887 [*sic*] Crichton-Browne left the Neurological Society he had helped found", as he was President of the organisation in the following year!

[98] Oppenheim's citation is "Bynum, 1985:96–97" but my reading of this passage differs from Oppenheim's.

[99] For example, a cursory examination of the 1894 NSL membership list shows the following to have been members: Ernest Birt (West Riding Asylum), Hubert Bristowe (County Asylum, Wells), Harry Corner (Bethlem Royal Hospital), E. Long Fox, Peter Macdonald (County Asylum, Dorchester), S.R. Macphail (Borough Asylum, Rowditch), William Menzies (County Asylum, Rainhill), W.J. Mickle (Grove Hall Asylum, Bow), David Nicolson (Broadmoor), Conolly Norman (Richmond Asylum, Dublin), Edmund Lewis Rowe (Borough Asylum, Ipswich), Percy Smith (Bethlem Royal Hospital), Henry Sutherland, Hack Tuke, Batty Tuke, Joseph Wiglesworth (County Asylum, Rainhill) , Ernest Wills (Claybury Asylum, Essex), and Guy Wood (County Asylum, Rainhill). Furthermore, one of the eight newly elected members in 1894 was asylum based: W. Lloyd Andriezen (West Riding Asylum).

[100] For example, my preliminary researches into the history of the Neurological Society of London (Larner 2026a) have indicated presentations by Wiglesworth in 1892 (*Brain* 1892;15(3–4):431) and Batty Tuke in 1894 (*Brain* 1894;17(2):179). Even in the early twentieth century (June 1901) the asylum-based clinicians Richard Rows and David Orr presented at an extraordinary NSL meeting held in Manchester (Larner 2024a).

latest neurological research", citing his final contribution to *Brain* published in 1887–1888.[101]

Whilst Crichton-Browne's name certainly did disappear from the NSL membership lists, I do not find the idea of a rupture convincing. Could this not simply have reflected redirection of his (finite) energies elsewhere, of being busier in other spheres? The case is, of course, flatly contradicted by his 1897 claim that neurology was his "own department".[102] Moreover, other names disappeared from the NSL membership lists (e.g. Allbutt, Clapham, Bevan-Lewis) without similar claims arising.

By the time of his death in 1938 Crichton-Browne's influence on the development of neurology was well recognised, indeed a given. His *BMJ* obituary stated that "Crichton-Browne established at Wakefield the first *neurological* research laboratory in the Kingdom, where Sir David Ferrier was enabled to carry out his experiments on cerebral localization".[103] Gordon Holmes's obituary notice for the Royal Society averred that, as pursued at WRA by Crichton-Browne, the "most promising line of study [of mental disease] was a *neurological* approach".[104]

The label of Crichton-Browne as neurologist may also be found in the secondary literature[105]: MacNalty described him as a "great pioneer in neurological research"[106] and was of the opinion that "The debt that modern neurology owed to this pioneer is immense"[107]; Neve and Turner categorised him as "alienist, neurologist and author"[108]; and Jellinek called him a "pioneer neurologist".[109]

Hence Crichton-Browne had a foot in both camps, migrating between psychiatry and neurology, by way of the greater scientific claims of the latter, in

---

[101] Oppenheim (1991:75), quoting from Crichton-Browne (1887–1888:105). Finn (2012:163) repeated this argument and citation.

[102] Crichton-Browne (1897:995). In retrospect, the absence of Ferrier's name from Crichton-Browne's listing here of "the genius and labours of a few great men" may be deemed surprising, and might perhaps speak to the concerns of Oppenheim (1991:74–75) and Finn (2012:163) regarding Crichton-Browne's departure from the Neurological Society of London.

[103] *BMJ* 1938;1:311 [my italics].

[104] Holmes (1939:519) [my italics].

[105] For example, Edwards (2014). Bone and Stone (2023) erroneously included him amongst the "glittering array of staff" at "Queens [*sic*] Square" along with Jackson, Ferrier, "Gower's [*sic*], and Brown Squared [*sic!*]".

[106] MacNalty (1957:912).

[107] MacNalty (1965:249). In MacNalty's account of "some pioneers of the past in neurology" both Hughlings Jackson and Ferrier also make the cut.

[108] Neve and Turner (1995:399).

[109] Jellinek (2005). I confess to being unable to grasp why Jellinek also characterised Crichton-Browne as a "scientific drop-out".

part established at WRA and in *WRLAMR* by Ferrier and Hughlings Jackson. Another possible driver may have related to the apparent view that for asylum doctors "prestige remained conspicuously low",[110] an accusation which could hardly be levelled at physicians as a professional group. Moreover, as a sociable man, the relative isolation of Wakefield and the West Riding may have palled in comparison to the lure of the metropolitan centre.

Clifford Allbutt

Clifford Allbutt's career moved between general medicine and psychiatry but he was essentially a physician (FRCP 1883; Honorary Member of the MPA 1896). His appointment as a Commissioner in Lunacy, perhaps engineered by Crichton-Browne, was something of a surprise and proved to be a relatively brief interlude (1889–1892) before he returned to medicine as the Regius Professor of Physic in Cambridge (1892–1925). Despite his many publications, including in *Brain* (Table 6.4), Allbutt did not contribute to the *Journal of Mental Science* (Table 6.5) although he was listed amongst the contributors to Hack Tuke's (1892) *Dictionary of psychological medicine* ("Insanity in children" I:202–205). One member of the WRA resident staff, Bevan-Lewis, later appeared in Allbutt's multi-volume *A System of Medicine* (1899). Almost 50 years after his death Allbutt was adjudged to have been amongst the "master mariners" of neurology in the century 1870–1970 along with Hughlings Jackson, Ferrier, William Gowers (1845–1915), Henry Head (1861–1940), Gordon Holmes, and Kinnier Wilson (1878–1937),[111] a judgment with which few would now concur, likewise perhaps his characterisation as a "neuropsychiatrist".[112]

David Ferrier

Aside from his attendance at the WRA pathological laboratory in Spring 1873 and the medical *conversazione* in November 1873, Ferrier had no other direct contact with the Asylum, or with asylum medicine, to my knowledge, but these contacts were highly significant (as discussed in Chap. 7). Ferrier was a physician and remained so throughout his long career (FRCP 1877, Honorary Member of the MPA 1895), playing a notable role in the inauguration of

---

[110] Scull (1979:176).
[111] Gibson (1971:290).
[112] Reynolds and Broussolle (2018).

Brain (Table 6.4) but never publishing in the *Journal of Mental Science* (Table 6.5).[113] He was an original member of the Neurological Society of London in 1886 and its President in 1894. He has on occasion been described as both neurologist and "psychologist".[114]

Charles Ballance described Ferrier as the "John Hunter of Neurology", no doubt as a recognition of his experimental orientation.[115] Rose perhaps summarised the general view of posterity that considers Ferrier as one of the "giants who established the unique superiority of British neurology".[116] However, Crichton-Browne's view, published shortly after his departure from WRA, was that "The great value of Ferriers' [*sic*] labours consists, I believe, in their having opened up for us a pathway to a concrete mental pathology, which will ultimately lead to a position where we shall be able to find the subjective equivalents of morbid appearances or, conversely, the anatomical substrata of subjective states",[117] an ambition which was ultimately to prove unfounded. In similar vein, the contribution of WRA to the development of Ferrier's discoveries was soon forgotten in some quarters: "King's College School and Hospital have had a long array of glorious names upon its staff. … Ferrier gained his laurels here".[118]

John Hughlings Jackson

Designated by the Critchleys as the "Father of English neurology",[119] one might accordingly imagine Hughlings Jackson's links to psychiatry to have

---

[113] Some comments made by Ferrier in August 1881 at the International Medical Congress, Section of Mental Diseases, following a lecture by Tamburini on "Cerebral Localization and Hallucinations", appeared in a subsequent report published in *J Ment Sci* 1881–1882;27(October 1881):464–465. He also appears in *J Ment Sci* 1907;53:606–607.

[114] Macmillan (2016:62). The Royal Society webpage for the Ferrier Medal and Lecture describes Ferrier as "neurologist and psychologist" (https://royalsociety.org/medals-and-prizes/ferrier-lecture/, accessed 30/03/2025).

[115] Ballance (1928).

[116] Rose (2010).

[117] Crichton-Browne (1878–1879:355).

[118] *BMJ* 1895;2:145 (20th July). In similar vein, "It was in 1873 that he [Ferrier] began at King's [College Hospital, London] his researches on the brain" (https://history.rcplondon.ac.uk/inspiring-physicians/sir-david-ferrier; accessed 05/12/2023).

[119] Critchley and Critchley (1998). Jackson was also called the "Father of Neurology" by Foster Kennedy (1935:480; cited by the Critchleys 1998:194) and the "father of modern English neurology" by Purves-Stewart (1939:41; I do not find this usage cited by the Critchleys). Macdonald Critchley designated Jackson as "the father of British neurology" (Critchley 1960:617). Wetherill (1961:266) noted that Jackson "has been called 'The Father of English Neurology'" but gave no reference. The earliest reference I have found dates to 1896 when the Neurological Society of London founded the Hughlings Jackson Lectureship, with Jackson appointed the first to give the named lecture: "It was believed that to succeed,

been slight. However, he was appointed to membership of the MPA in 1866, long before any of the other physicians involved with WRA (e.g. Ferrier, Allbutt), and before his election as FRCP in 1868. He attended at least one MPA meeting, at York in 1869,[120] and held the role of Auditor at the MPA (1869–1871). He did publish some papers in the *Journal of Mental Science* in the 1870s (Table 6.5) and his work was frequently referenced in its pages. Many years later, on 24th February 1888, he read a lecture to the MPA Quarterly meeting at Bethlem Hospital on the subject of post-epileptic states.[121]

Dewhurst later compiled a book entitled *Hughlings Jackson and Psychiatry*.[122] But any argument for Jackson as psychiatrist manqué must rest there. Hughlings Jackson himself stated that "*Not being an alienist physician*, I mostly see cases in which the mental symptoms after epileptic attacks are comparatively slight" (V:106–107) [my italics].[123] George Savage observed that Jackson tried to avoid seeing patients with mental health problems because he could not help them: "as for insanity, he disliked it, and, unlike the neurologist of to-day, he would have nothing to do with insane patients if he could help it.".[124] It is therefore not surprising that Jackson's contact with WRA *per se* was minimal, none of it direct in all likelihood (as argued in Chap. 7), albeit highly significant in terms of the contributions he made to *WRLAMR*.

Taylor & Marsh, in their report unveiling the true identity of the patient designated by Jackson as "Z" (their "Dr. Z"), stated of Jackson that:

Despite his avowed interest in the "organ of mind" his separation from the interests of the asylum doctors is total. Thus a case placed at the frontier (and at

---

as lecturer, the father of English neurology will be an incentive to all distinguished workers in this science, whether at home or abroad"; *BMJ* 1896;2:1463 (Hughlings Jackson Lectureship). For discussion, see Larner 2025u.

[120] This is known in part from a rare surviving example of Jackson's correspondence, a letter to his brother Tom in New Zealand, dated 18th June 1869, cited in Critchley and Critchley (1998:49): "In July I go to York to be present at a meeting of the Psychological Association which will be held there under Dr. Laycock's Presidency". See Chap. 7 for information about his presence at this meeting as reported in the medical press.

[121] *J Ment Sci* 1888–1889;34:145, which reported that amongst those in attendance were "H. Sutherland" and "H.R. Sankey". The subsequent paper (Jackson 1888–1889) was "an expansion" of the address, and is discussed by Greenblatt (2022:417–422).

[122] Dewhurst (1982), in which (105) he bemoaned the fact that Jackson had not been elected an Honorary member of the MPA, nor had an obituary published in the *Journal of Mental Science*, unlike Ferrier. For "Jackson as a psychiatrist", see also Riese and Gooddy (1955:233–234).

[123] The wording "Not being an alienist physician" also occurred in Jackson (1888–1889:490).

[124] Savage (1917:315–316).

the division) between neurology and psychiatry symbolises their subsequent parting to their mutual loss.[125]

Henry Sutherland

As the son (and grandson) of an asylum doctor, Henry Sutherland's career trajectory bore some relation to Crichton-Browne's but also manifested differences. He had the credentials of both a physician and an asylum doctor. The former included Membership of the Royal College of Physicians of London, achieved early in his career; appointments as "Physician to the St George's, Hanover Square, Dispensary"; and to a Lectureship at a London teaching hospital (Westminster). The latter included experience of asylum medicine from his time at WRA, proprietorship of private lunatic asylums, and his ongoing interests and publications in the field insanity, the latter extending for over almost 20 years from his time at WRA and including contribution to Hack Tuke's (1892) *Dictionary of psychological medicine*. Nevertheless, one cannot argue that he pursued any kind of dedicated research programme, founded any research school, or fostered younger clinicians to follow in his wake. He did become a member of the Neurological Society of London (1889),[126] but was not elected either FRCP or FRS.

Herbert Major

Major's training was in asylum medicine and exclusively at WRA. Nevertheless, his clinical work there brought him into contact with Allbutt and Milner Fothergill, and his research interests in the histology and pathology of the brain may have been known to neurologists, although it seems that his work was largely neglected in his own time (and by posterity).[127]

Crochley Clapham

Like Crichton-Browne and Sutherland, Crochley Clapham was essentially an asylum physician who also managed to plant a foot in the neurology camp.

---

[125] Taylor and Marsh (1980:758).

[126] *BMJ* 1901;2:1643. My preliminary researches into the history of the Neurological Society of London have not indicated that Sutherland made any presentations to this group, although the published details of the early meetings of the Society are limited.

[127] Larner and Triarhou (2024a, b).

He gained honorary appointments as a physician in Sheffield, many years after leaving WRA, the announcements of which credited him as "M.R.C.P.Ed." and "F.R.C.P.E." respectively, and he was denoted "F.R.C.P.Ed." in his obituary in the *Journal of Mental Science* in 1923.[128] He was described as "the British neurologist",[129] relating to a publication on the "noble forehead".

William Bevan-Lewis

The most robust claim for any of the WRA doctors to be a neurologist was made on behalf of Bevan-Lewis, notably by another asylum doctor, Joseph Shaw Bolton, who described him as "one of the greatest of neurologists" and, furthermore:

> He justly acquired a greater scientific reputation than that of any of his predecessors, and his position as a neurologist was never greater than it is at present [1928], when it is universally acknowledged that much of his best work waited a quarter of a century for confirmation and acceptance.[130]

This judgment most likely related to Bevan-Lewis's pathological work which had afforded many publications in *Brain* (Table 6.4). It might also refer to Bevan-Lewis's adherence to the ideas of cortical localisation promulgated by Ferrier, a subject on which he continued to publish (as did Bolton).[131] Bevan-Lewis was also an original member of the Neurological Society of London but he never presented material to the Society and indeed resigned from it sometime around October 1893.[132]

Professionally, therefore, Bevan-Lewis was never a neurologist but always an asylum doctor. He contributed to Hack Tuke's (1892) *Dictionary of psychological medicine*, and finished his career as President of the MPA in 1909. Many years later, he was adjudged amongst the "master mariners" of

---

[128] *Medical Press and Circular* 1891;52:696 (30th December; Appointments). *Medical Press and Circular* 1901;71:186 (13th February; Appointments). *J Ment Sci* 1923;69(October 1923):592–593 [at 592].

[129] See Harrington (1987:225n2), re Anon. (1881–1882).

[130] Bolton (1928:588 and 612). See also Larner and Triarhou (2023). Shorvon and Compston (2019:305) reported that "Neurology continued at the West Riding Lunatic Asylum ... especially under the direction of Joseph Shaw Bolton".

[131] Lewis (1877), Lewis and Clarke (1878), Bevan Lewis (1883) (which mentioned Hughlings Jackson, Herbert Spencer, and Ferrier). Bolton (1910).

[132] Neurological Society Council Minutes 1886–1898, Royal Society of Medicine (NS/A/1, p.70).

neuroanatomy in the century 1870–1970, along with A.W. Campbell, Grafton Elliott Smith and Horne Craigie.[133]

Journal

Publication of a dedicated journal may be construed as one measure of the emergence of a distinct clinical specialty, and indeed might be deemed a *sine qua non* for any aspiration to specialist clinical and scientific credibility. Although technically a house journal, *WRLAMR* clearly had aspirations to national and international dissemination, as evidenced by the multiple reviews which appeared in the medical literature (Table 6.2).

It may be argued as to whether or not *WRLAMR* was the first dedicated neurological journal, or merely a precursor for this development in the shape of *Brain*. Certainly, *WRLAMR* contained material which would be of interest to any physician pursuing neurological interests, be they merely a part or the sum total of his [*sic*] practice, but there was also much content that focussed on the interests of asylum doctors. Hence, in retrospect, it might be considered as a hybrid journal of psychiatry and neurology. At the time of its publication, the distinction between neurology and asylum medicine (or alienism, medical psychology, psychiatry) was still being negotiated, as made explicit in the "manifesto" for *Brain: a journal of neurology* published in *Mind*:

> The functions and diseases of the nervous system will be discussed both in their physiological and psychological aspects; but mental phenomena will be treated only in correlation with their anatomical substrata, and mental disease will be investigated as far as possible by the methods applicable to nervous diseases in general.[134]

This distinction was also being clarified elsewhere. For example, at the sixth annual meeting of the American Neurological Association held in New York in June 1880, at the evening meeting on the third day (18th June), it was resolved that "a distinction should no longer be made between the alienist and the neurologist … but that it should be recognized that the neurologist is one who is an expert in all diseases of the brain, the spinal cord, their membranes, and the peripheral nerves, whether those diseases eventuate in insanity or

---

[133] Gibson (1971:290). For Elliott Smith, see Triarhou (2020:2604–2606).

[134] *Mind* 1878;3:295. Also *Brain* 1878–1879;1:unpaginated (discussed in Chap. 6).

not".[135] Hence this may be an example of parallel or convergent evolution. In a later parlance it may also be characterised as a "turf war", one which was to determine the professional boundaries of neurology and psychiatry thereafter.[136]

The formulation of *WRLAMR* as a hybrid psychiatry/neurology journal, based on its contents, might also be applied to other "earliest" journals, such as the *Archiv für Psychiatrie und Nervenkrankheiten* established in Berlin by Griesinger in 1868 (it became *European Archives of Psychiatry and Clinical Neuroscience* in 1990) and the *Chicago Journal of Nervous and Mental Disease* which commenced publication in January 1874 (this was the forerunner of the *Journal of Nervous and Mental Disease*, dropping "Chicago" in 1876). Considering journals ostensibly devoted exclusively to neurology, the *Transactions of the American Neurological Association* was first published in 1875, the Association having been inaugurated at a meeting in December 1874. Charcot founded his first dedicated neurological journal, the *Archives de Neurologie*, in 1880. The *Neurologisches Centralblatt* first appeared in 1882; the *Deutsche Zeitschrift für Nervenheilkunde* first appeared in 1891 (later named renamed *Zeitschrift für Neurologie* in 1947, and the *Journal of Neurology* in 1971).

Contemporary judgments of *WRLAMR* included the view that it was the first of its kind (*British and Foreign Medico-Chirurgical Review* and the *Indian Medical Gazette*; see Chap. 6). Some retrospective judgments have also placed *WRLAMR* first, for example Easterbrook considered it to be "the first English journal of neurology and neuropathology",[137] and in similar vein Hurn noted that these "medical reports were far more neurologically oriented than the research output from asylums—indeed than the typical content of the <u>Journal of Mental Science</u>".[138] More commonly however, *Brain* has been adjudged to take the prize,[139] declaring itself unequivocally as "a journal of neurology", although this judgment of posterity was not the view of the inaugural editors who stated in Volume 1 that "On the Continent and in America there are many journals which treat specially of diseases of the Nervous System".[140] Of course, many papers on neurological subjects continued to appear in general

---

[135] *Trans Am Neurol Assoc* 1880;6:50

[136] This may require a qualifier, as "in the Anglophone world", since neuropsychiatry persisted in Germany.

[137] Easterbrook (1938:297).

[138] Hurn (1998:65) [underlining in original].

[139] For example, Jellinek (2005:429–430), Finn (2012:188), Casper (2014:12).

[140] *Brain* 1878–1879;1:unpaginated.

medical journals, and some neurologists did not publish in *Brain* (most notably William Gowers apparently boycotted the journal for many years[141]).

Meetings

Meetings at local, regional, national, and international level play an important role in the associational life of any profession, fulfilling both educational and social roles and perhaps bringing a sense of integration to practitioners otherwise geographically distant. Certainly, the medical *conversazione* at WRA were heralded by Crichton-Browne "as a means of bringing together the representatives of every branch of the profession in Yorkshire with a view to promote the interchange of experience and ideas on the scientific aspects of medicine".[142] The "scientific aspects" were provided by means of the lectures and demonstrations by renowned professional leaders external to the Asylum, as well as by display of materials generated within the Asylum itself. However, beyond the appeal to local practitioners and the articles written in the local popular press, the meetings were little noticed in the national medical journals of note (Table 8.1). They may have done a little to raise the profile of WRA, but as for providing any impetus to the origin of neurology as a distinct discipline their effect was probably nugatory.

Meetings specifically dedicated to the subject of neurology as a discipline in the United Kingdom date from the decade following the WRA *conversazione*, specifically those of the Neurological Society of London (NSL) whose first formal meeting was convened in January 1886. Both continuities and discontinuities between the format of NSL meetings and WRA *conversazione* have been noted (see Chap. 8), but as regards professional development it is of note that NSL meetings featured the participation not only of neurologists (or physicians with a major interest in, and a practice comprising patients with, diseases of the nervous system), as would be expected, but also of asylum doctors. In the NSL membership list (N = 132) published as an addendum to *Brain* in 1891,[143] four members had been or were resident WRA staff: Crichton-Browne and Bevan-Lewis were original members, Crochley Clapham (1887) and Sutherland (1889) were elected later. Another six NSL

---

[141] This was thought to be due to a falling out with the editor of *Brain*, Armand de Watteville (1846–1925). See Scott et al. (2012:169–170), Shorvon and Compston (2019:115 and n31), Larner and Triarhou (2025b).

[142] *Wakefield Journal and Examiner* 20th October 1871, p.2, col.7 (Medical Conversazione at the West Riding Asylum).

[143] *Brain* 1891;14(1):A8–A12 (A = addendum, after p.144).

members had links to WRA: Allbutt, Broadbent, Lauder Brunton, Ferrier and Hughlings Jackson (all original members), and Brudenell Carter (elected 1889).[144] During the 21-year existence of the Neurological Society, before its absorption into the Royal Society of Medicine as its Section of Neurology in 1907, at least four of its Presidents were or had been asylum-based: Crichton-Browne (1888), George Savage (1897), William Julius Mickle (1901), and John Batty Tuke (1905). This supports the argument that neurologists at this time were not seeking or promoting secession from general medicine.[145]

The Origins of British Neurology: Psychiatry and Neurology

With the sole exception of the West Riding, *no addition to our knowledge of insanity has been made in the memory of any man now living by the superintendent of any public asylum in this country.*[146]

This anonymous judgment, published in 1918, over 40 years after Crichton-Browne departed WRA and the cessation of *WRLAMR* and the medical *conversazione*, might be deemed overly harsh. Granted, the same author(s) did note the work of David Orr and Richard Rows in the first two decades of the twentieth century,[147] although opining that their work was "solely microscopical, and the experience of the last fifty years has shown plainly enough that the microscope is not the instrument by which a knowledge of insanity is to be attained".[148] The omission from this account of Alfred Walter Campbell (1868–1937), who worked at Rainhill Asylum in Lancashire between 1892 and 1905, is a notable oversight.[149] Campbell (elected MPA 1894) contributed to the understanding of cortical cytoarchitectonics, published papers in *Brain*, and collaborated with the distinguished neurologist Henry Head (1861–1940).[150] However, these exceptions aside, no other asylum-based research in basic neuroscience performed in the United Kingdom, similar to

---

[144] By 1897, Allbutt, Crichton-Browne, Clapham, and Bevan-Lewis no longer featured on the NSL membership list. *Brain* 1897;20(4):A13–A18 (A = addendum, after p.549).

[145] Casper (2014:37) (cf. Ophthalmology)

[146] Anon. (1918:386) [italics in original].

[147] For Orr and Rows, see Shephard (1996), Larner (2024a, 2025v).

[148] Anon. (1918:385–386).

[149] For Campbell, see Macmillan (2011–2012, 2016), Triarhou (2020:2598–2604). Bevan-Lewis was admired by Campbell according to Macmillan, 2011–2012:38 and 2016:92.

[150] Respectively, Campbell (1905a), Campbell, (1905b), and Head and Campbell (1900).

that occurring at WRA, springs to mind.[151] Hence, it may be inferred that WRA was unique in the period 1866 to 1876 which permitted it to "gain its later reputation as a birth-place for neurology rather than as a stimulant for psychiatry".[152]

Considered as a liminal period for neurology as a discipline, this was an era when professional boundaries were evolving, not yet fully established, and hence porous (as illustrated by some of the individual case studies of career trajectory discussed in the Faculty section, *vide supra*). Diseases of the brain which are now deemed "neurological" would inevitably have been dealt with by asylum doctors at this time, for example epilepsy (which may even have merited a dedicated ward at WRA for refractory cases), as well as by those like Hughlings Jackson forging a career in neurology.[153]

The factors underpinning clinical specialisation in the nineteenth century have been discussed by Weisz, some of which have been touched upon here (see Chap. 1: Introduction: Professionalisation and specialisation), such as a large and integrated community of doctors and the advancement of medical knowledge through rigorous empirical clinical research. In addition, this critical mass of individuals "made it possible to produce clinical knowledge based on large numbers of clinical cases, analysed quantitatively as well as qualitatively, and frequently complemented by data from postmortem dissections.".[154] Clearly all these factors were in place at WRA. Moreover, it was "the influence of localist organic thinking, based on pathological anatomy and subsequently on new technologies such as the ophthalmoscope and the laryngoscope, that created 'foci of interest' in organ systems around which specialties could develop.".[155] Contrary to the "localist organic" basis of neurology, however, "the original basis of psychiatry was the need to isolate and manage a uniquely troublesome class of patients"[156] based on their behaviour rather than their brain pathology.

---

[151] Walk (1976; 1990:27) suggested that "Hubert Bond was able … to attract to his hospital, Long Grove, a brilliant team, including Bernard Hart, Henry Devine, Ernest Jones, and the most junior, Edward Mapother" but I think these names will be unfamiliar or unknown to most neurologists.

[152] Hurn (1998:66). In this context, a later characterisation (by "GW" 1987) of Stanley Royd Hospital, as WRA was later renamed, as "the erstwhile 'Maudsley of the North'" seems entirely inapposite.

[153] This porosity of professional boundaries persisted into the early twentieth century, for example see the case of the asylum doctor Richard Rows (1866–1925) who presented at neurological meetings and published in neurological journals (Larner 2024a). Early in his medical career Rows was house physician to Henry Charlton Bastian at University College Hospital; Bastian, one of the earliest physicians at Queen Square, had himself served as an assistant medical officer at Broadmoor Hospital in the mid-1860s.

[154] Weisz (2006:18).

[155] Weisz (2006:10), explaining George Rosen's analysis of the development of specialisation.

[156] Idem.

In the context of specialisation, the interest of Allbutt, Aldridge, and particularly Hughlings Jackson in ophthalmoscopy may be of note. This instrument was at least in part responsible for the emergence of ophthalmology as a specialty, one with which Jackson was closely associated. Its own specialist forum, the Ophthalmological Society of the United Kingdom, was founded in 1880.[157] Jackson's Bowman Lecture to the Ophthalmological Society in November 1885 has been referred to as "a spirited defence of medical specialisation".[158] However, predating this by some years, Jackson's Oration delivered before the Medical Society of London in May 1877 "had first offered a spirited defense"[159] of specialisation. Therein Jackson noted that:

> There is no harm in studying a special subject; the harm is in doing any kind of work with a narrow aim and with a narrow mind. Differentiation of medical investigation has led to results of inestimable value. If, in the smallest degree, I succeed in furthering the integration which should quickly follow this necessary differentiation, I shall feel that my address will be of some little value.[160]

Moreover, "for the sake of scientific discipline, a study of ophthalmology is most important". Allbutt's work[161] was cited as having "done more than any other work towards what I would call the integration of ophthalmology with general medicine".[162]

However, it was not until 1886 that a similar society was founded for neurology, the Neurological Society of London, with Hughlings Jackson as its first President. Presumably, the desired integration following on from the necessary differentiation had retarded any earlier move to the specialisation of neurology. Even then, this organisation, which became the Neurological Society of the United Kingdom in 1903, did not aspire to specialist status, although it did "acquire" *Brain* in 1888. It was assimilated easily into the Royal Society of Medicine (RSM) when the latter was founded in 1907.[163] Not until 1932 was an organisation "limited to those actively engaged in any

---

[157] Casper (2014:31–37). Jackson was subsequently President of the Ophthalmological Society, in 1888–1889.

[158] Casper (2014:33). On Jackson's Bowman Lecture, see also Greenblatt (2022:377–378).

[159] Greenblatt (2022:377).

[160] Jackson (1877:575). The language of differentiation and integration as complementary puts one in mind of the fundamental theorem of calculus.

[161] Specifically, Allbutt (1871a).

[162] Jackson (1877:575).

[163] A dedicated Section of Psychiatry at the RSM was not initiated until 1912.

branch of neurology", the Association of British Neurologists (ABN), founded.[164]

If we accept Andrew Scull's view to the effect that:

"Psychiatry" did not emerge on the historical stage fully formed … It was, on the contrary, the product of a long and complex series of changes[165]

then it follows logically, by simple syllogism, that "Neurology" too (as per Stephen Casper's quote which forms the epigraph of this chapter) emerged as a "long and complex series of changes". But as with any biography, personal or institutional, periods of rapid development and change may be discerned. These may perhaps be understood by recourse to a symbiotic model.

A Symbiotic Approach

The philosopher Graham Harman adopted the biological model of Serial Endosymbiosis Theory (SET), initially developed by Lynn Sagan (later Lynn Margulis; 1938–2011), to support his object-oriented ontology. Sagan had proposed in 1967 that the organelles of eukaryotic cells originated as independent creatures which then became subordinate components of the cell, an idea which is now largely accepted in biology.[166] Harman envisaged symbiosis as a special type of relation that changed the reality of one of its relata, change leading to an object/subject different in kind from what had gone before. He suggested that perhaps two symbioses should be sought amongst each of the categories of persons, places, and things to explain processes of change.[167]

Places

Considering the origins of British neurology, I would suggest that two symbioses in the "places" category are obvious: the National Hospital for the Paralysed and Epileptic in Queen Square, London; and WRA.

---

[164] For the history of the ABN, see Casper (2007, 2011 and 2014:118–121, 125–131). The use of the word "limited" is of note.

[165] Scull (2006:87).

[166] Harman (2016:45–46). Sagan (1967). I am grateful to Thomas Larner for introducing me to the work of Graham Harman.

[167] For an attempt to apply these ideas to medical biography, see Larner (2023e). Incidentally, for a possible inadvertent precedent, in his history of Wakefield, J.W. Walker (1934, 1939) divided his indexing into Persons, Places, and Subjects.

The standard claim of "Queen Square" as the birthplace of British neurology rests on the date of its foundation, 1860, thus predating any similar institution, and the undeniable quality of its distinguished faculty in its early years, including Brown-Séquard (appointed 1860), Hughlings Jackson (1862), and William Gowers (medical registrar from 1870, physician 1872).[168] In many ways, Hughlings Jackson and Gowers defined the idiom of neurology as a clinical discipline. But any exclusive claim for Queen Square as the origin of British neurology is simply not sufficient.

Even though some Queen Square clinicians were elected as Fellows of the Royal Society in the nineteenth century (e.g. Hughlings Jackson, Bastian, Gowers, Horsley[169]), no experimental animal work of any note was performed at or emerged from the institution during its early years, up to and including the period encompassed by the present study. To be sure, Charles Brown-Séquard (1817–1894), an "advocate of experimental physiology as a means of providing a rational basis for medical care", was on the staff between 1860 and 1863, but the impression gained from his biography is that he was overwhelmed with clinical work and indeed left following the realisation "that he was wasting his time in medical practice rather than pursuing scientific studies".[170] Moreover, Charles Bland Radcliffe, chosen as Brown-Séquard's replacement as physician at Queen Square,[171] in preference to Jackson, had published "research" which was committed to the idea that the active phase of muscle action was relaxation, based on the apparent similarities of rigor mortis and muscle contraction, a proposal which Radcliffe held to but which went nowhere over the next 20 years.[172] Neither Hughlings Jackson nor Gowers were experimentalists in the manner pursued by Ferrier.[173]

---

[168] For biographical material on Gowers, see Scott et al. (2012). Ferrier is not included in this list since he was not appointed to the staff at Queen Square until 1880.

[169] Ferrier is not included in this list since he was not appointed at Queen Square when elected FRS in 1876, that distinction only came in 1880.

[170] Aminoff (1993:2, 49). See also Shorvon and Compston (2019:105).

[171] Lyons (1966:41–42).

[172] Eadie (2007), Larner and Triarhou (2024c). I presume he is the "Dr. Radcliffe" referred to by Mitchell (II:86, 95). A similar proposal to Radcliffe's, to the effect that muscular contraction and rigor mortis were essentially one and the same, seems to have been developed independently by Ludimar Hermann (1838–1914) in the 1860s whilst he was working in du Bois-Reymond's laboratory in Berlin, an idea dismissed by du Bois-Reymond (Finkelstein 2013:182–185). Hermann was later Professor of Physiology in Zürich.

[173] To qualify this remark: it was certainly the case Gowers undertook clinico-pathological work, for example describing what later became known as Gowers tract in the spinal cord (ventral spinocerebellar tract). He also performed some clinical experiments, for example related to the innervation of the anal sphincter, communicated to the Royal Society by Burdon Sanderson in 1877 (Gowers 1877), and the knee jerk in 1879 (described in Lazar 2022). However, if Gowers did any animal experimental work it was collaborative (e.g. Gowers and Sankey 1877).

Victor Horsley (1857–1916) was the Queen Square clinician, other than Ferrier, most inclined to pursue animal experimentation in the later nineteenth century, although not appointed to the hospital until 1886. He "set aside Thursday afternoons and Saturday mornings for experimental work",[174] and was a "brilliant and original experimenter and physiologist".[175] His research work may have occurred at the Brown Animal Sanatory Institution in South London where he was Superintendent from 1884–1890,[176] or later in a sky-lighted workshop at his house. Much of his work was devoted to mapping of the cerebral cortex, hence extending the work of Ferrier. Moreover, he collaborated with other Queen Square colleagues, such as Felix Semon and Charles Beevor,[177] although neither of them set up independent research programmes.[178]

Queen Square had neither laboratory nor animal facilities in the nineteenth century,[179] and those clinicians who did undertake experimental work, such as Ferrier, did so elsewhere and in their own time. As Shorvon and Compston have shown. "Until the first decade of the twentieth century, there had been no question of the National Hospital financing research". Not until 1903 were the first steps taken in the research funding history of the National Hospital with the establishment of the Nervous Diseases Research Fund (NDRF); appointment of a whole-time director of the NDRF was approved in 1904. Gordon Holmes resigned as resident medical officer in 1905 to occupy this post, holding it until 1909.[180] Hence this appears to have been a relatively junior post, as this appointment occurred before Holmes gained the MRCP (1908) and was appointed as physician (1909). Indeed, it was not until the 1930s that, courtesy of funding from the Rockefeller Foundation, a dedicated research programme was inaugurated at Queen Square, led by Arnold Carmichael (1896–1978). Even the proposal for this research institute has been characterised as "genuinely remarkable" and "unprecedented in Britain".[181]

---

[174] MacNalty (1957:913).

[175] Purves Stewart (1939:45).

[176] Ferrier may have worked at the Brown Institution in the 1870s with John Burdon Sanderson (Romano 2002:182).

[177] Shorvon and Compston (2019:156–157), Aminoff (2022:42–46).

[178] Charles Scott Sherrington (1857–1952) also later undertook cortical mapping studies, following Ferrier and Horsley.

[179] Shorvon and Compston (2019:105–106).

[180] Ibid., 2019: 176, 178–179. Elsewhere (2019:217–218) they stated that Holmes was "director of research" from 1906.

[181] Casper (2014:113). See also Shorvon and Compston (2019:190–193).

Furthermore, in addition to these institutional defects, neither a dedicated journal akin to *WRLAMR* nor meetings akin to the WRA *conversazione* were associated with Queen Square during its early years. To my knowledge, the only Queen Square physician to publish in *WRLAMR* was Hughlings Jackson, whose affiliation was given as "Physician to the London Hospital and to the Hospital for the Epileptic and Paralysed" (with the exception of VI:266–309, in which no affiliation was noted), whereas many WRA personnel appeared in the early volumes of *Brain* (Table 6.4). Unlike *WRLAMR*, *Brain* was not under the aegis of any institution or organisation when first published.

Whilst Queen Square may have hosted internal meetings to consider clinical cases, for example for the benefit of medical students from University College London, I am not aware that any public meetings similar to those at WRA, inviting external local practitioners, were sponsored by Queen Square in its early years. No Queen Square physician had attended the WRA medical *conversazione*. The constituency of the subsequently founded Neurological Society of London included both physicians and psychiatrists, but not other, general medical, practitioners.

Evidently then, the experimental research ethos established at WRA predated that at Queen Square by several decades. Hence, the symbiosis of clinical and experimental approaches to neurology, forged respectively at Queen Square and WRA, may be held to account for the bipartite nature of the discipline handed on to future generations of neurologists.

Persons

Proceeding to the "persons" category, I would suggest that once again two symbioses are obvious: John Hughlings Jackson and David Ferrier.

They were, by Ferrier's later account,[182] acquainted from an early stage of Ferrier's career in London, hence from about 1870–1871. Their collaboration appears to have been informal, in that they never published a substantive paper together[183] but may well have shared ideas and information. Ferrier had undertaken his experiments at WRA at least in part to test the views of Jackson on the pathology of epilepsy as a discharging lesion, and the evidence indicates that Jackson was aware of Ferrier's experimental findings at an early

---

[182] Ferrier (1892:884).

[183] They did both appear amongst the authors of letters to the medical press in August 1900 during the dispute between medical staff and the management at the National Hospital: *BMJ* 1900;2:333 and 392; *Lancet* 1900;2:351–352 and 463.

stage, and hence able to comment upon them.[184] Hence Jackson brought the clinical skills and philosophical inferences (the "Socrates of neurology"[185]), Ferrier the experimental techniques of the physiological laboratory, to the understanding of neurological questions, with fruitful results, establishing empirically the concept of cortical localisation.

A case might also be made, of course, for William Gowers. Certainly, his writings, in particular his *Manual of diseases of the nervous system* dating from the 1880s, "the Bible of neurology",[186] were more accessible than Jackson's and influenced generations of trainees in the field. But even Gowers, Jackson's only rival in terms of clinical acumen, when speaking at the unveiling of the bust of Jackson when he retired from the staff at Queen Square in 1906 stated "Let us look upon this bust and then turn to the living counterpart—our master!".[187] Furthermore, as Gowers was not an experimentalist he could not bring the methods of laboratory science to the study of neurological questions.

Things

Defining symbioses in the category of "things" pertinent to the origins of British neurology is perhaps more difficult. Odious though it may be to characterise patients as "things", their diseased nervous systems were the raw material upon which observation at the clinical and pathological level was based.[188] It might be argued that the case books and postmortem books at WRA and the medical records at Queen Square constitute symbiotic "things" but this is surely the same argument at one remove, as is their replacement by the papers based on such material which were published in *WRLAMR* and later in *Brain*. Likewise for experimental animals, the subjects of Ferrier's vivisections, which garnered not only physiological knowledge but the opprobrium of the antivivisection movement and galvanised the processes which led to the passage of the Cruelty to Animals Act of 1876.

In his account of symbioses, Harman did not specify whether "things" should be either concrete or abstract. Accordingly, it might be suggested that

---

[184] Greenblatt (2022:166–168).

[185] Ballance (1928).

[186] Eadie et al. (2012).

[187] Critchley (1949:91), Scott et al. (2012:236–237).

[188] In a different context, specifically the career of Matthew Baillie (1761–1823), the pathological anatomist and physician (Muqit and Larner 2022), cadavers have been suggested in the category of symbiotic things (Larner 2023e). Finn (2012:19) argued "that patients were a fundamental element in the [Wakefield] asylum's programme of research" and considered "The Patient as Material" (2012:89).

the conceptualisation of science engendered by these clinical and experimental researches themselves constituted a symbiosis:

> Every science begins by accumulating observations, and presently generalises these empirically; but only when it reaches the stage at which its empirical generalisations are included in a rational generalisation, *does it become a developed science.*[189]

For neurology, the rational generalisation which emerged was cortical localisation and the validity of the clinico-anatomical method. Unlike phrenology, this was based on an accumulation of observations, clinical and experimental, which were empirically generalised. Finn argued that WRA imported and institutionalised the idea of cerebral localisation[190] and Star repeatedly characterised *Brain* as a "localizationalist journal".[191] That both clinical and experimental approaches, exemplified respectively by the work of Hughlings Jackson and Ferrier, should converge was both remarkable and empowering. The adoption of this methodology into clinical practice was prompt and facilitated the emergence not only of neurology as a discipline but also, eventually, of neurosurgery and neuropsychology. In the case of the former, the most powerful attribute of a scientific model, that of accurate prediction, was most clearly manifest, in that the modelling of neurological processes by cortical localisation permitted accurate prediction of lesion site for the purposes of operative intervention.[192]

Lesion localisation remains a canonical idea, integral to the practice of clinical neurology today. There are anomalies, such as "false-localising signs", but these are rarely encountered in clinical practice and can be accommodated mechanistically.[193] It is therefore something of a surprise that one of the key didactic texts devoted to localisation in clinical neurology published in the past 30 years, that by Brazis, Masdeu and Biller, makes no mention of Ferrier, neither in the editions used during my training,[194] nor in more recent

---

[189] Jackson (1881:329) [italics in original], quoting "'Data of Ethics,' p.61, Herbert Spencer".

[190] Finn (2012:151, 155).

[191] Star (1989:32, 49, 102, 167).

[192] Hughes Bennett and Godlee (1884). Ferrier was present at this landmark operation, but not Hughlings Jackson (Greenblatt 2022:366–369), although others have claimed he was present (e.g. MacNalty 1957:914; Spillane 1974a:705 and 1981:398; Star 1989:59). Spillane (1981:397) was of the opinion that this operation "marked the highlight of Ferrier's career". Star (1989) argued that attempts at clinical localisation often failed, necessitating various strategies to accommodate or paper over these anomalies.

[193] Larner 2003b, 2025w

[194] Larner (2002).

editions, although "A brief history of localization: aphasia as an example" appeared in the fifth edition.[195]

Summary

Hence, this symbiotic explication of the origins of British neurology engenders not an either/or formulation, either general medicine or psychiatry, but rather a both/and conjunction or reconciliation.[196] The interaction of the clinical expertise developed at Queen Square, through the concentration of many patients in one site and the expertise developed by the clinicians working there, particularly by Jackson, and the experimental approaches to brain physiology developed at WRA, particularly by Ferrier, are the ultimate antecedents which have resulted in the bipartite, two-fold nature of the profession of neurology in Great Britain.

The criteria relating to the characterisation of professions, based on a reading of Flexner, and to the development of specialisation, based on a reading of Weisz (both discussed in Chap. 1),[197] were all fulfilled at WRA during the period 1866–1876. In contrast, at this time at Queen Square, whilst some of the institutional and faculty requirements may have been in place, there was neither laboratory, nor in house journal, nor public meetings for the purposes of acquiring and disseminating specialised knowledge, unlike the situation at WRA. All the necessary elements for a nascent profession of neurology as a clinical and research discipline were in place at WRA in the early 1870s.

Wakefield is not a location immediately associated with medical innovation unlike, say, the "golden triangle" of Cambridge, Oxford, or London.[198] Nevertheless, as has been shown, for a brief period in its history WRA was at the forefront of developments in neuroscience. Thus, I would argue that it is

---

[195] Brazis et al. (2007:1–3). I thank Dr. Lauren Fratalia for bringing this edition to my attention.

[196] Experimentalists might prefer to characterize these conditions in terms of necessity and sufficiency, or loss of function and gain of function, respectively: necessity/loss prevents a particular event or development from occurring, whereas sufficiency/gain permits it.

[197] Weisz (2006:11, 15).

[198] Some authors have written of the "Wakefield triangle" (Bewley 2008:35) or the "golden triad" (Rollin and Reynolds 2018) referring to York, Wakefield, and Leeds as centres of psychiatric research in the latter half of the nineteenth century. (Wakefield is, of course, part of the "Rhubarb triangle", that area of West Yorkshire famous for producing forced rhubarb, a form of agriculture dating from the late nineteenth century.) Oxonians might be aware that John Radcliffe (1652–1714), the benefactor commemorated in the former Radcliffe Infirmary, the Radcliffe Lunatic Asylum (later the Warneford Hospital), the John Radcliffe Hospital, the Radcliffe Science Library, and the Radcliffe Observatory, was born in Wakefield and had his early education there before moving to University College, Oxford, in 1666 at the age of 13 (Fitzherbert Jones 2014:28). His memorial in the University Church of St Mary does not mention his Wakefield origin.

indeed the case that, as E.D. Adrian stated in 1939, this was "a classical period in the history of medicine, the period when neurology became a science".[199]

Conclusion/Epilogue: Endings

Only seldom are peripheral locations examined as zones of the production and shaping of knowledge.[200]

The beginnings initiated by James Crichton-Browne at WRA proved fragile, partially disintegrating almost as soon as he had departed from Wakefield: no more *conversazione*; only one further issue of *WRLAMR*; no further visiting staff availing themselves of the clinical or research opportunities of the Asylum. To be sure, some further research publications emerged under the auspices of his successors as superintendent, Herbert Major and William Bevan-Lewis, mostly microscopical studies, and oriented towards the priorities of asylum medicine rather than neurology.[201] Some patients admitted during the Crichton-Browne decade eventually found their way into the medical literature.[202]

During Bevan-Lewis's long superintendency (1884–1910), the infrastructure of WRA underwent further significant changes: an outpatient department was opened (1889) and the pathology department was reconstructed to include a complete outfit of laboratories (1895), as well as the planning and building of a new acute hospital on the site (opened in 1900). During these years, the founding of further branches of the West Riding Asylum occurred, at Menston (1888) and Storthes Hall, Huddersfield (1904).

Bevan-Lewis's successor, Joseph Shaw Bolton (1867–1946), continued to pursue research, and was able to straddle the psychiatrist/physician divide: he was FRCP (1909) and Gulstonian Lecturer at the RCP in 1910, speaking on cerebral localisation,[203] and eventually became MPA President (1928), his Presidential lecture devoted to an historical account of WRA.[204] With Bolton's retirement in 1933, somewhat under the shadow of an embezzlement scandal perpetrated by two Asylum employees, the power of the superintendent was

---

[199] Adrian (1939:433).

[200] Borch (2018:120).

[201] Wallis (2017a), documented some of the research developments at WRA in the period after Crichton-Browne. Also Larner (2026d).

[202] For example, "George W-, admitted Jan. 16th, 1875", by Reynolds (1886–1887).

[203] Bolton (1910).

[204] Bolton (1928).

severely curtailed.[205] With the advent of the National Health Service in 1948, WRA was renamed Stanley Royd Hospital. In August 1984, an outbreak of salmonella food poisoning at the hospital made the national news headlines, as the infection affected many patients and staff and caused the deaths of 19 patients.[206] With the implementation of the Care in the Community policy for patients with mental health problems, Stanley Royd Hospital finally closed in 1995.

A museum had been opened at the hospital in 1975, named the Stephen G. Beaumont Museum after the Chairman of the committee who funded the project, but the principal mover was the former hospital secretary (1961–1973) and Asylum historian A.L. (Lawrence) Ashworth (ca. 1913–2001)[207] who had "prevented the 'destruction' of some of the older records, including those that dated back to the hospital's early years when it opened as the West Riding Pauper Lunatic Asylum in 1818".[208] When Stanley Royd Hospital closed, the museum transferred to the Fieldhead Hospital site.[209] The records of the Asylum were thankfully saved, and now constitute an unparalleled resource for the study of WRA. They are held by the West Yorkshire Archive Service and are inscribed on the UNESCO memory of the world register. Using these records, various historical works relating to WRA have been written.[210]

WRA was originally located at "some distance from the nearest habitation",[211] but the city of Wakefield, as it became in 1888, eventually encroached on its environs. The surviving physical remains of the Asylum may be reached on foot, a somewhat uphill walk from the centre of town which demonstrates to the twenty-first century traveller that ease of access to WRA cannot have been straightforward in an age when transportation was by foot, horse, and railway. The walk serves to make manifest the importance of the postal service and the railways as key vectors of the nineteenth century system for the communication of scientific research.

---

[205] Ashworth (1975:75).

[206] Anon. (1986b), Department of Health and Social Security (1986). Difficulties in tracing the source recall the investigations of the cholera outbreak in 1849 (Wright 1850). I first heard of the Stanley Royd Hospital at the time of the salmonella outbreak, an event which coincided with my time as a clinical medical student.

[207] According to material at www.wakefieldasylum.co.uk (accessed 05/02/2025), Ashworth was first employed at WRA in 1929 when aged 16 and gave 72 years of service, hence these approximate dates of birth and death. I have not found an obituary.

[208] Ellis (2015:335). Ashworth's (1975) book was published to coincide with the opening of the museum.

[209] Fieldhead Hospital, opened 1972, now houses the Mental Health Museum containing artefacts from WRA (Ellis 2015).

[210] For example, Bolton (1928), Ashworth (1975), Todd and Ashworth (1991, n.d.), Finn (2012), Scrimgeour (2015), Wallis (2017a).

[211] Todd and Ashworth (1991:389).

The original 1818 block still stands and has been converted into flats, and the recreation hall currently serves as a church. Now, instead of walls to keep patients in, there are fences to keep non-residents out, and numbered wards have given way to numbered parking spots. The local street names commemorate Tuke, who had no connection with the Asylum other than design suggestions, and Ashworth, a long-time administrator, but there is no memorial to the pioneers of the 1860s and 1870s, James Crichton-Browne, David Ferrier, or John Hughlings Jackson, individuals with whom this place is indelibly linked in intellectual history. A stanza in the poem "1818–1996" written by Ronald Ayres recalls some of them:

Tuke, Ellis and Corsellis,

Ferrier, Crichton-Brown [*sic*] and Bevan-Lewis,

Bolton and their fellows,

Brought wisdom, energy enlightenment.[212]

The purpose of the current work has in part been to redress this imbalance.

> To Wakefield people, the words "Stanley Royd" have that dark resonance that always used to come with a passing reference to the local mental asylum. Possibly anyone from anywhere could name a similar place and recall, in the old unreformed days when spades were called spades, an equivalent mental institution.[213]

Whilst this may be true for "Stanley Royd", at least to the older generation, "West Riding Pauper Lunatic Asylum" seems to have impinged little, if at all, on the collective memory of Wakefield. The current doyen of popular local history books, Paul Dawson, has little to say on the subject.[214] In his *A-Z of*

---

[212] The poem appeared in Grainger (1996:94–98, quoted stanza at 94). It was written "for the Thanksgiving Service at St. Faiths [*sic*] Church, Stanley Royd Hospital. Sunday April 21st 1996".

[213] Wade (2016:125), where the actual wording is "and equivalent mental institutions" which I presume to be incorrect, hence the substitution of my reading in this quotation. Growing up in Cirencester, Gloucestershire, in the 1960s and 1970s, my "equivalent mental institution" was Coney Hill Hospital, outside Gloucester, some 15 miles away. My paternal grandfather, Herbert Edward Larner (born 1895), died there in 1968. A common taunt for any oddity of behaviour manifested by one's contemporaries in my childhood was "you're going to (end up in) Coney Hill" or "they're going to come and take you to Coney Hill". Professor Andrew Lees (personal communication, 21/10/2024) has informed me that when he lived in Leeds "naughty small children were threatened with admission to Menston". Susan Fogarty (personal communication, 04/11/2024) grew up in St Helens and gave me a similar account regarding Rainhill Asylum. I suspect that many people of a certain age have similar recollections.

[214] I find no mention in Dawson (2003, 2005, 2015a, 2015b, 2020).

Wakefield, he stated that "By the mid-twentieth century the city could boast five hospitals as well as the West Riding Lunatic Asylum, which was established in the first half of the nineteenth century – possibly earlier."[215] This overt uncertainty about the foundation date of the institution is also evident in a subsequent comment:

> Pinderfields General Hospital originated as part of the West Riding Pauper Lunatic Asylum (established 1818) through the efforts of Dr William Bevan Lewis in 1867 [*sic*] to provide separate accommodation for the recently diagnosed mentally ill. The hospital was expanded in 1899, with the new buildings being opened on 8 March 1900 at a total cost of £69,000."[216]

Dawson is not alone: other local historians have also erred in their comments, however brief, on the Asylum and its personnel. Even Mark Davis, specifically looking at WRA, characterised Crichton-Browne as "a gifted and enthusiastic Director, gathering in an eminent team of neuropsychiatrists including Hughling [*sic*] Jackson and David Ferrier".[217] Neither Wakefield Historical Publications nor its *Wakefield Historical Journal* (16 volumes published between 1974–2012) contain any material devoted to the Asylum, as far as I can ascertain.[218]

WRA was thus a place apart, marginal, peripheral, decentred, isolated,[219] with respect not only to the country but also to the town, and not only geographically but also culturally and historically, hence not only figuratively but also metaphorically. Yet this marginality may have been one of the keys to its success, however transient, in that it permitted innovations and developments in the short-term, at the price of allowing their origins to be forgotten or ignored in the long-term. Scientific knowledge was not created solely in centres of power and then appropriated and reworked in the periphery[220]—the intellectual traffic could move in the opposite direction. Speaking of the

---

[215] Dawson (2019:9).

[216] Idem. Repeated verbatim in Dawson (2022:75). As shown in Chap. 5, Bevan-Lewis did not arrive at WRA until 1875, and then in a very junior capacity, and he did not become superintendent until 1884 in which role he oversaw the developments mentioned by Dawson.

[217] Davis (2013a:25).

[218] Based on material accessed in https://www.wakefieldhistoricalsociety.org.uk

[219] The title of Bannister's (2005) history of Menston Asylum/High Royds Hospital, "*In splendid isolation*", might also be applicable to WRA during the period 1866–1876.

[220] Gavroglu et al. (2008).

German-language universities of the nineteenth century, Otis noted that "One important consequence of … [their] decentralization was the creation of new scientific fields",[221] a comment which I suggest is equally applicable to WRA in the period 1866–1876 and hence to the origins of the experimental scientific strand within the tradition of British neurology. To paraphrase E.D. Adrian, it was the locus where neurology became a science.

FINIS.

---

[221] Otis (2007a:12).

Appendix

Possible Funding Sources for *WRLAMR*

In Chap. 6, in the section on Funding, I suggested that money to fund the publication of *WRLAMR* might come from three possible sources documented in each Annual Asylum *Report*, viz. "Stationery, Printing, and Advertising"; "Books, Periodicals, and Music"; and "Incidentals". The available figures for the full years of Crichton-Browne, superintendency, 1867–1875, are tabulated in Table A1.

Just eyeballing these figures, it is evident that between 1870 and 1871 there was an increase in all three categories, and whilst there is then a fall to approximately 1870 levels of expenditure in "Stationery, Printing, and Advertising" (by 1872) and "Books, Periodicals, and Music" (by 1873), the fall back in "Incidentals" is much less, and never approximates the 1870 level.

Another way to look at the costs in each category is to analyse them using the cumulative sum (cusum) method, an elementary mathematical method which may be used to illustrate trends in serial data. As per the method used previously (Larner 2011; derived from Kinsey et al. 1989), the first-year datum (1867) was used as a reference point, with subtraction of this reference point from successive annual data points and the remainder added to the previous sum (for ease of calculation, costs were rounded to the nearest pound for each year). Using this method, if successive datapoints are the same as the reference point, the cusum plot remains at zero; if successive datapoints rise or fall, then the cusum plot does likewise.

© The Editor(s) (if applicable) and The Author(s), under exclusive license to Springer Nature
Switzerland AG 2026

A. J. Larner, *The West Riding Asylum and the Origins of British Neurology 1866-1876*,
https://doi.org/10.1007/978-3-032-12591-0

Table A1 Costs taken from "Balance Sheet for the Year" printed in the Annual Reports of the Committee of Visitors and Medical Superintendents Report[a]

For the year	Stationery, printing, and advertising	Books, periodicals, and music	Incidentals
1867	£202 17s 9d	£102 13s 2d	£91 2s 7d
1868	£161 6s 7d	£75 16s 2d	£87 2s 3d
1869	–	–	–
1870	£252 14s 11d	£115 9s 4d	£89 6s 7d
1871	£302 11s 0d	£158 6s 2d	£169 10s 3d
1872	£255 6s 2d	£163 7s 5d	£135 16s 0d
1873	£264 18s 1d	£127 7s 8d	£143 7s 3d
1874	–	–	–
1875	–	–	–

[a]Figures are taken from the Balance Sheets, which are not paginated, of *Report*, respectively 1868, 1869, 1871, 1872, 1873, and 1874 (each *Report* refers to the expenditure of the previous year)

Table A2 Cusum points for "Stationery, Printing, and Advertising"

Year	Cost (rounded to the nearest pound)	Calculation	Cusum point
1867	203	203	0
1868	161	(161–203) + 203 = 161	−42
1870	253	(253–203) + 161 = 211	+8
1871	303	(303–203) + 211 = 311	+108
1872	255	(255–203) + 311 = 363	+160
1873	265	(265–203) + 363 = 425	+222

The calculation of cusum points is shown in the following tables: "Stationery, Printing, and Advertising" (Table A2); "Books, Periodicals, and Music" (Table A3); and "Incidentals" (Table A4). These results are then illustrated graphically (Fig. A1).

Whilst it is evident that the slope of all three plots increases between 1870 and 1871, this is steepest for "Stationery, Printing, and Advertising", followed by "Incidentals", followed by "Books, Periodicals, and Music".

Of course, this analysis cannot prove that funding for *WRLAMR* came from any one or more of these sources, but it is perhaps suggestive. Confounders may have been a general increase in the costs of these materials, perhaps related to inflation. Another point to consider is that the figures presented in Table A1, prepared by the Clerk and Steward of the Asylum, involved three different individuals: George Appleyard (1867), Henry S. Roxby (1868 and 1870), and M. Cairns (1871, 1872, 1873). If each used a different method to calculate costs it might invalidate any inferences about funding sources of *WRLAMR* based on these figures.

Table A3 Cusum points for "Books, Periodicals, and Music"

Year	Cost (rounded to the nearest pound)	Calculation	Cusum point
1867	103	103	0
1868	76	(76–103) + 103 = 76	−27
1870	115	(115–103) + 76 = 88	−15
1871	158	(158–103) + 88 = 143	+40
1872	163	(163–103) + 143 = 203	+100
1873	127	(127–103) + 203 = 227	+124

Table A4 Cusum points for "Incidentals"

Year	Cost (rounded to the nearest pound)	Calculation	Cusum point
1867	91	91	0
1868	87	(87–91) + 91 = 87	−4
1870	89	(89–91) + 87 = 85	−6
1871	170	(170–91) + 85 = 164	+73
1872	136	(136–91) + 164 = 209	+118
1873	143	(143–91) + 209 = 261	+170

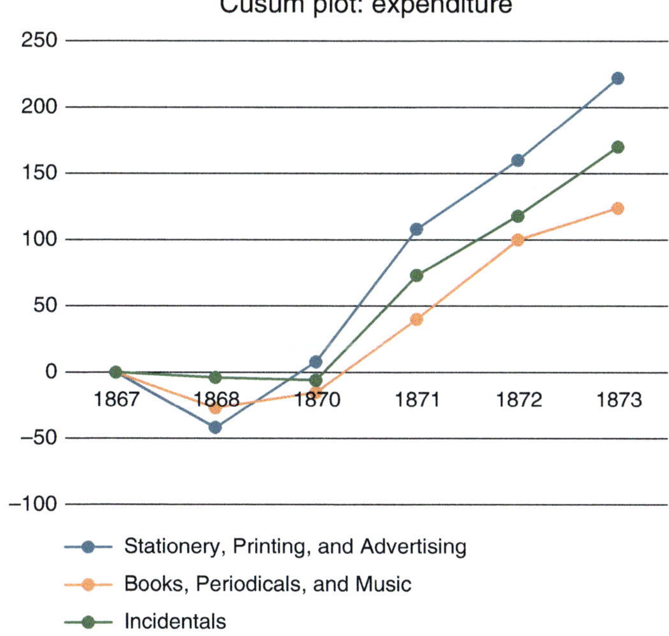

Fig. A1 Cusum plots for expenditure in different categories, 1867–1873

Finn (2012:84–85) reached similar conclusions, increased spending in 1871–1872, but using different base figures and methods.

Appendix References

Kinsey SE, Giles FJ, Holton J. Cusum plotting of temperature charts for assessing antimicrobial treatment in neutropenic patients. BMJ 1989; 299: 775–776.

Larner AJ. Teleneurology by internet and telephone. A study of medical self-help. London: Springer, 2011.

Bibliography

A number of points about this bibliography need to be made explicit from the outset.

Papers published in the *West Riding Lunatic Asylum Medical Reports* are not included in this bibliography. For a complete listing of these 80 papers, see Chap. 6, Table 6.1. Likewise, published reviews of the various volumes of *WRLAMR* are not included here as these are listed in Chap. 6, Table 6.2. Likewise, those papers published in *Brain* by *WRLAMR* staff, present or former, in the first six years of its publication, 1878–1879 to 1883–1884, are not included here as these are listed in Chap. 6, Table 6.4.

Some authors of works of history elect to separate references into categories, such as unpublished theses versus published works, or primary versus secondary publications, even sometimes subdividing these into primary books, primary papers, secondary books and secondary papers. As I find such arrangements cumbersome, I have preferred to lump all references of whatever type into one alphabetical list, believing this to be easier for the reader when searching for a reference.

Many references in the text refer to news items, obituaries, reviews, etc., all of which are uncredited as to authorship in their original form. To avoid an overwhelming number of entries under "[Anon.]", references to items published in the notes or news columns of Journals or newspapers, such as individual appointments or reports of meetings, and likewise obituaries (unless signed), are simply listed in the appropriate footnotes rather than in this Bibliography (despite which it may still appear over-documented!). Sufficient information is presented in the footnotes to permit the reader to track down these references if required.

[?] = unknown; [??] = uncertain.

Adams CE. James Crichton Browne [*sic*] and controlled evaluation of drug treatment for mental illness. J R Soc Med. 2010;103(4):160–1.

A. J. Larner, *The West Riding Asylum and the Origins of British Neurology 1866-1876*,
https://doi.org/10.1007/978-3-032-12591-0

Adams R. Flighty, melancholic and wild: 250 years of mental health care in York. A history of Bootham Park Hospital previously known as The York Asylum. York: Quacks Books; 2025.

Adan G, Larner AJ. Sesquicentenary of the knee jerk reflex: the contributions of Hughlings Jackson, Horsley, and Sherrington. J Hist Neurosci. 2025;34(3):509–16.

Adrian ED. Ferrier Lecture. The localization of activity in the brain. Proc R Soc Lond B Biol Sci. 1939;126:433–49.

Akkermans R. David Ferrier. Lancet Neurol. 2016;15(7):666.

Alberti SJMM. Conversaziones and the experience of science in Victorian England. Journal of Victorian Culture. 2003;8:208–30.

Aldren Turner W. The late Sir David Ferrier. BMJ. 1928;1(3508):574–5. (31st March)

Allbutt TC. On the state of the optic nerves and retinae as seen in the insane. Med Chir Trans. 1868a;51:97–142.

Allbutt TC. On the state of the optic nerves and retinae as seen in the insane. BMJ. 1868b;1(376):257. (14th March)

Allbutt TC. On the state of the optic nerves and retinae as seen in the insane. Lancet. 1868c;1(2325):377–8. (21st March)

Allbutt TC. The state of the optic nerves and retinae as seen in the insane. Med Times Gaz. 1868d;1:328. (21st March)

Allbutt TC. Case of cerebral disease in a syphilitic patient. St George's Hosp Rep. 1868e;3:55–65.

Allbutt TC. On the use of the ophthalmoscope in diseases of the nervous system and of the kidneys and also in certain general disorders. London: MacMillan and Co.; 1871a.

Allbutt TC. Electro-therapy. Br Foreign Med Chir Rev. 1871b;48(95):38–57.

Allbutt TC. Syphilitic disease of the small arteries of the encephalon. Trans Pathol Soc Lond. 1872;23:16.

Allbutt TC. Discussion on visceral syphilis, especially of the central nervous system and cardiovascular system. BMJ. 1921;2(3162):177–83. (6th August)

Allbutt[TC], Teale[??TP]. Review IX. Medical ophthalmoscopy. Br Foreign Med Chir Rev 1868; 41 (81): 126–150.

Alphabetical list of graduates of the University of Edinburgh from 1859 to 1888 (both years included) with historical appendix (including present and past office bearers) and separate lists of honorary graduates and graduates with honours; information as to University Library, Museum, Laboratories, benefactions to the University, etc. Edinburgh: James Thin, 1889.

Aminoff MJ. Brown-Séquard. A visionary of science. New York: Raven Press; 1993.

Aminoff MJ. Victor Horsley. The world's first neurosurgeon and his conscience. Cambridge: Cambridge University Press; 2022.

Andrews ES. Senility before Alzheimer: old age in British psychiatry, c.1835–1912. Unpublished PhD thesis, University of Warwick, 2014. http://go.warwick.ac.uk/wrap/65690

Anning ST, Walls WKJ. A history of the Leeds School of Medicine. One and a half centuries 1831–1981. Leeds: Leeds University Press; 1982.

[Anon.]. The cholera at the Wakefield Lunatic Asylum. Lond Med Gaz. 1849;9:865. (16th November)

[Anon.]. The Association of Medical Officers of Asylums and Hospitals for the Insane. J Psychol Med Ment Pathol. 1853;6(23):453–5.

[Anon.]. The Medico-Psychological Association. Lancet. 1865;2(2186):97. (22nd July)

[Anon.]. The education, position, and pay of Assistant Medical Officers of County Asylums. J Ment Sci 1868–1869; 14. (October 1868): 376–381.

[Anon.]. The sanitary condition of Wakefield. Med Times Gaz. 1870;1:36–7. (8th January)

[Anon.]. My friend the mad-doctor. All the Year Round. 1873;10(250):469–76. (13th September)

[Anon.]. The treatment of insanity. J Ment Sci. 1874–1875;20(July 1874):224–35.

[Anon.]. Report of the Lancet Commission on Lunatic Asylums. Lancet. 1876;1(2755):891–3. (17th June); 2 (2757): 17–19 (1st July)

[Anon.]. Publisher's notice. Br Foreign Med Chir Rev. 1877;60(120):512.

[Anon.]. The noble forehead. J Ment Sci. 1881–1882;27(January 1882):623–24.

[Anon.]. Promotion in the asylum service. The greatest hardship of the Assistant Medical Officer. Hospital (Lond 1886). 1918;64(1678):385–6. (3rd August)

[Anon.]. Queen Square and the National Hospital 1860–1960. London: Edward Arnold; 1960.

[Anon.]. The years of Lennox Browne. J Laryngol Otol Suppl. 1986a;22:10–25.

[Anon.]. Stanley Royd: the epidemiological lesson. BMJ. 1986b;292(6521):644–5. (8th March)

Anstie FE. Insane patients in London workhouses. J Ment Sci. 1865–1866;11(October 1865):327–36.

Anstie FE. Lectures on the prognosis and treatment of certain acute diseases, with special reference to the indications afforded by the graphic study of the pulse. Delivered at the Royal College of Physicians of London. Lancet. 1867;2:35–6. (13th July), 63–65 (20th July), 123–124 (3rd August), 189–191 (17th August), 385–387 (28th September)

Anstie FE. On certain modifications of Marey's sphygmograph. Lancet. 1868;1:783–4. (20th June)

Anstie F. On the hereditary connections between certain nervous diseases. J Ment Sci. 1871–1872;17(January 1872):471–84.

Arbuckle JH. Ocular cases. BMJ. 1876a;1(806):720–1. (10th June)

Arbuckle JH. A rapid and simple method of staining and mounting fresh brain for microscopic examination. Glasgow Med J. 1876b;8(2):207–12.

Arbuckle JH. A case of intra-cranial tumour. Glasgow Med J. 1876c;8(3):327–33.

Arlidge JT. The growth of lunacy. Br Foreign Med Chir Rev. 1870;45(90):407–28.

Ashworth AL. Stanley Royd Hospital, Wakefield. One hundred and fifty years. A history. Wakefield: Wakefield Area Health Authority; 1975.

Ashworth B. The Bramwells of Edinburgh. A medical dynasty. Edinburgh: Royal College of Physicians of Edinburgh; 1986.

Bailey JB. The medical institutions of London. The medical societies of London. BMJ. 1895;2(1802):100–3. (13th July)

Balfour Browne JH. On the method of the study of mind. J Ment Sci. 1870–1871;16(July 1870):233–47.

Balfour Browne JH. The medical jurisprudence of insanity. London: J. & A. Churchill; 1871a.

Balfour Browne JH. Partial moral mania—kleptomania. Br Foreign Med Chir Rev. 1871b;47(94):498–514.

Balfour Browne JH. Hegelian law, mathematics and physiology. J Ment Sci. 1872–1873;18(January 1873):561–78.

Balfour Browne JH. Responsibility and disease. An essay. London: Baillière, Tindall, and Cox; 1873a.

Balfour Browne JH. "Eugene Aram", a psychological study. J Ment Sci. 1873b-1874;19(July 1873):247–55.

Ballance C. The late Sir David Ferrier. BMJ. 1928;1(3508):574. (31st March)

Bannister A. In splendid isolation: a short history of High Royds Hospital, the former West Riding Pauper Lunatic Asylum at Menston. Leeds: Leeds Mental Health; 2005.

Barclay J. A caring community. A centenary history of the National Society for Epilepsy and the Chalfont Centre, 1892–1992. London: National Society for Epilepsy; 1992.

Barlow N, editor. The autobiography of Charles Darwin 1809–1882. With original omissions restored. Edited with Appendix and Notes by his grand-daughter. London: Collins; 1958.

Bartholow R. Experimental investigations into the functions of the human brain. Am J Med Sci. 1874;67:305–13.

Batty Tuke J. On the morbid histology of the brain and spinal cord as observed in the insane. Br Foreign Med Chir Rev. 1873;51(102):450–60.

Batty Tuke J. The teaching and practice of psychological medicine. Lancet. 1874;1(2629):108–9. (17th January)

Bearn AG. Sir Clifford Allbutt. Scholar and physician. London: Royal College of Physicians; 2007.

Benham WT. On the value of the corpus luteum as a proof of impregnation; with a case in which an unimpregnated ovum was found in the virgin uterus. Edinb Med J. 1873;19(2):127–34.

Benham WT. The result of a post-mortem examination on a hydrocephalic idiot (congenital). J Ment Sci. 1874–1875;20(July 1874):259–62.

Bevan Lewis W. A case of disseminated cerebral sclerosis. J Ment Sci. 1877–1878;23(January 1878):564–5.

Bevan Lewis W. Teachings of the sphygmograph in general paralysis of the insane. J Ment Sci. 1881–1882;27(April 1881):1–11.

Bevan Lewis W. The human brain. Histological and coarse methods of research. A manual for students and Asylum Officers. London: J. & A. Churchill; 1882.

Bevan Lewis W. Cerebral localisation in its relationships to psychological medicine. BMJ. 1883;2(1187):624–8. (29th September)

Bevan Lewis W. A text-book of mental diseases: with special reference to the pathological aspects of insanity. London: Charles Griffin; 1889.

Bevan Lewis W. General pathology of the nervous system. In: Allbutt C, editor. A system of medicine. Volume VI. London: Macmillan and Co.; 1899. p. 490–510.

Bevan-Lewis W. The Presidential Address on the biological factor in heredity, delivered at the Sixty-eighth Annual Meeting of the Medico-Psychological Association, held at Wakefield on July 22nd and 23rd, 1909. J Ment Sci. 1909;55:591–630.

Beveridge A. Thomas Clouston and the Edinburgh School of psychiatry. In: Berrios GE, Freeman H, editors. 150 years of British Psychiatry 1841–1991. London: Royal College of Psychiatrists; 1991. p. 359–88.

Beveridge A. The odd couple: the partnership of J.C. Bucknill and D.H. Tuke. Psychiatr Bull. 1998;22(1):52–6.

Beveridge AW, Renvoize EB. Electricity: a history of its use in the treatment of mental illness in the second half of the nineteenth century. Br J Psychiatry. 1988;153:157–62.

Bewley T. Madness to mental illness. A history of the Royal College of Psychiatrists. London: Royal College of Psychiatrists; 2008.

Bickford JAR. The old Hull Borough Asylum (1849–1883). Hull: Self-published; 1981.

Bickford JAR. De la Pole Hospital (1883–1983). Hull: Self-published; 1983.

Bickford JAR, Bickford ME. The private lunatic asylums of the East Riding. Hull: East Yorkshire Local History Society; 1976.

Bickford JAR, Bickford ME. The medical profession in Hull 1400–1900. A biographical dictionary. Hull: Kingston upon Hull City Council; 1983.

Biographies of Medical Lunacy Commissioners 1828–1912. http://studymore.org.uk/6biom.htm.

Birt E. On certain questions relating to the urinology of the insane. Brain. 1886–1887;9(3):362–84.

Bodington GF. On the past and present treatment of insanity. BMJ. 1876;2(813):140–4. (29th July)

Bolton JS. On a contribution to the localisation of cerebral function, based on the clinico-pathological study of mental disease. Lancet. 1910;1(4519):980–7. (9th April)

Bolton JS. The evolution of a mental hospital—Wakefield, 1818–1928. The Presidential address at the eighty-seventh annual meeting of the Royal Medico-Psychological Association held at the West Riding Mental Hospital, Wakefield, July 11, 1928. J Ment Sci. 1928;74(October 1928):587–633.

Bone I, Larner AJ. The trial of David Ferrier, November 1881: context, proceedings, and aftermath. J Hist Neurosci. 2024;33(4):333–54.

Bone I, Stone JL. The advent of epilepsy directed neurosurgery: the early pioneers and who was first. J Hist Neurosci. 2023;32(4):470–90.

Borch C (trans: Hentschel AM). Brainwaves. A cultural history of electroencephalography. London: Routledge, 2018.

Bowditch HP. Report on physiology. Boston Med Surg J. 1873;88:79–82.

Bradley J. "A certain instability of mind": Herbert Mayo, 1796–1852, surgeon and physiologist. J Med Biogr. 2017;25(2):122–30.

Bramwell B. The Edinburgh Medical School and its professors in my student days (1865–1869). Edinb Med J. 1923;30(4):133–56.

Brazier MAB. A history of the electrical activity of the brain. The first half-century. London: Pitman; 1961.

Brazis PW, Masdeu JC, Biller J. Localization in clinical neurology. 5th ed. Philadelphia: Lippincott Williams & Wilkins; 2007.

Breathnach C. Eduard Hitzig, neurophysiologist and psychiatrist. Hist Psychiatry. 1992;3(11):329–38.

Breathnach CS. The house: Wakefield Asylum, 1818…. Ir J Psychol Med. 1996;13(1):42.

Broadbent WH. An attempt to remove the difficulties attending the application of Dr. Carpenter's theory of the function of the sensori-motor ganglia to the common form of hemiplegia. Br Foreign Med Chir Rev. 1866;37:468–81.

Broadbent WH. On the cerebral convolutions of a deaf and dumb woman. J Anat Physiol. 1870;4(2):218–348.27.

Broadbent WH. The structure of the cerebral hemisphere. J Ment Sci. 1870–1871;16(April 1870):1–24.

Broadbent WH. On the cerebral mechanism of speech and thought. Med Chir Trans. 1872a;55:145–94.

Broadbent WH. On the causation and significance of the choked disc in intracranial diseases. BMJ. 1872b;1(598):633–5. (15th June)

Broadbent WH. A lecture on the theory of construction of the nervous system. Delivered at a Conversazione at the West Riding Asylum, Wakefield. BMJ. 1876;1(795):371–3. (25th March); 1 (796): 401–403 (1st April); 1 (797): 433–436 (8th April)

Broadbent W. Hughlings Jackson as pioneer in nervous physiology and pathology. Brain. 1903;26(3):305–66.

Broadbent ME, editor. Life of Sir William Broadbent Bart., K.C.V.O. London: John Murray; 1909.

Brown M. Rethinking early nineteenth-century asylum reform. Hist J. 2006;49(2):425–52.

Browne WAF. Derangements of the faculty of language from injury to the anterior lobe of the cerebrum. Lancet. 1833;2(510):330–3. (8th June)

Browne WAF. What asylums were, are, and ought to be: being the substance of five lectures delivered before the managers of the Montrose Royal Lunatic Asylum. Edinburgh: Adam and Charles Black; 1837.

Browne WAF. Epileptics: their mental condition. J Ment Sci. 1865–1866;11(October 1865):336–63.

Browne WAF. Address; on Medico-psychology. J Ment Sci. 1866–1867;12(October 1866):309–27.

Browne WAF. On anaesthesia, hyperaesthesia, pseudo-aesthesia, chiefly as met with in the insane. The substance of a lecture delivered to the members of Professor Laycock's class of psychological medicine, on their clinical visit to the Crichton Institution for the Insane, 26th July, 1873. Br Foreign Med Chir Rev. 1873;52(104):441–63.

Browne J. Darwin and the face of madness. In: Bynum WF, Porter R, Shepherd M, editors. The anatomy of madness. Essays in the history of psychiatry. Volume I. People and ideas. London: Routledge; 1985. [2004]. p. 151–64.

Brunton TL, Ferrier D. Report on the progress of physiology. J Anat Physiol. 1871;6(1):218–48.

Brunton TL, Ferrier D. Report on physiology. J Anat Physiol. 1872;7(1):175–91.

[Bucknill JC]. Prospectus. Asylum Journal. 1853;1:1–7.

Bucknill JC. An address on the law of murder in its medical aspects. Read to an audience of medical men assembled at the West Riding Asylum, November 20th, 1874. BMJ. 1874;2(726):667–72. (28th November)

Burdett HC. Hospitals and asylums of the world: their origin, history, construction, administration, management, and legislation; with plans of the chief medical institutions accurately drawn to a uniform scale, in addition to those of all the hospitals of London in the jubilee year of Queen Victoria's reign. Volume II. Asylum construction, with plans and bibliography. London: J. & A. Churchill; 1891.

Burdon Sanderson J. Handbook of the sphygmograph. London: Hardwicke; 1867.

Burman JW. Two cases of sudden death from unusual causes. Lancet. 1870;2(2466):778–9. (3rd December)

Burman JW. Gangrene of the lung in asylum practice. BMJ. 1871;1(530):195. (25th February)

Burman JW. On larceny, as committed by patients in the earlier stages of general paralysis. J Ment Sci. 1872–1873;18(January 1873):536–43.

Burman JW. Some results from the use of chloral hydrate. Lancet. 1872a;1(2533):356–7. (16th March)

Burman JW. On the treatment of acute mania by the subcutaneous injection of the combined acetates of conia and morphia. Practitioner. 1872b;9:335–47.

Burman JW. West Riding Lunatic Asylum. Case of Bright's disease, diagnosed in the first instance by means of the ophthalmoscope—death from convulsions—interesting autopsy. Med Times Gaz. 1873;1:62–3. (18th January)

Burman JW. Four departmental asylums in the north-west of France. J Ment Sci. 1873-1874;19(January 1874):541–52.

Burman JW. The cooling of the body after death. BMJ. 1874;1(691):408. (28th March)

Burman JW. Four departmental asylums in the north-west of France. J Ment Sci. 1874-1875a;20(April 1874):74–81.

Burman JW. Some further cases of general paralytics committed to prison for larceny; with remarks. J Ment Sci. 1874-1875b;20(July 1874):246–54.

Burman JW. Typhoid fever and sewage. BMJ. 1879a;2(987):876. (29th November)

Burman JW. Pulmonary apoplexy and emphysema as a *post mortem* appearance in cases of death from epilepsy. BMJ. 1879b;2(989):936. (13th December)

Burman JW. Constant and inconstant tinctures. BMJ. 1885;1(1275):1149–50. (6th June)

Burnham J. The British Medical Journal in America. In: Bynum WF, Lock S, Porter R, editors. Medical journals and medical knowledge. Historical essays. London: Routledge; 1992. p. 165–87.

Buzzard T. Clinical aspects of syphilitic nervous affections. London: J. & A. Churchill; 1874.

Buzzard T. The late Dr. Anstie. Practitioner. 1876;16:1–43.

Bynum WF. The nervous patient in eighteenth- and nineteenth-century Britain: the psychiatric origins of British neurology. In: Bynum WF, Porter R, Shepherd M, editors. The anatomy of madness. Essays in the history of psychiatry. Volume I. People and ideas. London: Routledge, 1985 [2004]: 89–102. [Reprinted in: Murray RM, Turner TH, editors. Lectures on the history of psychiatry. The Squibb Series. London: Gaskell, 1990: 115–127.]

Bynum WF, Neve M. Hamlet on the couch. In: Bynum WF, Porter R, Shepherd M, editors. The anatomy of madness. Essays in the history of psychiatry. Volume I. People and ideas. London: Routledge; 1985. [2004]. p. 289–303.

Bynum WF, Wilson JC. Periodical knowledge: medical journals and their editors in nineteenth-century Britain. In: Bynum WF, Lock S, Porter R, editors. Medical journals and medical knowledge. Historical essays. London: Routledge; 1992. p. 29–48.

Cade JF. John Frederick Joseph Cade: family memories on the occasion of the 50th anniversary of his discovery of the use of lithium in mania. 1949. Aust N Z J Psychiatry. 1999;33(5):615–8. and 4 pages following

Cambiaghi M. James Crichton-Browne (1840–1938). J Neurol. 2019;266(7):1819–20.

Campbell AW. Histological studies on the localisation of cerebral function. Cambridge: Cambridge University Press; 1905a.

Campbell AW. Cerebral sclerosis. Brain. 1905b;28(3–4):367–437.

Carlson C, Devinsky O. The excitable cerebral cortex. Fritsch G, Hitzig E. Über die elektrische Erregbarkeit des Grosshirns. Arch Anat Physiol Wissen 1870; 37:300–32. Epilepsy Behav. 2009;15(2):131–2.

Carmichael A. A memoir of the life and philosophy of Spurzheim. Dublin: W.F. Wakeman; 1833.

Carpenter WB. Principles of mental physiology, with their applications to the training and discipline of the mind, and the study of its morbid conditions. London: Henry S. King; 1874.

Carpenter M. Asylum nursing before 1914: a chapter in the history of labour. In: Davies C, editor. Rewriting nursing history. London/Sydney: Croom Helm; 1980. p. 123–45.

Carr EH. What is history? Harmondsworth: Penguin Books; 1961. [1981]

Carter RB. The ophthalmoscope: its varieties and its use. Trans: from the German of Dr. Adolf. Zander. With notes and additions by the translator. London: Robert Hardwicke; 1864.

Carter RB. Medical ophthalmology. In: Allbutt C, editor. A system of medicine. Volume VI. London: Macmillan and Co.; 1899. p. 826–53.

Cashman B. A Proper House. Bedford Lunatic Asylum: 1812–1860. Bedford: North Bedfordshire Health Authority; 1992.

Casper ST. "Then why not an Association of British Neurologists?": British neurologists and the founding of an elite medical society. Adv Clin Neurosci Rehabil. 2007;7(5):16–7.

Casper ST. One hundred members of the Association of British Neurologists: a collective biography for 1933–1960. J Hist Neurosci. 2011;20(4):338–56.

Casper ST. The neurologists. A history of a medical specialty in modern Britain, c.1789–2000. Manchester: Manchester University Press; 2014.

Cavanaugh R. James Crichton-Browne. Lancet Neurol. 2018;17(1):31.

Celestin L-C. Charles-Edouard Brown-Séquard. The biography of a tormented genius. Cham: Springer; 2014.

Chalmers I. Comparing like with like: some historical milestones in the evolution of methods to create unbiased comparison groups in therapeutic experiments. Int J Epidemiol. 2001;30:1156–64.

Charcot JM, Pitres A. Contribution a l'étude des localisations dans l'écorce des hémisphères du cerveau. Observations relatives aux paralysies et aux convulsions d'origine corticale. Revue Mensuelle de Médecine et de Chirurgie. 1877;1:1–18.

Clapham C. Nitrite of amyl in sea-sickness. Lancet. 1875;2(2712):276. (21st August)

Clapham C. On the brainweights of some Chinese and Pelew Islanders. J Anthropol Inst G B Irel. 1878;7:89–94.

Clapham C. Brain, weight of, in the insane. In: Tuke DH, editor. A dictionary of psychological medicine giving the definition, etymology and synonyms of the terms used in medical psychology with the symptoms, treatment, and pathology of insanity and the law of lunacy in Great Britain and Ireland, vol. I. London: J. & A. Churchill; 1892a. p. 164–8.

Clapham C. Head, size and shape of, in the insane. In: Tuke DH, editor. A dictionary of psychological medicine giving the definition, etymology and synonyms of the terms used in medical psychology with the symptoms, treatment, and pathology of insanity and the law of lunacy in Great Britain and Ireland, vol. I. London: J. & A. Churchill; 1892b. p. 574–80.

Clapham C. Sir John Charles Bucknill, M.D., F.R.C.P., F.R.S., citizen-soldier and psychologist. J Ment Sci. 1897;43(October 1897):885–9.

Clapham C. The out-patient treatment of insanity in general hospitals. BMJ. 1898a;1(1947):1067–8. (23rd April)

Clapham C. A note on the comparative intellectual value of the anterior and posterior cerebral lobes. J Ment Sci. 1898b;44(April 1898):290–5.

Clark MJ. The rejection of psychological approaches to mental disorder in late nineteenth century British psychiatry. In: Scull A, editor. Madhouses, mad-doctors, and madmen. The social history of psychiatry in the Victorian era. Philadelphia: University of Pennsylvania Press; 1981. p. 271–312.

Clarke H. Drawings of Wakefield. Being the fourth volume of the Journal of the Wakefield Historical Society. Wakefield: Wakefield Historical Society; 1977.

Clarkson H. Memories of Merry Wakefield. An octogenarian's recollections: being personal reminiscences, anecdotes, and impressions during the greater part of the nineteenth century. Wakefield: W.H. Milnes; 1887.

Clouston TS. Tuberculosis and insanity. J Ment Sci. 1863–1864;9(April 1863):36–65.

Clouston TS. Experiments to determine the precise effect of bromide of potassium in epilepsy. J Ment Sci. 1868–1869;14(October 1868):305–21.

Clouston TS. Skae's classification of mental disease. J Ment Sci. 1875–1876;21(January 1876):532–50.

Cobbold CWS. Haematoma auris. BMJ. 1873;2(668):457–8. (18th October).

Cohen, Lord, of Birkenhead. The Rt. Hon. Sir Thomas Clifford Allbutt, F.R.S. (1836–1925). In: Rook A, editor. Cambridge and its contribution to medicine, Proceedings of the Seventh British Congress on the History of Medicine University of Cambridge, 10–13 September, 1969. London: Wellcome Institute for the History of Medicine; 1971. p. 173–92

Collins K. Ernest Hart: editor of the British Medical Journal, 1866–1898. J Med Biogr. 2024;32(1):145–52.

Coote S. Oliver Goldsmith. The vicar of Wakefield. London: Penguin Classics; 1766. [1986]

Cooter RJ. Phrenology and British alienists, c. 1825–1845. Part I: converts to a doctrine. Med Hist. 1976a;20(1):1–21.

Cooter RJ. Phrenology: the provocation of progress. Hist Sci. 1976b;14(4):211–34.

Courtenay EM. Case of foreign body in the oesophagus. J Ment Sci. 1889;34(January 1889):539–41.

Cox C, Marland H. Disorder contained. Mental breakdown and the modern prison in England and Ireland, 1840–1900. Cambridge: Cambridge University Press; 2022.

Crammer JL. Training and education in British psychiatry 1770–1970. In: Freeman H, Berrios GE, editors. 150 years of British Psychiatry Volume II: The Aftermath. London: Athlone Press; 1996. p. 209–42.

Crichton BJ. The history and progress of psychological medicine. J Ment Sci. 1860–1861;7(April 1861):19–31.

Crichton Browne J. Personal identity, and its morbid modifications. J Ment Sci 1862–1863; 8 (October 1862): 385–395; 8 (January 1863): 535–545.

Crichton Browne J. Mania ephemera. Med Crit Psychol J. 1863;3(9):45–59.

Crichton Browne J. The actions of bromide of potassium upon the nervous system. Edinb Med J. 1865;10(12):1085–104.

Crichton Browne J. The etiology [*sic*] of insanity. Br Foreign Med Chir Rev. 1867;40:169–203.

Crichton Browne J. The education, position, and pay of Assistant Medical Officers of County Asylums. J Ment Sci. 1868–1869;14(January 1869):599–601.

Crichton Browne J. A case of gangrene of the lung: with remarks. BMJ. 1871a;1(528):141–3. (11th February)

Crichton Browne J. Laburnum poisoning. Med Press Circ. 1871b;11:222–3. (15th March)

Crichton Browne J. Chloral hydrate: its inconveniences and dangers. Lancet. 1871c;1(2483):440–1. (1st April); 1 (2484): 473–475 (8th April)

Crichton Browne J. Clinical lectures on mental and cerebral diseases. BMJ. 1871d;1(539):441–2. (29th April); 1 (540): 467–468 (6th May)

Crichton Browne J. Ergot of rye in the treatment of mental diseases. Practitioner. 1871e;6:321–36.

Crichton Browne J. Clinical lectures on mental and cerebral diseases. BMJ. 1871f;2(552):113–4. (29th July); 2 (553): 145–146 (5th August)

Crichton Browne J. Conium in the treatment of acute mania. Lancet. 1872a;1(2527):143–4. (3rd February); 1 (2528): 182–183 (10th February); 1 (2529): 217–218 (17th February). [Also published in American Journal of Insanity 1872; 29 (July): 118–132.]

Crichton Browne J. Clinical lectures on mental and cerebral diseases. BMJ. 1872b;2(615):403–6. (12th October); 2 (616): 429–431 (19th October)

Crichton Browne J. Clinical lectures on mental and cerebral diseases. BMJ. 1873;1(642):425–7. (19th April); 1 (643): 455–457 (26th April)

Crichton Browne J. Notes on epilepsy, and its pathological consequences. J Ment Sci. 1873–1874;19(April 1873):19–46.

Crichton Browne J. Clinical lectures on mental and cerebral diseases. BMJ. 1874a;1(697):601–3. (9th May); 1 (698): 640–643 (16th May)

Crichton Browne J. Notes on the nitrite of amyl. Practitioner. 1874b;13:179–84.

Crichton Browne J. Two cases of general paralysis treated by Calabar bean. BMJ. 1874c;2(721):522–3. (24th October)

Crichton Browne J. On the actions of picrotoxine and the antagonism between picrotoxine and chloral hydrate. BMJ. 1875a;1(743):409–11. (27th March); 1 (744): 442–444 (3rd April); 1 (745): 476–478 (10th April); 1 (746): 506–507 (17th April); 1 (747): 540–542 (24th April)

Crichton Browne J. Correspondence. J Ment Sci. 1875-1876a;21(April 1875):152.

Crichton Browne J. Arachnoid cysts. J Psychol Med Ment Pathol (Lond). 1875b;1(2):167–81.

Crichton Browne J. Skae's classification of mental disease. A critique. J Ment Sci. 1875-1876b;21(October 1875):339–65.

Crichton Browne J. Les fonctions des couches optiques. Revue Scientifique de la France et de l'étranger. 1876;5(41):345–54.

Crichton-Browne J. Presidential address, delivered at the Royal College of Physicians, London, on Friday, July 26th, 1878. J Ment Sci. 1878–1879;24(October 1878):345–73.

Crichton-Browne J. Discussion [of Bastian's presentation "The 'muscular sense': its nature and cortical localisation" to the Neurological Society of London]. Brain. 1887–1888;10(1):103–6.

Crichton-Browne J. The Cavendish Lecture on dreamy mental states. Delivered before the West London Medico-Chirurgical Society on June 20th, 1895. Lancet. 1895;2(3750):73–5. (13th July)

Crichton-Browne J. Ethics and individualism in medicine. BMJ. 1897;2(1919):990–7. (9th October)

Crichton-Browne J. The first Maudsley Lecture. J Ment Sci. 1920;66(July 1920):199–225.

Crichton-Browne J. The story of the brain. Edinburgh: Oliver and Boyd; 1924.

Crichton-Browne J. Victorian jottings from an old commonplace book. London: Etchells and Macdonald; 1926.

Crichton-Browne J. Stray leaves from a physician's portfolio. London: Hodder and Stoughton; 1927.

Crichton-Browne J. What the doctor thought. London: Ernest Benn; 1930.

Crichton-Browne J. The doctor's second thoughts. London: Ernest Benn; 1931.

Crichton-Browne J. The doctor's after thoughts. London: Ernest Benn; 1932.

Crichton-Browne J. From the doctor's notebook. London: Duckworth; 1937.

Crichton-Browne J. The doctor remembers. London: Duckworth; 1938.

Critchley M. Sir William Gowers 1845–1915: a biographical appreciation. London: William Heinemann Medical Books; 1949.

Critchley M. Hughlings Jackson, the man; and the early days of the National Hospital. Proc R Soc Med. 1960;53(8):613–8.

Critchley M, Critchley EA. John Hughlings Jackson. Father of English neurology. Oxford: Oxford University Press; 1998.

Crowther C. Some observations respecting the management of the Pauper Lunatic Asylum, at Wakefield. Wakefield: A. Hurst; 1830.

Crowther A. Administration and the asylum in Victoria, 1860s–1880s. In: Coleborne C, MacKinnon D, editors. "Madness" in Australia: histories, heritage and the asylum. St Lucia: University of Queensland Press; 2003. p. 85–95.

Crowther A. *Pygmalion* at the Asylum. WS Gilbert Soc J. 2013;5(32):5–21.

Dahlquist C, Kinderman P. "Picture imperfect": the motives and uses of patient photography in the asylum. Hist Psychiatry. 2023;34(2):130–45.

Davis M. West Riding Pauper Lunatic Asylum through time. Stroud: Amberley Publishing; 2013a.

Davis M. Voices from the asylum. West Riding Pauper Lunatic Asylum. Stroud: Amberley Publishing; 2013b.

Dawson PL. Wakefield revisited. Stroud: Tempus; 2003.

Dawson P. Wakefield memories. Stroud: Sutton Publishing; 2005.

Dawson PL. Changing Wakefield. Stroud: Fonthill Media; 2015a.

Dawson PL. Secret Wakefield. Stroud: Amberley Publishing; 2015b.

Dawson PL. A-Z of Wakefield. People, places, history. Stroud: Amberley Publishing; 2019.

Dawson PL. Wakefield at work. People and industries through the years. Stroud: Amberley Publishing; 2020.

Dawson PL. Wakefield. A potted history. Stroud: Amberley Publishing; 2022.

Department of Health and Social Security. The report of the committee of enquiry into an outbreak of food poisoning at Stanley Royd Hospital. London: HMSO; 1986.

Dewhurst K. Hughlings Jackson on psychiatry. Oxford: Sandford Publications; 1982.

Diamond S. Wundt before Leipzig. In: Rieber RW, editor. Wilhelm Wundt and the making of a scientific psychology. New York/London: Plenum Press; 1980. p. 3–70.

Didi-Huberman G. Invention d'hysterie. Charcot et l'iconographie photographique de la Salpêtrière. Paris: Macula; 1982.

Digby A. Changes in the asylum: the case of York, 1777–1815. Econ Hist Rev. 1983;36(2):218–39.

Digby A. Madness, morality and medicine. A study of the York Retreat, 1796–1914. Cambridge: Cambridge University Press; 1985.

Dodds[?], Strahan[?], Greenlees[?]. Assistant Medical Officers in Asylums: their status in the speciality. J Ment Sci 1890; 36 (January 1890): 43–50.

Doyle D. John Thomson (1765–1846). J R Coll Physicians Edinb. 2009;39:190.

Draaisma D. (trans: Fasting B) Disturbances of the mind. Cambridge: Cambridge University Press; 2009.

Duncan JF. President's Address at the Annual Meeting of the Medico-Psychological Association, held August 11th, 1875, at the Royal College of Physicians, Dublin. J Ment Sci. 1875–1876;21(October 1875):313–38.

Eadie MJ. *Rigor mortis* and the epileptology of Charles Bland Radcliffe (1822–1889). J Clin Neurosci. 2007;14(3):201–7.

Eadie M. Sir Charles Locock and potassium bromide. J R Coll Physicians Edinb. 2012;42:274–9.

Eadie M. William Henry Broadbent (1835–1907) as a neurologist. J Hist Neurosci. 2015;24:137–47.

Eadie MJ, Scott AEM, Lees AJ, Woodward M. William Gowers: the never completed third edition of the "Bible" of neurology. Brain. 2012;135(10):3178–88.

Earle P. A visit to thirteen asylums for the insane in Europe; to which are added a brief notice of similar institutions in transatlantic countries and in the United

States, and an essay on the causes, duration, termination and moral treatment of insanity. With copious statistics. Philadelphia: J. Dobson; 1841. p. 10–5.

Easterbrook CC. The chronicle of Crichton Royal. Dumfries: Courier Press; 1937.

Easterbrook CC. Sir James Crichton-Browne. Edinb Med J. 1938;45(4):294–301.

Easterbrook CC. The chronicle of Crichton Royal (1833–1936). Being the story of a famous mental hospital during its first century, and illustrating the evolution of the hospital care and treatment of mental invalids in Scotland. Dumfries: Courier Press, 1940.

Edwards S. The naturalist and the neurologist. On Charles Darwin and James Crichton-Browne. 2014 (28th May). https://publicdomainreview.org/essay/the-naturalist-and-the-neurologist-on-charles-darwin-and-james-crichton-browne.

Ellis R. A field of practise or a mere house of detention? The asylum and its integration, with special reference to the county asylums of Yorkshire, c.1844–1888. Unpublished PhD thesis, University of Huddersfield, 2001. https://eprints.hud.ac.uk/id/eprint/4670/.

Ellis R. "Without decontextualization": the Stanley Royd Museum and the progressive history of mental health care. Hist Psychiatry. 2015;26(3):332–47.

Feindel W. Thomas Willis (1621–1675)—the founder of neurology. CMAJ. 1962;87:289–96.

Ferrier D. Experimental researches in cerebral physiology and pathology. BMJ. 1873a;1(643):457. (26th April)

Ferrier D. Experimental researches in cerebral physiology and pathology. J Anat Physiol. 1873b;8(1):152–5.

Ferrier D. Hitzig on experiments on the brain. Lond Med Rec. 1874a;2:399–402.

Ferrier D. The localization [*sic*] of function in the brain (Abstract). Proc R Soc Lond. 1874b;22:229–32.

Ferrier D. Experiments on the brain of monkeys—No. 1. Proc R Soc Lond. 1874c;23:409–30.

Ferrier D. The Croonian Lecture. Experiments on the brain of monkeys (Second Series). Philos Trans R Soc Lond. 1875a;165:433–88.

Ferrier D. The Croonian Lecture, "Experiments on the brain of monkeys" (Second Series). Proc R Soc Lond. 1875b;23:431–2.

Ferrier D. Experiments on the brain of monkeys, with especial reference to the localisation of sensory centres in the convolutions. BMJ. 1875c;2(765):277. (28th August)

Ferrier D. The functions of the brain. London: Smith, Elder & Co.; 1876.

Ferrier D. The localisation of cerebral disease being the Gulstonian [*sic*] Lectures of the Royal College of Physicians for 1878. London: Smith, Elder & Co.; 1878a.

Ferrier D. The Goulstonian Lectures on the localisation of cerebral disease. Br Med J. 1878b;1(901):471–6. (6th April)

Ferrier D. The Goulstonian Lectures on the localisation of cerebral disease. Br Med J. 1878c;1(902):515–9. (13th April)

Ferrier D (trans: Obersteiner H). Die Functionen des Gehirnes. Braunschweig: Druck und Verlag von Friedrich Vieweg und Sohn, 1879.

Ferrier D. The functions of the brain. 2nd ed. London: Smith, Elder & Co.; 1886.

Ferrier D. Cerebral localisation in relation to therapeutics: being the Cameron Lecture of the University of Edinburgh, delivered February 26, 1892. Edinb Med J. 1892;37(10):881–97.

Ferrier D. The regional diagnosis of cerebral disease. In: Allbutt C, editor. A system of medicine. Volume VII, Diseases of the nervous system (Continued). London: Macmillan and Co.; 1899. p. 271–394.

Ferrier D. The regional diagnosis of cerebral disease. In: Allbutt C, Rolleston HD, editors. A system of medicine. Volume VIII, Diseases of the brain and mental diseases. 2nd ed. London: Macmillan and Co.; 1911. p. 37–162.

Ferrier [D]. The localisation of the functions in the brain. Nature. 1873c;8:477–8.

Finger S. David Ferrier and Eduard Hitzig: the experimentalists map the cerebral cortex. In: Finger S, editor. Minds behind the brain. A history of the pioneers and their discoveries. Oxford: Oxford University Press; 2000. p. 155–75.

Finkelstein G. Emil du Bois-Reymond. Neuroscience, self, and society in nineteenth-century Germany. Cambridge: MIT Press; 2013.

Finn MA. The West Riding Lunatic Asylum and the making of the modern brain sciences in the nineteenth century. Unpublished PhD thesis, University of Leeds, 2012. https://etheses.whiterose.ac.uk/3412/.

Finn MA, Stark JF. Medical science and the Cruelty to Animals Act 1876: a re-examination of anti-vivisectionism in provincial Britain. Stud Hist Phil Biol Biomed Sci. 2015;49:12–23.

Fitzherbert Jones R. Oxford's medical heritage. The people behind the names. Oxford: University of Oxford Medical Informatics Unit; 2014.

Folsom CF. Disease of the mind. Notes on the early management, European and American progress, modern methods, etc., in the treatment of insanity, with especial reference to the needs of Massachusetts and the United States. Boston: A. Williams & Co.; 1877.

Foster BW. On the use of the sphygmograph in the investigation of disease. London: T. Richards; 1866.

Foucault M. History of madness [Folie et déraison: Histoire de la folie à l'âge classique]. London: Routledge; 1961. [2006]

Fournier J-A. De l'ataxie locomotrice d'origine syphilitique. Annales de Dermatologie et de Syphilologie. 1875;7:187–97.

Fraser TR, Brunton TL, Ferrier D. Report on the progress of physiology: from 1st January to 1st April, 1871. J Anat Physiol. 1871;5(2):389–411.

Freidson E. Profession of medicine. A study of the sociology of applied knowledge. New York: Dodd, Mead & Co.; 1970. [1975]

French RD. Antivivisection and medical science in Victorian society. Princeton: Princeton University Press; 1975.

Fritsch G, Hitzig E. Über die elektrische Erregbarkeit des Grosshirns [On the electrical excitability of the cerebrum]. Archiv für Anatomie, Physiologie und Wissenschaftliche Medicin. 1870;37:300–32.

Fritsch G, Hitzig E. The electrical excitability of the cerebrum. J Neurosurg. 1963;20(10):905–16.

Fritsch G, Hitzig E. Electric excitability of the cerebrum (Über die elektrische Erregbarkeit des Grosshirns). Epilepsy Behav. 2009;15(2):123–30.

Fryer C. Case of caries of hard palate from the abuse of mercury. Med Press Circ. 1870;9:490. (22nd June)

Fürbringer M. Friedrich Arnold. In: Heidelberger Professoren aus dem 19. Jahrhundert; Festschrift der Universität zur zentenarfeier ihrer Erneuerung durch Karl Friedrich. Zweiter band. Heidelberg: Carl Winter's Universitätsbuchhandlung; 1903. p. 1–110.

Fye WB. T. Lauder Brunton and amyl nitrite: a Victorian vasodilator. Circulation. 1986;74(2):222–9.

Fye WB. T. Lauder Brunton, 1844–1916. Clin Cardiol. 1989;12:675–6. [Reprinted in: Hurst JW, Conti CR, Fye WB, editors. Profiles in cardiology. Mahwah: Foundation for Advances in Medicine and Science, Inc., 2003: 156–157.]

Fye WB. J. Milner Fothergill. Clin Cardiol. 1992;15:220–2. [Reprinted in: Hurst JW, Conti CR, Fye WB, editors. Profiles in cardiology. Mahwah: Foundation for Advances in Medicine and Science, Inc., 2003: 154–155.]

Fye WB. William Henry Broadbent. Clin Cardiol. 1990;13:62–4. [Reprinted in: Hurst JW, Conti CR, Fye WB, editors. Profiles in cardiology. Mahwah: Foundation for Advances in Medicine and Science, Inc., 2003: 146–147.]

Galton JC. Muscles of the fore and hind limbs in *Dasypus sexcinctus*. Trans Linn Soc Lond. 1869a;26(3):523–65.

Galton JC. The myology of the upper and lower extremities of *Orycteropus Capensis*. Trans Linn Soc Lond. 1869b;26(3):567–608.

Galton JC. Note of an abnormality in the human dental series. J Anat Physiol. 1872;6(2):428–30.

Galton JC. The human homologue of the "moderator band" of Reil. BMJ. 1873;2(656):83. (26th July)

Galton JC. On the epitrochleo-anconeus or anconeus sextus (Gruber). J Anat Physiol. 1874;9(1):168.2–175.

Gardner D. James Bell Pettigrew (1832–1908) MD, LLD, FRS, comparative anatomist, physiologist and aerobiologist. J Med Biogr. 2017;25(3):169–78.

Gatehouse CA. The West Riding Lunatic Asylum: the history of a medical research laboratory, 1871–1876. Unpublished MSc thesis. University of Manchester; 1981.

Gavroglu K, Patiniotis M, Papanelopoulu F, Simões A, Carneiro A, Diogo MP, Bertomeu Sánchez JR, García Belmar A, Nieto GA. Science and technology in the European periphery: some historiographical reflections. Hist Sci. 2008;46(2):153–75.

Geison GL. Michael Foster and the Cambridge School of Physiology. The scientific enterprise in Late Victorian Society. Princeton: Princeton University Press; 1978.

George MS. *Brain Stimulation's* expanding impact—now immediately free to download by anyone, anywhere and at anytime. Brain Stimul. 2020;13:277–9.

George MS, Trimble MR. The changing nineteenth-century view of epilepsy as reflected in the West Riding Lunatic Asylum Medical Reports, 1871–1876, vols 1–6. Neurology. 1992;42(1):246–9.

Gibson WC. Early contributions to the study of the nervous system. In: Gibson WC, editor. British contributions to medical science. The Woodward-Wellcome Symposium University of British Columbia 1970. London: Wellcome Institute for the History of Medicine; 1971. p. 283–91.

Gilby WH. On the dysentery which occurred in the Wakefield Lunatic Asylum in the years 1826, 1827, 1828, and 1829. North Engl Med Surg J. 1830–1831;1(1):91–101.

Gill HC. On the action and use of hyoscyamine. Practitioner. 1878;20:85–93. [Reprinted in: Braithwaite's Retrospect 1878; 77 (January–June): 326–328.]

Gill HC. Twins suffering from mania. J Ment Sci. 1882–1883;28(January 1883):540–4.

Gilman SL, editor. The face of madness. Hugh W. Diamond and the origin of psychiatric photography. New York: Brunner/Mazel; 1976.

Gilman S. Seeing the insane. New York: Brunner/Mazel; 1982.

Goetz CG, Bonduelle M, Gelfand T. Charcot. Constructing neurology. New York: Oxford University Press; 1995.

Goffman E. Asylums. Essays on the social situation of mental patients and other inmates. London: Penguin; 1961. [2022]

Golding R. West Riding Asylum: Music and theatre in the large-scale pauper asylum. In: Music and moral management in the Nineteenth-Century English lunatic asylum. Cham: Palgrave Macmillan; 2021. p. 129–56.

Goodbody F. Liverpool's medical community 1930–1998: social, knowledge and business networks. Unpublished PhD thesis, University of Liverpool, 2020. https://livrepository.ac.uk/3093988/1/200871054_Jun2020.pdf

Gowers WR. The automatic action of the sphincter ani. Proc R Soc Lond. 1877;26:77–84.

Gowers WR. A manual and atlas of medical ophthalmoscopy. London: J. & A. Churchill; 1879.

Gowers WR, Sankey HRO. The pathological anatomy of canine "chorea". Med Chir Trans. 1877;60:229–48.

Grainger R. Asylum. Memories of a local institution. Wakefield: Eastmoor Books; 1996.

Greaves I, editor. Jonathan Miller. One thing and another. Selected writings 1954–2016. London: Oberon Books; 2017.

Greenblatt SH. John Hughlings Jackson. Clinical neurology, evolution, and Victorian brain science. Oxford: Oxford University Press; 2022.

GW. John Todd, formerly Consultant Psychiatrist, High Royds Hospital, Menston. Bull Royal Coll Psychiatrists. 1987;11(7):248.

Hack Tuke D. The past and present provision for the insane poor in Yorkshire. BMJ. 1889a;2(1494):367–71. (17th August)

Hack Tuke D. The past and present provision for the insane poor in Yorkshire, with suggestions for the future provision for this class. (Read at the Leeds Meeting of the British Medical Association). London: J. & A. Churchill, 1889b.

Hack Tuke D, editor. A dictionary of psychological medicine giving the definition, etymology and synonyms of the terms used in medical psychology with the symptoms, treatment, and pathology of insanity and the law of lunacy in Great Britain and Ireland. London: J. & A. Churchill; 1892.

Hacking I. Mad travellers. Reflections on the reality of transient mental illnesses. London: Free Association Books; 1998.

Haig M. How to stop time. Edinburgh: Canongate; 2017.

Hare EH. 1878. D. Hack Tuke MD. Insanity in ancient and modern life with chapters on its prevention. Chapter VII Facts and figures in regard to the increase in insanity. London, Macmillan & Co. In: Thompson C, editor. The origins of modern psychiatry. Chichester: John Wiley; 1987. p. 49–58.

Hare EH. The origin and spread of dementia paralytica. J Ment Sci. 1959;105:594–626.

Hare E. Old familiar faces: some aspects of the asylum era in Britain. In: Murray RM, Turner TH, editors. Lectures on the history of psychiatry. The Squibb Series. London: Gaskell; 1990. p. 82–100.

Harman G. Immaterialism. Cambridge: Polity Press; 2016.

Harper J. Dr. W.A.F. Browne. Proc R Soc Med. 1955;48(8):590–3.

Harrington Tuke T. Address delivered at the Annual Meeting of the Medico-Psychological Association, held at the Royal College of Physicians, August 6th, 1873. Lancet. 1873a;2(2613):446–8. (27th September)

Harrington Tuke T. The Medico-Psychological Association. The President's Address for 1873. J Ment Sci. 1873b–1874;19(October 1873):327–40.

Harrington A. Medicine, mind, and the double brain. A study in Nineteenth-Century thought. Princeton: Princeton University Press; 1987.

Harris LJ, Almerigi JB. Probing the human brain with stimulating electrodes: the story of Roberts Bartholow's (1874) experiment on Mary Rafferty. Brain Cogn. 2009;70:92–115.

Head H. Obituary. John Hughlings Jackson, M.D., F.R.C.P., F.R.S. BMJ. 1911;2(2650):953. (14th October)

Head H, Campbell AW. The pathology herpes zoster and its bearing on sensory localisation. Brain. 1900;23(3):353–523.

Heaman EA. St Mary's. The history of a London teaching hospital. Montreal: McGill-Queen's University Press; 2003.

Henson RA. The editors of *Brain*. Practitioner. 1978;221:639–44.

Hervey N. A slavish bowing down: the Lunacy Commission and the psychiatric profession 1845–1860. In: Bynum WF, Porter R, Shepherd M, editors. The anatomy of madness. Essays in the history of psychiatry. Volume II. Institutions and society. London: Routledge, 1985 [2004]:98–131.

Higgins G. Rules for the management of the Pauper Lunatic Asylum for the West Riding of the County of York, erected at Wakefield. Wakefield; 1821.

Hill SA, Laugharne R. Mania, dementia and melancholia in the 1870s: admissions to a Cornwall asylum. J R Soc Med. 2003;96(7):361–3.

Hitzig E. Untersuchungen uber das Gehirns. Neue folge. Archiv für Anatomie, Physiologie und wissenschaftliche Medicin. 1874;41:392–441.

Hollander B. In search of the soul, and the mechanism of thought, emotion, and conduct. Volume I. The history of philosophy and science from ancient times to the present day. London/New York: Kegan Paul, Trench, Trubner & Co./EP Dutton & Co.; 1921.

Holmes GM. Sir James Crichton-Browne 1840–1938. Obit Not Fell R Soc. 1939;2:519–21.

Holtby W. South Riding. London: Virago Modern Classics; 1936. [2010]

Hoole DDJ. William Bevan Lewis and the scientific asylum. Newsletter R Coll Psychiatr. 2013;10:1–2.

Hornsby A. Unfeeling brutes? The 1875 Royal Commission on Vivisection and the Science of Suffering. Victorian Review. 2019;45:97–115.

Horsley V. Note on the patellar knee-jerk. Brain. 1883–1884;6(3):369–71.

Horwitz NH. Historical perspective. David Ferrier (1843–1928). Neurosurgery. 1994;35(4):793–4.

Howden T. Scheme for pensioning lunatic asylum attendants. Lancet. 1871;1(2478):291. (25th February)

Howden T. Pensions to attendants. J Ment Sci. 1872–1873;18(October 1872):471–2.

Howe AJ. The resignation of Sir William Charles Ellis. J Med Biogr. 2017;25(4):245–51.

Hubel DH, Wiesel TN. Brain and visual perception. The story of a 25-year collaboration. Oxford: Oxford University Press; 2005.

Hughes Bennett [A], Godlee RJ. Excision of a tumour from the brain. Lancet. 1884;2(3199):1090–1. (20th December)

Hunting P. The history of the Royal Society of Medicine. London: RSM Press; 2002.

Hunting P. The Medical Society of London 1773–2003. London: Medical Society of London; 2003.

Hunting P. Sir Thomas Lauder Brunton Bt FRCP FRS (1844–1916). J Med Biogr. 2016;24(4):433–9.

Hurn JD. The history of general paralysis of the insane in Britain, 1830–1950. Unpublished PhD thesis, University of London, 1998. https://discovery.ucl.ac.uk/1349281/1/339949.pdf.

Iniesta I, Larner AJ. John Hughlings Jackson (1835–1911): his major contributions on epilepsy and European influence. Eur J Neurol. 2011;18(Suppl 2):449. (abstract P2303)

Ireland WW. Daniel Hack Tuke, M.R.C.S., M.D., LL.D. J Ment Sci. 1895;41(July 1895):377–86.

Jackson JH. On the anatomical and physiological localisation of movements in the brain. Lancet. 1873a;1(2577):84–5. (18th January); 1 (2579): 162–164 (1st February)

Jackson JH. On the anatomical investigation of epilepsy and epileptiform convulsions. BMJ. 1873b;1(645):531–3. (10th May)

Jackson JH. A series of cases illustrative of cerebral pathology: cases of intra-cranial tumour. Med Times Gaz. 1873c;2:33–5. (12th July)

Jackson JH. London Hospital. Remarks on limited convulsive seizures, and on the after-effects of strong nervous discharges. Lancet. 1873d;2(2624):840–1. (13th December)

Jackson JH. An address on ophthalmology in its relation to general medicine. BMJ. 1877;1(854):575–7. (12th May)

Jackson JH. Remarks on dissolution of the nervous system as exemplified by certain post-epileptic conditions. Med Press Circ. 1881;31:329–32. (20th April)

Jackson JH. On post-epileptic states. A contribution to the comparative study of insanities. J Ment Sci 1888–1889; 34 (October 1888): 349–365; 34 (January 1889): 490–500.

Jackson JH, Colman WS. Case of epilepsy with tasting movements and "dreamy state" – very small patch of softening in the left uncinate gyrus. Brain. 1898;21:580–90.

Jackson MJ, Hughlings J. In: Bynum WF, Bynum H, editors. Dictionary of Medical Biography. Westport: Greenwood Press; 2007. p. 694–6.

Jacob A, Larner AJ. Clifford Allbutt (1836–1925). J Neurol. 2013;260(1):346–7.

James RR. Robert Brudenell Carter. Br J Ophthalmol. 1941;25(7):330–9.

James FE. The life and work of Thomas Laycock (1812–1876). Unpublished PhD thesis, University of London, 1996. https://discovery.ucl.ac.uk/id/eprint/1318051/.

Jefferson G. The prodromes to cortical localization. J Neurol Neurosurg Psychiatry. 1953;16(2):59–72.

Jellinek EH. The Kinnier Wilson library in Edinburgh. J Neurol Neurosurg Psychiatry. 2004;75(6):933–5.

Jellinek EH. Sir James Crichton-Browne (1840–1938): pioneer neurologist and scientific drop-out. J R Soc Med. 2005;98(9):428–30.

Kennedy F. John Hughlings Jackson. Bull N Y Acad Med. 1935;11(8):479–80.

Johnson A. The diary of Thomas Giordani Wright: apprentice doctor in Newcastle upon Tyne, 1824–29. Med Hist. 1999;43(4):468–84.

Johnston W. Roll of the Graduates of the University of Aberdeen 1860–1900. Aberdeen: Aberdeen University Press; 1906.

Jones K. Asylums and after. A revised history of the mental health services: from the early eighteenth century to the 1990s. London/Atlantic Highlands: Athlone Press; 1993.

Jones CL. The Medical Trade Catalogue in Britain, 1870–1914. Pittsburgh: University of Pittsburgh Press; 2013.

Kasper BS, Taylor DC, Janz D, Kasper EM, Maier M, Williams MR, Crow TJ. Neuropathology of epilepsy and psychosis: the contributions of J.A.N. Corsellis. Brain. 2010;133(12):3795–805.

Keeler CR. The ophthalmoscope in the lifetime of Hermann von Helmholtz. Arch Ophthalmol. 2002;120(2):194–201.

Kesteven WB. Remarks on the use of the bromides in the treatment of epilepsy and other neuroses. J Ment Sci. 1869–1870;15(July 1869):205–13.

Keynes M, Butterfield J. Sir Clifford Allbutt: physician and Regius Professor 1892–1925. J Med Biogr. 1993;1(2):67–75.

Kropotkin P. The conquest of bread. [Amazon], 1892.

Kullmann DM. Editorial. Brain. 2019;142(1):1.

Langley GE. Sir John Charles Bucknill 1817–1897: our founder. Br J Psychiatry. 1980;137:105–10.

Larner AJ. Hermann Ludwig Ferdinand von Helmholtz (1821–1894). Eye (Lond). 1994;8:717.

Larner AJ. *Localization in clinical neurology* (4th edition) by PW Brazis, JC Masdeu, J Biller. Adv Clin Neurosci Rehabil. 2002;2(3):32.

Larner AJ. Jenner, on the intellect. Adv Clin Neurosci Rehabil. 2003a;3(2):29.

Larner AJ. False localising signs. J Neurol Neurosurg Psychiatry. 2003b;74(4):415–8.

Larner AJ. The place of the ice pack test in the diagnosis of myasthenia gravis. Int J Clin Pract. 2004;58:887–8.

Larner AJ. Has Shakespeare's Iago deceived again? http://bmj.com/cgi/eletters/333/7582/1335, 2007 (2nd January).

Larner AJ. Dr. Samuel Gaskell (1807–1886): a brief biography, and thoughts on his possible influence on Elizabeth Gaskell's writings. Gaskell Soc Newsletter. 2016;62:11–8.

Larner AJ. *Queen Square. A history of the National Hospital and its Institute of Neurology* by S Shorvon and A Compston. Adv Clin Neurosci Rehabil. 2019a;18(3):19.

Larner AJ. Neuroliterature. Patients, doctors, diseases. Literary perspectives on disorders of the nervous system. Gloucester: Choir Press; 2019b.

Larner AJ. Neuroliterature 2. Biography, semiology, miscellany. Further literary perspectives on disorders of the nervous system. Gloucester: Choir Press; 2023a.

Larner AJ. The *West Riding Lunatic Asylum Medical Reports*: the precursor of *Brain*? Brain. 2023b;146(11):4437–45.

Larner AJ. A month in the country: the sesquicentenary of David Ferrier's classical cerebral localisation researches of 1873. J R Coll Physicians Edinb. 2023c;53(2):128–31.

Larner AJ. Neuroliterature: David Ferrier (1843–1928). Adv Clin Neurosci Rehabil. 2023d;22(2):20–2.

Larner AJ. Medical biography: a symbiotic methodology? J Med Biogr. 2023e;31(2):76–7.

Larner AJ. Richard Gundry Rows (1866–1925). J Neurol. 2024a;271(10):7059–60.

Larner AJ. Winifred Holtby (1898–1935): a mental hospital visit, early 1930s—Psychiatry in literature. Br J Psychiatry. 2024b;225(3):400.

Larner AJ. Herbert Coddington Major (1850–1921). J Neurol. 2024c;271(4):2144–6.

Larner AJ. Liminality analysis: a conceptual framework applicable to medical biography? J Med Biogr. 2024d;32(4):357–8.

Larner AJ. John Hughlings Jackson (1835–1911): an addition to his published writings? Adv Clin Neurosci Rehabil. 2024e;23(1):24–5.

Larner AJ. Arnold Pick (1851–1924): a centenary appreciation. Adv Clin Neurosci Rehabil. 2024f;22(4):14–5.

Larner AJ. William Aldren Turner (1864–1945). J Neurol. 2024g;271(8):5699–701.

Larner AJ. The origins of "neurology" and "neurologist". Adv Clin Neurosci Rehabil. 2025a;23(3):22–3. https://doi.org/10.47795/MTRH2044.

Larner AJ. George Eliot, *Middlemarch*, and the West Riding Asylum at Wakefield. In: Larner AJ. Neuroliterature 3. Biography, Semiology, Miscellany. More perspectives on the nervous system and its disorders. Gloucester: Choir Press; 2025b. p. 174–9.

Larner AJ. Robert Wilfred Skeffington Lutwidge (1802–1873). In: Larner AJ. Neuroliterature 3. Biography, Semiology, Miscellany. More perspectives on the nervous system and its disorders. Gloucester: Choir Press; 2025c. p. 30–3.

Larner AJ. Winifred Holtby (1898–1935): vignettes of mental health, early 1930s. In: Larner AJ. Neuroliterature 3. Biography, Semiology, Miscellany. More perspectives on the nervous system and its disorders. Gloucester: Choir Press; 2025d. p. 197–200.

Larner AJ. Dickens, 'Horniblow', and James Crichton-Browne (1840–1938). The Dickensian. 2025e;121(1):23–7.

Larner AJ. Prosopography versus biography in the history of neurology: a clinician's viewpoint. In: Larner AJ. Neuroliterature 3. Biography, Semiology, Miscellany. More perspectives on the nervous system and its disorders. Gloucester: Choir Press; 2025f. p. 26–9.

Larner AJ. Alexander Ecker (1816–1887). J Neurol. 2025g;272(4):301.

Larner AJ. Late nineteenth-century connections between Irish psychological medicine and the West Riding Asylum, Wakefield, England. 2025h: submitted.

Larner AJ. When and how did the ophthalmoscope reach England? In: Larner AJ. Neuroliterature 3. Biography, Semiology, Miscellany. More perspectives on the nervous system and its disorders. Gloucester: Choir Press; 2025i. p. 167–9.

Larner AJ. David Ferrier (1843–1928): *annus mirabilis* 1873. In: Larner AJ. Neuroliterature 3. Biography, Semiology, Miscellany. More perspectives on the nervous system and its disorders. Gloucester: Choir Press; 2025j. p. 56–68.

Larner AJ. Neuroliterature: David Ferrier (1843–1928). In: Larner AJ. Neuroliterature 3. Biaphy, Semiology, Miscellany. More perspectives on the nervous system and its disorders. Gloucester: Choir Press; 2025k. p. 180–7.

Larner AJ. David Ferrier's lectures on "Sleep and Dreaming" (1876): context and content considered. In: Larner AJ. Neuroliterature 3. Biography, Semiology,

Miscellany. More perspectives on the nervous system and its disorders. Gloucester: Choir Press; 2025l. p. 188–96.

Larner AJ. John Hughlings Jackson (1835–1911): Discovery of further publications for inclusion in the Catalogue Raisonné. Adv Clin Neurosci Rehabil. 2025m; https://doi.org/10.47795/TEKI7506

Larner AJ. Retrodiagnosis: the ontological, the epistemic, and the ethical. In: Larner AJ. Neuroliterature 3. Biography, Semiology, Miscellany. More perspectives on the nervous system and its disorders. Gloucester: Choir Press; 2025n. p. 9–18.

Larner AJ. Aphantasia avant le nom: historical perspectives on the absence or loss of visual imagery. Neuropsychologia. 2025o;218:109254.

Larner AJ. Dumfries and Galloway: three neuro-history vignettes. In: Larner AJ. Neuroliterature 3. Biography, Semiology, Miscellany. More perspectives on the nervous system and its disorders. Gloucester: Choir Press; 2025p. p. 204–7.

Larner AJ. Arthur Thomas Myers (1851–1894): "Quaerens", "Z", and "Dr. Z" revisited. In: Larner AJ. Neuroliterature 3. Biography, Semiology, Miscellany. More perspectives on the nervous system and its disorders. Gloucester: Choir Press; 2025q. p. 77–89.

Larner AJ. John Charles Bucknill (1817–1897): pioneer in neurology? In: Larner AJ. Neuroliterature 3. Biography, Semiology, Miscellany. More perspectives on the nervous system and its disorders. Gloucester: Choir Press; 2025r. p. 34–7.

Larner AJ. "To discuss and exchange views upon professional topics": *conversazione* at the West Riding Asylum, 1871–1875. Hist Psychiatry 2025s;36(4):225-40.

Larner AJ. William Henry Broadbent (1835–1907). J Neurol. 2025t;272(5):376.

Larner AJ. John Hughlings Jackson (1835–1911): When did he become the "father of English/British neurology"? Adv Clin Neurosci Rehabil. 2025u; https://doi.org/10.47795/JQUP4220

Larner AJ. Richard Rows (1866–1925) and "functional mental illness": the interface between psychiatry and neurology, 1912–1926. Hist Psychiatry. 2025v;36(4):250-68.

Larner AJ. False localising signs: a topographical anatomy. In: Larner AJ. Neuroliterature 3. Biography, Semiology, Miscellany. More perspectives on the nervous system and its disorders. Gloucester: Choir Press; 2025w. p. 125–31.

Larner AJ. The Neurological Society: 1885–1907. 2026a.; submitted.

Larner AJ. David Ferrier's 1874 Royal Society Croonian Lecture. 2026b.; in preparation.

Larner AJ. Friedrich Arnold (1803–1890). 2026c.; submitted.

Larner AJ. Neuropathology research at the West Riding Asylum, 1884–1903. 2026d.; in preparation.

Larner AJ, Gardner-Thorpe C. Robert Lawson (?1846–1896). J Neurol. 2012;259(4):792–3.

Larner AJ, Gardner-Thorpe C. John Charles Bucknill (1817–1897). J Neurol. 2023;270(8):4154–5.

Larner AJ, Griffiths TD. David Ferrier's 2nd monkey ("monkey F"): the inaugural experimental studies of the auditory cortex. J Hist Neurosci. 2025;34(3):495–508.

Larner AJ, Mbizvo GK. John Todd (1914–1987). J Neurol. 2025;272(1):76.

Larner AJ, Swash M. Hughlings Jackson's second thoughts on mental states in epilepsy. Neurology. 2024;103:e209959.

Larner AJ, Triarhou LC. William Bevan-Lewis (1847–1929). J Neurol. 2023;270(2):1190–1.

Larner AJ, Triarhou LC. Herbert Major on the insula: an early depiction of von Economo neurones? J Chem Neuroanat. 2024a;138:102435.

Larner AJ, Triarhou LC. Pioneers of cortical cytoarchitectonics: the forgotten contribution of Herbert Major. Brain Struct Funct. 2024b;229(7):1655–63.

Larner AJ, Triarhou LC. Charles Bland Radcliffe (1822–1889). J Neurol. 2024c;271(8):5702–3.

Larner AJ, Triarhou LC. Heinrich Obersteiner (1847–1922). J Neurol. 2025a;272(3):227.

Larner AJ, Triarhou LC. Armand de Watteville (1846–1925). J Neurol. 2025b;272(2):136.

Latour B. On the partial existence of existing and non-existing objects. In: Daston LJ, editor. Biographies of scientific objects. Chicago: University of Chicago Press; 2000. p. 247–69.

Lauder Brunton T. On the use of nitrite of amyl in angina pectoris. Lancet. 1867;2(2291):97–8. (27th July)

Lauder Brunton T. Nitrite of amyl in angina pectoris. Trans Clin Soc Lond. 1870a;3:191–200.

Lauder Brunton T. On the action of nitrite of amyl on the circulation. J Anat Physiol. 1870b;5(1):92–101.

Lauder Brunton T. The physiological action of alcohol. Practitioner. 1876;16:57–64, 118–35.

Lauder Brunton T. A presidential address on medical science forty years ago: a retrospect and a forecast. Delivered before the Medical Society of London on Oct. 9th, 1905. Lancet. 1905;2(4285):1087–9. (14th October)

Lauder Brunton T. Vascular troubles in later life. Birm Med Rev. 1909;66:191–212.

Lawson R. Neurotic medicines; with special reference to camphor and its monobromide. Practitioner. 1874;13:324–37.

Lawson R. On the monobromide of camphor. Practitioner. 1875a;14:262–70.

Lawson R. Brains and intellect. Lancet. 1875b;2(2713):306–8. (28th August)

Lawson R. Notes on asylum surgery. J Psychol Med Ment Pathol (Lond). 1875c;1:275–7.

Lawson R. On meningitis and allied changes in the meninges of the insane. Br Foreign Med Chir Rev. 1876a;57:413–39.

Lawson R. A contribution to the investigation of the therapeutic actions of hyoscyamine. Practitioner. 1876b;17:7–19.

Lawson R. On the symptomatology of alcoholic brain disorders. Brain. 1878–1879;1(2):182–94.

Lawson R. The epilepsy of Othello. J Ment Sci. 1880–1881;26(April 1880):1–11.

Laycock T. The objects and organization of the Medico-Psychological Association; the anniversary address. J Ment Sci. 1869–1870;15(October 1869):327–43.

Laycock T. The teaching and practice of psychological medicine as influenced by classifications of insanity. Lancet. 1874;1(2627):4–6. (3rd January); 1 (2628):48–50 (10th January)

Laycock [T]. A memorandum on the pay, position, and education of Assistant Medical Officers of Asylums. J Ment Sci. 1867–1868;13(January 1868):587–8.

Lazar JW. Anglo-American interest in cerebral physiology. J Hist Neurosci. 2009;18(3):304–11.

Lazar JW. David Ferrier: brain drawings and brain maps. Prog Brain Res. 2013;203:95–113.

Lazar JW. The early history of the knee-jerk reflex in neurology. J Hist Neurosci. 2022;31(4):409–24.

Leblanc R. Fearful asymmetry. Bouillaud, Dax, Broca, and the localization of language, Paris, 1825–1879. McGill-Queen's Univeristy Press; 2017.

Lennox WG, Lennox MA. Epilepsy and related disorders. London: J. & A. Churchill; 1960.

Levine-Clark M. Dysfunctional domesticity: female insanity and family relationships among the West Riding poor in the mid-nineteenth century. J Fam Hist. 2000;25(3):341–61.

Levine-Clark M. "Embarrassed circumstance": gender, poverty, and insanity in the West Riding of England in the early-Victorian years. Clio Med. 2004;73:123–48.

Levinge EG. Organic dementia; loss of vertical equilibrium and other motor phenomena; tumour of left temporo-sphenoidal lobe of brain. BMJ. 1878;2(915):52–3. (13th July)

Lewis B. On the preparation of sections of fresh brain for immediate microscopical examination. Med Times Gaz. 1876a;1:247–8. (4th March)

Lewis B. Case of hemiplegia with great depression of temperature. Lancet. 1876b;2(2771):502–3. (7th October)

Lewis B. Case of epileptiform convulsions in general paralysis of the insane, with localisation of discharging lesions. Lancet. 1877;1(2798):529–31. (14th April)

Lewis A. The Twenty-Fifth Maudsley Lecture – Henry Maudsley: his work and influence. J Ment Sci. 1951;97(April 1951):259–77.

Lewis B, Clarke H. The cortical lamination of the motor area of the brain. Proc R Soc Lond. 1878;27:38–49.

Leyland J, editor. Contemporary medical men and their professional work: biographies of leading physicians and surgeons, with portraits, from the "Provincial Medical Journal". Volume I and Volume II. Leicester: Office of the Provincial Medical Journal, 1888.

Lipson SE, Montes JA, Devinsky O. Epilepsy in *The Alienist and Neurologist*, 1880 and 1920. Epilepsia. 2002;43(8):912–9.

Littlewood A. Storthes Hall remembered. Huddersfield: University of Huddersfield; 2003.

Lock S. Ferrier, David. In: Bynum WF, Bynum H, editors. Dictionary of Medical Biography. Westport: Greenwood Press; 2007. p. 490.

Lord JR. Obituary. Alexander Lawrence, M.A., M.D. Aberd., once Medical Superintendent, Cheshire County Mental Hospital, Upton, Chester. Ordinary Member since 1870. J Ment Sci. 1928;74(April 1928):362–3.

Loughran T. Shell-shock and medical culture in First World War Britain. Cambridge: Cambridge University Press; 2017.

Low J. Dr. Charles Frederick Newcombe. The alienist who became collector of the native art treasures of the Pacific Northwest. Beaver (Magazine of the North). 1982;Spring:32–9.

Lowe J. Case of rupture of the heart. Lancet. 1872;2(2563):524. (12th October)

Luria AR. The working brain. An introduction to neuropsychology. Harmondsworth: Penguin; 1973.

Lyons JB. The citizen surgeon. A biography of Sir Victor Horsley F.R.S., F.R.C.S. 1857–1916. London: Peter Dawnay; 1966.

Macmillan M. An odd kind of fame. Stories of Phineas Gage. Cambridge: MIT Press; 2000.

Macmillan M. Alfred Walter Campbell's Rainhill days. Medical Historian (Bulletin of the Liverpool Medical History Society). 2011–2012;23:29–52.

Macmillan M. Snowy Campbell. Australian pioneer investigator of the brain. Melbourne: Australian Scholarly Publishing; 2016.

MacNalty A. Sir Victor Horsley: his life and work. BMJ. 1957;1(5024):910–6. (20th April)

MacNalty A. Some pioneers of the past in neurology. Med Hist. 1965;9(3):249–59.

Madden TM. On puerperal mania. Br Foreign Med Chir Rev. 1871;48(96):477–95.

Magnello E. The introduction of mathematical statistics into medical research: the roles of Karl Pearson, Major Greenwood and Austin Bradford Hill. In: Magnello E, Hardy A, editors. The road to medical statistics. Amsterdam/New York: Rodopi; 2002. p. 95–123.

Major HC. The value of the staining process in the histology of the morbid brain. Lancet. 1874;1(2636):333–4. (7th March)

Major HC. Histology of the brain in apes. Unpublished MD thesis, University of Edinburgh, 1875. https://era.ed.ac.uk/handle/1842/32031.

Major H. Note on the histology of the human brain. J Ment Sci. 1875-1876a;21(July 1875):276–7.

Major HC. Observations on the brain of the Chacma Baboon. J Ment Sci. 1875–1876b;21(January 1876):498–512.

Major HC. The structure of the island of Reil in apes. Lancet. 1877a;2(2811):45–6. (14th July); 2 (2812): 84–85 (21st July)

Major HC. On statistical tables of the causes of insanity. J Psychol Med Ment Pathol (Lond). 1877b;3:260–4.

Major HC. Adulteration of beer. Lancet. 1877c;2(2829):753. (17th November)

Major HC. Observations on the structure of the brain of the white whale (*Delphinapterus leucas*). J Anat Physiol. 1879;13(2):127–138.1.

Major HC. Case of paralytic idiocy with right-sided hemiplegia; epilepsy; atrophy with sclerosis of the left hemisphere of the cerebrum and of the right lobe of the cerebellum. J Ment Sci. 1879–1880;25(July 1879):161–5.

Major HC. Atrophy and sclerosis of the cerebellum occurring in a case of epileptic imbecility. J Ment Sci. 1882–1883;28(January 1883):532–5.

Major HC. Remarks on the results of the collective record of the causation of insanity. J Ment Sci. 1884–1885;30((April 1884):1–7.

Malcolm E. 'Ireland's crowded madhouses': the institutional confinement of the insane in nineteenth- and twentieth-century Ireland. In: Porter R, Wright D, editors. The confinement of the insane. International perspectives, 1800–1965. Cambridge: Cambridge University Press; 2003. p. 315–33.

Manning HJ. A note concerning the hydrate of chloral. Lancet. 1873;1(2594):695–6. (17th May)

Marland H. Medicine and society in Wakefield and Huddersfield 1780–1870. Cambridge: Cambridge University Press; 1987.

Maudsley H. Body and mind. An inquiry into their connection and mutual influence, specially in reference to mental disorders; being the Gulstonian Lectures for 1870, delivered before the Royal College of Physicians. With Appendix. Cambridge: Cambridge University Press; 1870a. [2017]

Maudsley H. Gulstonian Lectures on the relations between body and mind, and between mental and other disorders of the nervous system. Lancet. 1870b;1(2435):609–12. (30th April)

Maudsley H. Insanity and its treatment. J Ment Sci. 1871–1872;17(October 1871):311–34.

Maudsley H. Stealing as a symptom of general paralysis. Lancet. 1875;2(2724):693–5. (13th November)

Maudsley H. A Mental Hospital—its aims and uses. Arch Neurol Psychiatry Pathol Lab Lond County Asylums. 1909;4:1–12.

McCandless P. "Build! Build!" The controversy over the care of the chronically insane in England 1855–1870. Bull Hist Med. 1979;53(4):553–74.

McCrae M. Simpson. The turbulent life of a medical pioneer. Edinburgh: Birlinn; 2010.

McDowall TW. Asylum notes on scarlet fever. J Ment Sci. 1871–1872;17(July 1871):210–20.

McDowall TW. Cases in which mental derangement appeared in patients suffering from progressive muscular atrophy. J Ment Sci. 1872–1873;18(October 1872):390–7.

McDowall W. [*sic*]. Notes on guarana. Practitioner. 1873;11:161–75.

McDowall TW. Antiquarian scraps relating to insanity. J Ment Sci. 1873–1874;19(October 1873):386–98.

McEniery DF. The "Scientific" phrenologist—Bernard Hollander (1864–1934). J Med Biogr. 2021;29(2):95–101.

McGilchrist I. The master and his emissary. The divided brain and the making of the Western World (New expanded edition). New Haven/London: Yale University Press, 2019.

Mellett DJ. Bureaucracy and mental illness: the Commissioners in Lunacy 1845–90. Med Hist. 1981;25:221–50.

Merrington WR. University College Hospital and its Medical School: a history. London: Heinemann; 1976.

Millett D. Illustrating a revolution: an unrecognized contribution to the "Golden Era" of cerebral localization. Notes Rec R Soc Lond. 1998;52(2):283–305.

Milner Fothergill J. The depressants of the circulation and their use. BMJ. 1874;1(681):77–9. (17th January)

Milner Fothergill J. The mental aspects of ordinary disease. J Ment Sci. 1874–1875;20(October 1874):387–409.

Mindham RHS. The West Riding of Yorkshire pauper Lunatic Asylum at Wakefield, 1814–1995. Br J Psychiatry. 2020;217(3):534.

Morrell JB. The chemist breeders: the research schools of Liebig and Thomas Thomson. Ambix. 1972;19:1–46.

Morris H. Who really owns the history of medicine? Topics Hist Med. 2021;1:3–5.

Morriss-Kay G. The *Journal of Anatomy*: origin and evolution. J Anat. 2016;229:2–31.

Muqit MMK, Larner AJ. Matthew Baillie (1761–1823): from Shotts to Duntisbourne Abbots. Scott Med J. 2022;67(3):129–33.

Murphy TD. Medical knowledge and statistical methods in early nineteenth-century France. Med Hist. 1981;25(3):301–19.

Murphy S. The best is yet to be. 175th anniversary history of the West Cheshire Hospital, with memories from the Moston and Manor hospitals. Chester: C.C. Publishing; 2004.

Neve M, Turner T. What the Doctor thought and did: Sir James Crichton-Browne (1840–1938). Med Hist. 1995;39(4):399–432.

Nicol P. On cutaneous diseases in the insane. J Cutaneous Med Dis Skin. 1870a;4(15):197–203.

Nicol P. Othaematoma, or the asylum ear. Br Foreign Med Chir Rev. 1870b;46(91):191–8.

Nicol P, Mossop I. On the action of certain neurotics on the cerebral circulation. Br Foreign Med Chir Rev. 1872;50(99):200–5.

Noguchi H, Moore JW. A demonstration of Treponema pallidum in the brain in cases of general paralysis. J Exp Med. 1913;17(2):232–8.

Nolan P. Mental health nursing in Great Britain. In: Freeman H, Berrios GE, editors. 150 years of British Psychiatry Volume II: The Aftermath. London: Athlone Press; 1996. p. 171–92.

Nuttall AD. Dead from the waist down. Scholars and scholarship in literature and the popular imagination. New Haven and. London: Yale University Press; 2003.

O'Connor WJ. Founders of British physiology. A biographical dictionary, 1820–1885. Manchester/New York: Manchester University Press; 1988.

O'Connor WJ. British physiologists 1885–1914. A biographical dictionary. Manchester/New York: Manchester University Press; 1991.

Ogle JW. On the use of the ophthalmoscope as a help to diagnosis in diseases of the nervous system. Med Times Gaz. 1860;1:572–4. (9th June)

Oppenheim J. Shattered nerves. Doctors, patients, and depression in Victorian England. New York: Oxford University Press; 1991.

Ormerod W. Richard Caton (1842–1926): pioneer electrophysiologist and cardiologist. J Med Biogr. 2006;14(1):30–5.

Otis L. Müller's lab. Oxford: Oxford University Press; 2007a.

Otis L. Howled out of the Country: Wilkie Collins and H.G. Wells retry David Ferrier. In: Stiles A, editor. Neurology and literature, 1860–1920. Basingstoke: Palgrave Macmillan; 2007b. p. 27–51.

Outterson Wood T. The early history of the Medico-Psychological Association. J Ment Sci. 1896;42(April 1896):241–60.

Ozer MN. The British vivisection controversy. Bull Hist Med. 1966;40(2):158–67.

Paget GE. The Harveian Oration 1866. Cambridge: Deighton, Bell, and Co.; 1866.

Parenti M. The assassination of Julius Caesar. A people's history of ancient Rome. New York: The New Press; 2003.

Paris A, Lake L, Joseph A, et al. Nitrous oxide-induced subacute combined degeneration of the cord: diagnosis and treatment. Pract Neurol. 2023;23(3):222–8.

Parker RR, Dutta A, Barnes R, Fleet T. County of Lancaster Asylum, Rainhill: 100 years ago and now. Hist Psychiatry. 1993;4:95–105.

Parry-Jones B. The Warneford Hospital, Oxford, 1826–1976. Oxford: Holywell Press; 1976.

Pearce JMS. The West Riding Lunatic Asylum. J Neurol Neurosurg Psychiatry. 2003a;74(8):1141.

Pearce JMS. Sir Thomas Clifford Allbutt. J Neurol Neurosurg Psychiatry. 2003b;74(10):1443.

Pearce JMS. Sir David Ferrier MD, FRS. J Neurol Neurosurg Psychiatry. 2003c;74(6):787.

Pearce JMS. Brain disease leading to mental illness: a concept initiated by the discovery of general paralysis of the insane. Eur Neurol. 2012;67:272–8.

Pearce JMS, Lees AJ. Yorkshire's influence on the foundation of British Neurology. J Neurol Neurosurg Psychiatry. 2013;84(1):6–9.

Pearn AM. "This excellent observer …": the correspondence between Charles Darwin and James Crichton-Browne, 1869–75. Hist Psychiatry. 2010;21:160–75.

Pedlar V. Experimentation or exploitation? The investigations of David Ferrier, Dr. Benjulia, and Dr. Seward. Interdiscip Sci Rev. 2003;28:169–74.

Peterson D, editor. A mad people's history of madness. Pittsburgh: University of Pittsburgh; 1982.

Pickstone JV, Marland H. Medicine in industrial Britain: the uses of local studies. Soc Hist Med. 1989;2(2):198–203.

Plaxton JW. An account of two cases of locomotor ataxia, with mental symptoms simulating those of General Paralysis. J Ment Sci. 1878–1879;24(July 1878):274–8.

Plaxton JW. Notes of cases in the Ceylon Lunatic Asylum. J Ment Sci. 1880–1881;26(January 1881):559–63.

Plaxton JW. Criminal insane in Ceylon. J Ment Sci. 1881–1882;27(April 1881):44–6.

Plaxton JW. Note on shrinkage of a hemisphere and subsequent pachymeningitis. J Ment Sci. 1888–1889;34(January 1889):531–3.

Porter R. The patient's view: doing medical history from below. Theory Soc. 1985;14(2):175–98.

Pressman JD. Last resort. Psychosurgery and the limits of medicine. Cambridge: Cambridge University Press; 1998.

Purves-Stewart J. Sands of time. Recollections of a physician in peace and war. London: Hutchinson & Co.; 1939.

Quétel C. History of syphilis. Baltimore: Johns Hopkins University Press; 1990.

Quick T. From phrenology to the laboratory: physiological psychology and the institution of science in Britain (c.1830–80). Hist Hum Sci. 2014;27(5):54–73.

Rabagliati A. On relapsing fever; with special reference to the epidemic in Bradford in 1869–70. Edinb Med J. 1873;19(6):497–515.

Rabagliati AH. Are there laws of therapeutics? Practitioner. 1877;19:165–73, 329–36.

Rabagliati A. The classification and nomenclature of diseases. BMJ. 1880;2(1026):333. (28th August)

Rabagliati A. Some remarks on the classification and nomenclature of diseases. BMJ. 1881;2(1073):114–7. (23rd July)

Rabagliati A. Reviews and Notices of Books. Brain. 1887–1888;10(4):512–24.

Ravetz JR. Scientific knowledge and its social problems. Oxford: Oxford University Press; 1971.

Rawling KDB. "She sits all day in the attitude depicted in the photo": photography and the psychiatric patient in the late nineteenth century. Med Humanit. 2017;43(2):99–110.

Rawling KDB. "The annexed photos were taken today": photographing patients in the late-nineteenth-century asylum. Soc Hist Med. 2021;34(1):256–84.

Reader NLM. An ancient practice alive and well today. The story of Westgate End House. Practitioner. 1971;206:691–7.

Regan M. A caring society. A study of lunacy in Liverpool and south west Lancashire from 1650 to 1948. Rainhill: St Helens and Knowsley Health Authority; 1986.

Regulations and orders of the Committee of Visitors, for the management and conduct of the Asylum. Female Department. West Riding Pauper Lunatic Asylum, Wakefield. Wakefield: B.W. Allen, 1873.

Renvoize E. The Association of Medical Officers of Asylums and Hospitals for the Insane, the Medico-Psychological Association, and their Presidents. In: Berrios GE, Freeman H, editors. 150 years of British Psychiatry 1841–1991. London: Royal College of Psychiatrists; 1991. p. 29–78.

[The] Report of the Medical Superintendent and Director of the West Riding Pauper Lunatic Asylum. Wakefield: Hicks and Allen, 1861.

Report of the Committee of Visitors and of the Medical Superintendent of the West Riding Pauper Lunatic Asylum for the year 1867. Wakefield: Hicks and Allen, 1868.

Report of the Committee of Visitors and of the Medical Superintendent of the West Riding Pauper Lunatic Asylum for the year 1868. Wakefield: Hicks and Allen, 1869.

Report of the Committee of Visitors and of the Medical Superintendent of the West Riding Pauper Lunatic Asylum for the year 1870. Wakefield: B.W. Allen, 1871.

Report of the Committee of Visitors and of the Medical Superintendent of the West Riding Pauper Lunatic Asylum for the year 1871. Wakefield: B.W. Allen, 1872.

Report of the Committee of Visitors and of the Medical Superintendent of the West Riding Pauper Lunatic Asylum for the year 1872. Wakefield: B.W. Allen, 1873.

Report of the Committee of Visitors and of the Medical Superintendent of the West Riding Pauper Lunatic Asylum for the year 1873. Wakefield: B.W. Allen, 1874.

Reynolds ES. On changes in the nervous system after amputation of limbs, with bibliography and recent case. Brain. 1886–1887;9(4):494–509.

Reynolds EH. Robert Bentley Todd (1809–1860). J Neurol. 2005;252(4):500–1.

Reynolds EH. John Hughlings Jackson and Thomas Laycock: brain and mind. Brain. 2020;143(2):711–4.

Reynolds EH, Broussolle E. Allbutt of Leeds and Duchenne de Boulogne: newly discovered insights on Duchenne by a British neuropsychiatrist. Rev Neurol. 2018;174(5):308–12.

Reynolds EH, Broussolle E. Anglo-French neurological interactions in the 19th and 20th centuries: Societies and journals. Rev Neurol. 2022;178(4):291–7.

Richards S. Vicarious suffering, necessary pain: physiological method in late nineteenth-century Britain. In: Rupke NA, editor. Vivisection in historical perspective. London/New York: Routledge; 1987. p. 125–48.

Richardson R. "Notorious abominations": architecture and the public health in *The Builder* 1843–83. In: Bynum WF, Lock S, Porter R, editors. Medical journals and medical knowledge. Historical essays. London: Routledge, 1992: 90–107.

Riese W, Gooddy W. An original clinical record of Hughlings Jackson with an interpretation. Bull Hist Med. 1955;29(3):230–8.

Ritch A. Workhouse or asylum? Accommodating pauper lunatics in nineteenth-century England. Med Hist. 2023;67(2):109–27.

Robertson CL. On the several means of providing for the yearly increase of pauper lunatics. J Ment Sci. 1864–1865;10(January 1865):471–91.

Rolleston HD. The Right Honourable Sir Thomas Clifford Allbutt K.C.B. A Memoir. London: MacMillan and Co.; 1929.

Rollin HR. Sir James Crichton-Browne. Psychiatric Bull. 2003;27(5):195.

Rollin HR, Reynolds EH. Yorkshire's influence on the understanding and treatment of mental diseases in Victorian Britain: the golden triad of York, Wakefield, and Leeds. J Hist Neurosci. 2018;27(1):72–84.

Romano TM. Making medicine scientific. John Burdon Sanderson and the culture of Victorian science. Baltimore/London: Johns Hopkins University Press; 2002.

Ropper AH, Burrell BD. How the brain lost its mind. Sex, hysteria and the riddle of mental illness. London: Atlantic Books; 2019. [2021]

Rose FC, editor. A short history of neurology. The British contribution 1660–1910. Oxford: Butterworth Heinemann; 1999.

Rose FC. Chapter 39: an historical overview of British neurology. Handb Clin Neurol. 2010;95:613–28.

Rose FC. History of British neurology. London: Imperial College Press; 2012.

Roth M. The Royal College of Psychiatrists: our immediate tasks and aims. Br J Psychiatry. 1972;120(557):359–66.

Rows RG. Proposal by Dr. Rows on behalf of the Medical Officer and Psychiatry Committee. J Ment Sci. 1914;60:654–5.

Rules for the management of the Pauper Lunatic Asylum, for the West Riding of the County of York, erected in the township of Stanley-cum-Wrenthorpe, in the parish of Wakefield. Wakefield: John Stanfield, 1847.

Russell R. Mental physicians and their patients: Psychological medicine in the English pauper lunatic asylums of the later nineteenth century. Unpublished PhD thesis, University of Sheffield, 1983. https://etheses.whiterose.ac.uk/2952/.

Russell R. The lunacy profession and its staff in the second half of the nineteenth century, with special reference to the West Riding Lunatic Asylum. In: Bynum WF, Porter R, Shepherd M, editors. The anatomy of madness. Essays in the history of psychiatry. Volume III. The asylum and its psychiatry. London: Routledge; 1988. [2004]. p. 297–315.

Rutherford W. An address on recent advances in anatomy and physiology. Delivered in the Subsection of Anatomy and Physiology at the Annual Meeting of the British Association, 1873. BMJ. 1873;2(666):391–3. (4th October)

Rutherford W. Address to the Department of Anatomy and Physiology by Professor Rutherford. In: Report of the forty-third meeting of the British Association for the Advancement of Science held at Bradford in September 1873. Notices and abstracts of miscellaneous communications to the sections. London: John Murray; 1874. p. 119–23.

Rutherford W, Fraser T, Brunton TL, Ferrier D. Report on the progress of physiology. J Anat Physiol. 1872;6(2):450–502.

Ryan AH. History of the British Act of 1876: an act to amend the law relating to cruelty to animals. J Med Educ. 1963;38:182–94.

Sabben JT. Two cases of atheroma of the blood vessels at the base of the brain, with remarks upon the symptoms, diagnosis, prognosis, and pathological condition in that affection. J Ment Sci. 1870–1871;16(April 1870):52–8.

Sabben JT, Balfour Browne JH. Handbook of law and lunacy; or, the medical practitioners complete guide in all matters relating to lunacy practice. London: J. & A. Churchill; 1872.

Sagan L. On the origin of mitosing cells. J Theoret Biol. 1967;14(3):255–74.

Sander JWAS, Barclay J, Shorvon SD. The neurological founding fathers of the National Society for Epilepsy and of the Chalfont Centre for Epilepsy. J Neurol Neurosurg Psychiatry. 1993;56(6):599–604.

Sandrone S, Zanin E. David Ferrier (1843–1928). J Neurol. 2014;261(6):1247–8.

"Sane Patient, A" [Merivale HC]. My experiences in a lunatic asylum. London: Chatto and Windus, 1879.

Sankey WHO. The Medico-Psychological Association: the President's address for 1868. J Ment Sci. 1868;14(October 1868):297–304.

Savage GH. Dr. Hughlings Jackson on mental disorders. J Ment Sci. 1917;63(July 1917):315–28.

Schäfer EA. On the functions of the temporal and occipital lobes: a reply to Dr. Ferrier. Brain. 1888–1889;11(2):145–65.

Schneck JM. Tertius Lydgate in Middlemarch and Thomas Clifford Allbutt. N Y State J Med. 1970;70:1086–90.

Schurr PH. Outline of the history of the Section of Neurology of the Royal Society of Medicine. J R Soc Med. 1985;78(2):146–8.

Scott A, Eadie M, Lees A. William Richard Gowers 1845–1915. Exploring the Victorian brain: a biography. Oxford: Oxford University Press; 2012.

Scrimgeour D. Proper people. Early asylum life in the words of those who were there. York: York Publishing; 2015.

Scull A. Museums of madness. The social organization of insanity in nineteenth-century England. London: Allen Lane; 1979.

Scull A. A Victorian alienist: John Conolly, FRCP, DCL (1794–1866). In: Bynum WF, Porter R, Shepherd M, editors. The anatomy of madness. Essays in the history of psychiatry. Volume I. People and ideas. London: Routledge; 1985. [2004]. p. 103–49.

Scull A. The insanity of place/The place of insanity. Essays on the history of psychiatry. London: Routledge; 2006.

Scull A. Psychiatry and its discontents. Oakland: University of California Press; 2019.

Scull A, Mackenzie C, Hervey N. Masters of Bedlam. The transformation of the mad-doctoring trade. Princeton: Princeton University Press; 1996.

Seguin EC. Clinical lecture on hemiplegic epilepsy. Boston Med Surg J. 1881;105:49–51.

Sharpey-Schafer E. History of the Physiological Society, 1876–1926. J Physiol. 1927;64(3 Suppl):1–181.

Sheehan J. The role and rewards of asylum attendants in Victorian England. Int Hist Nurs J. 1998;3(4):25–33.

Shephard B. "The early treatment of Mental Disorders": R.G. Rows and Maghull 1914–1918. In: Freeman H, Berrios GE, editors. 150 years of British Psychiatry Volume II: The Aftermath. London: Athlone Press; 1996. p. 434–64.

Shepherd JA. Lawson Tait. The rebellious surgeon (1845–1899). Lawrence: Coronado Press; 1980.

Shepherd M. Psychiatric journals and the evolution of psychological medicine. In: Bynum WF, Lock S, Porter R, editors. Medical journals and medical knowledge. Historical essays. London: Routledge, 1992:188–206.

Sherman SE. The history of the ophthalmoscope. In: Henkes HE, Zrenner C, editors. History of Ophthalmology. History of Ophthalmology, vol. 2. Dordrecht: Springer; 1989. p. 221–8.

Sherrington CS. Sir David Ferrier, 1843–1928. Proc R Soc Lond B Biol Sci. 1928;103:viii–xvi.

Shorter E, Healy D. Shock therapy. A history of electroconvulsive treatment in mental illness. Toronto: University of Toronto Press; 2007.

Shorvon SD. The idea of epilepsy. A medical and social history of epilepsy in the modern era (1860–2020). Cambridge: Cambridge University Press; 2023.

Shorvon S, Compston A. Queen Square. A history of the National Hospital and its Institute of Neurology. Cambridge: Cambridge University Press; 2019.

Shuttleton DE. An Account of … William Cullen: John Thomson and the making of a medical biography. Clio Med. 2014;94:240–66.

Silverman ME. Etienne-Jules Marey: nineteenth century cardiovascular physiologist and inventor of cinematography. Clin Cardiol. 1996;19:339–41. [Reprinted in: Hurst JW, Conti CR, Fye WB, editors. Profiles in cardiology. Mahwah, N.J.: Foundation for Advances in Medicine and Science, Inc., 2003: 143–145.]

Sloffer CA. From farmers to scientists: the West Riding Pauper Lunatic Asylum as a research institution. Unpublished MA thesis,. Johns Hopkins University; 2023.

Smith LD. "Cure, comfort and safe custody". Public lunatic asylums in early nineteenth-century England. London/New York: Leicester University Press; 1999.

Smith L. A gentleman's mad-doctor in Georgian England: Edward Long Fox and Brislington House. Hist Psychiatry. 2008;19(2):163–84.

Snaith RP. Images in psychiatry. The West Riding Pauper Lunatic Asylum. Am J Psychiatry. 1998;155:456.

Snow CP. Foreword. In: Hardy GH. A mathematician's apology. Cambridge: Cambridge University Press; 1967. [2019].

Snow SJ. Blessed days of anaesthesia. How anaesthetics changed the world. Oxford: Oxford University Press; 2008.

Spillane JD. A memorable decade in the history of neurology 1874–84. I. BMJ. 1974a;4(5946):701–6. (21st December)

Spillane JD. A memorable decade in the history of neurology 1874–84. II. BMJ. 1974b;4(5947):757–9. (28th December)

Spillane JD. The doctrine of the nerves. Chapters in the history of neurology. Oxford: Oxford University Press; 1981.

Spurzheim JG. Phrenology, in connexion with the study of physiognomy. Illustration of characters. With thirty-five plates. To which is prefixed a biography of the author by Nahum Capen. Boston: Marsh, Capen & Lyon; 1836.

Stahnisch FW. The use of animal experimentation in the history of neurology. In: Finger S, Boller F, Tyler KL, editors. History of neurology, Handbook of Clinical Neurology, volume 95, 3rd series. Edinburgh/Amsterdam: Elsevier; 2010. p. 129–48.

Star SL. Regions of the mind: brain research and the quest for scientific certainty. Stanford: Stanford University Press; 1989.

Stratmann L. Chloroform. The quest for oblivion. Stroud: Sutton Publishing; 2003.

Sutherland H. Forcible feeding of the insane. BMJ. 1872;1(595):555. (25th May)

Sutherland H. On the histology of the blood of the insane. BMJ. 1873;1(645):547. (10th May)

Sutherland H. The asylums of Paris, in 1872. J Ment Sci. 1873–1874;19(April 1873):87–92.

Sutherland H. Alcoholism in private practice. BMJ. 1874;2(724):610–1. (14th November)

Sutherland H. On the artificial feeding of the insane. J Psychol Med Ment Pathol (Lond). 1875a;1(1):98–115.

Sutherland H. Notes on a case of insanity indirectly caused by phimosis. BMJ. 1875b;1(756):845–6. (26th June)

Sutherland H. Ferrier on Labyrinthine vertigo – Menière's disease. London Medical Record. 1876;4:68–9. (15th February)

Sutherland H. Two cases of delusion as a premonitory symptom—in the one case not followed by insanity, and in the other followed by symptoms necessitating the detention of the patient in an asylum. J Ment Sci. 1877–1878;23(July 1877):248–9.

Sutherland H. The post-mortem on Harriet Staunton. Lancet. 1877a;2(2823):512–3. (6th October)

Sutherland H. On "agoraphobia". J Psychol Med Ment Pathol (Lond). 1877b;3(2):265–9.

Sutherland H. Note on the mixture of character found in epilepsy. Med Times Gaz. 1878;1:389. (13th April)

Sutherland H. Cases of general paralysis illustrating the influence which the previous life of the patient exercises upon his delusions. Med Times Gaz. 1879a;1:62–3. (18th January)

Sutherland H. Premonitory symptoms of insanity improved by medical and moral treatment. Med Times Gaz. 1879b;2:609. (29th November)

Sutherland H. Lectures on insanity. Med Times Gaz. 1883;2(255–257):565–7.

Sutherland H. Prognosis in cases of food refusal. J Ment Sci. 1883–1884;29(July 1883):178–88.

Sutherland H. To the Editors of the "Journal of Mental Science". J Ment Sci. 1885–1886;31(April 1885):147–8.

Sutherland H. The premonitory symptoms of insanity. BMJ. 1886;1(1309):188–90. (30th January)

Sutherland H. Cysts of the dura mater. Illus Med News. 1889;4:49–50. (20th July)

Sutherland H. A directory of justices in England and Wales, appointed under the Lunacy Act, 1890, to make orders for the reception of private patients. 1890–91. London: John Bale & Sons; 1890.

Sutherland H. Feeding (Forcible) of the insane. In: Tuke DH, editor. A dictionary of psychological medicine giving the definition, etymology and synonyms of the terms used in medical psychology with the symptoms, treatment, and pathology of insanity and the law of lunacy in Great Britain and Ireland, vol. I. London: J. & A. Churchill; 1892. p. 494–502.

Swash M. John Hughlings-Jackson [*sic*]: a sesquicentennial tribute. J Neurol Neurosurg Psychiatry. 1986;49(9):981–5.

Swash M. John Hughlings Jackson (1835–1911). J Neurol. 2005;252(6):745–6.

Swash M. John Hughlings Jackson (1835–1911): an adornment to the London Hospital. J Med Biogr. 2015;23(1):2–8.

Swash M. Medical specialisation at the London Hospital. The great awakening. Newcastle-upon-Tyne: Cambridge Scholars Publishing; 2024.

Tait L. The influence of milk in the propagation of contagious diseases. BMJ. 1870;2(508):344. (24th September)

Tait L. On the myoidema [*sic*] of phthisis. Dublin J Med Sci. 1871;52:316–53.

Tait AC. History of Crichton Royal. Med Hist. 1972;16(2):178–84.

Taylor K. Not so merry Wakefield. Barnsley: Wharncliffe Books; 2005.

Taylor DC, Marsh SM. Hughlings Jackson's Dr. Z: the paradigm of temporal lobe epilepsy revealed. J Neurol Neurosurg Psychiatry. 1980;43(9):758–67.

Taylor J, Holmes G, Walshe FMR, editors. John Hughlings Jackson. Selected Writings. Volume 1. On epilepsy and epileptiform convulsions. Nijmegen: Arts and Boeve; 1931. [1996]

Temkin O. The falling sickness. A history of epilepsy from the Greeks to the beginnings of modern neurology. (2nd ed, revised). Baltimore/London: The Johns Hopkins University Press; 1971.

Thompson G. Clinical memoranda. J Ment Sci. 1873–1874;19(January 1874):565.

Thompson G. On the physiology of general paralysis of the insane, and of epilepsy. J Ment Sci. 1874–1875b;20(January 1875):579–86.

Thompson G. On the physiology of general paralysis of the insane and of epilepsy. J Ment Sci. 1875–1876;21(April 1875):67–74.

Thompson G. On the use of the hydrobromate of hyoscine in the treatment of recurrent and acute mania. Lancet. 1888;1(3362):218. (4th February)

Thompson EP. History from below. Times Lit Suppl. 1966.; 7th April:279–80.

Thompson G, Clinical memoranda. A case of apoplectiform congestion of the brain. Death. Autopsy. J Ment Sci. 1874–1875a;20(April 1874):94–6.

Thomson J. An account of the life, lectures, and writings of William Cullen, M.D., Professor of the Practice of Physic in the University of Edinburgh. Edinburgh/London: William Blackwood and Sons; 1832. [1849]

Thornton EM. Hypnotism, hysteria and epilepsy: an historical synthesis. London: William Heinemann Medical Books; 1976.

Thorpe FT. A history of Middlewood Psychiatric Hospital, 1872-centenary-1972. Sheffield: Middlewood Hospital; 1972.

Tobia P. The patients of the Bristol Lunatic Asylum in the nineteenth century 1861–1900. Unpublished PhD thesis,. University of the West of England; 2017.

Todd J. The syndrome of Alice in Wonderland. CMAJ. 1955;73:701–4.

Todd J, Ashworth L. The West Riding Asylum and James Crichton-Browne, 1818–76. In: Berrios GE, Freeman H, editors. 150 years of British Psychiatry 1841–1991. London: Royal College of Psychiatrists; 1991. p. 389–418.

Todd J, Ashworth L. "The House": Wakefield Asylum, 1818 ….. Bradford: Double 'S' Printers, not dated [n.d.; *circa* 1995/6??].

Triarhou LC. Pre-Brodmann pioneers of cortical cytoarchitectonics II: Carl Hammarberg, Alfred Walter Campbell and Grafton Elliot Smith. Brain Struct Funct. 2020;225:2591–614.

Triarhou LC. Pre-Brodmann pioneers of cortical cytoarchitectonics I: Theodor Meynert, Vladimir Betz and William Bevan-Lewis. Brain Struct Funct. 2021;226:49–67.

Triarhou LC, Larner AJ. James Taylor (1859–1946). J Neurol. 2024;271(12):7636–7.

Trimble M. The intentional brain. Motion, emotion, and the development of modern neuropsychiatry. Baltimore: Johns Hopkins University Press; 2016.

Tuke S. Practical hints on the construction and economy of pauper lunatic asylums; including instructions to the architects who offered plans for the Wakefield Asylum, and a sketch of the most approved design. London: W. Alexander; 1815.

Turner W. The convolutions of the human cerebrum topographically considered. Edinb Med J. 1866;11(12):1105–22.

Turner T. Henry Maudsley: psychiatrist, philosopher, and entrepreneur. In: Bynum WF, Porter R, Shepherd M, editors. The anatomy of madness. Essays in the history of psychiatry. Volume III. The asylum and its psychiatry. London: Routledge; 1988. [2004]. p. 151–89.

Turner T. "Not worth powder and shot": the public profile of the Medico-Psychological Association, c. 1851–1914. In: Berrios GE, Freeman H, editors. 150 years of British Psychiatry 1841–1991. London: Royal College of Psychiatrists; 1991. p. 3–16.

Turner [W.]. A human cerebrum imperfectly divided into two hemispheres. J Anat Physiol. 1878;12(2):241–53.

Tyrer P, Craddock N. The bicentennial volume of the *British Journal of Psychiatry*: the winding pathway of mental science. Br J Psychiatry. 2012;200(1):1–4.

Underwood EA. Clifford Allbutt, scholar-physician and historian. Proc R Soc Med. 1963;56(Suppl 1):11–9.

van Gijn J. The Babinski sign: a centenary. Utrecht: Universiteit Utrecht; 1996.

Viets HR. West Riding, 1871–1876. Bull Hist Med. 1938;6:477–87.

Voisin A. Analysis and pathological physiology of the troubles of speech in the general paralysis of the insane. BMJ. 1875;1(755):807–8. (19th June)

Von Bonin G (trans). Some papers on the cerebral cortex. Springfield, Ill., Charles C. Thomas, 1960.

Waddington K. Brunton, Thomas Lauder. In: Bynum WF, Bynum H, editors. Dictionary of Medical Biography. Westport: Greenwood Press; 2007. p. 274–5.

Wade NJ. The emergence of neuroscience in the nineteenth century. Volume 7. Ferrier D. The functions of the brain with a note on the author by Nicholas J. Wade. London: Routledge/Thoemmes Press; 2000.

Wade S. Yorkshire curious and surprising. Amazing tales from the County, past and present. Wellington: Halsgrove; 2016.

"WAH". Dr Ferrier's experiments on the brain. Examiner. 1873;3426:966–7. (27th September)

Walk A. The centenary of the *Journal of Mental Science*. J Ment Sci. 1953;99:633–7.

Walk A. The history of mental nursing. J Ment Sci. 1961;107(January 1961):1–17.

Walk A. Medico-psychologists, Maudsley and The Maudsley. Br J Psychiatry. 1976;128:19–30. [Reprinted in: Murray RM, Turner TH, editors. Lectures on the history of psychiatry. The Squibb Series. London: Gaskell, 1990: 12–27.]

Walk A, Walker DL. Gloucester and the beginnings of the R.M.P.A. J Ment Sci. 1961;107(July 1961):603–32.

Walker JW. Wakefield. Its history and people. Wakefield: West Yorkshire Printing Co. Ltd.; 1934.

Walker JW. Wakefield. Its history and people. 2nd ed. Wakefield: Privately printed; 1939.

Wallis JA. On the separate treatment of recent and curable cases of insanity in special detached hospitals, with plan and description of buildings about to be erected for this purpose at the Lancaster County Asylum, Whittingham. J Ment Sci. 1894;40(July 1894):335–44.

Wallis J. Investigating the body in the Victorian Asylum. Doctors, patients, and practices. London: Palgrave Macmillan; 2017a.

Wallis J. Bloody technology: the sphygmograph in asylum practice. Hist Psychiatry. 2017b;28:297–310.

Walmsley T. Crichton-Browne's biological psychiatry. Psychiatr Bull. 2003;27(1):20–2.

Walton J. The treatment of pauper lunatics in Victorian England: the case of Lancaster Asylum, 1816–1870. In: Scull A, editor. Madhouses, mad-doctors, and madmen. The social history of psychiatry in the Victorian era. Philadelphia: University of Pennsylvania Press; 1981. p. 166–97.

Ward FH. Pathological work in county asylums. BMJ. 1877;1(838):93. (20th January)

Weisz G. Divide and conquer: a comparative history of medical specialization. New York: Oxford University Press; 2006.

Wesley J. Primitive physic or an easy and natural method of curing most diseases. London: The Epworth Press; 1960. p. 1747–80.

Wessels Q, Correia JC, Taylor AM. Sir William Turner (1832–1916)—Lancastrian, anatomist and champion of the Victorian era. J Med Biogr. 2016;24(4):500–6.

Wetherill JH. The York Medical School. Med Hist. 1961;5(3):253–69.

WFN Research Group on the History of the Neurosciences, Levy I. The West Riding Lunatic Asylum—birthplace of modern British neurology. J Neurol Sci. 1997;150(Suppl1):S172–3. (abstract 3-22-02)

White W. Directory and topography of the Boroughs of Leeds, Halifax, Huddersfield, and Wakefield; Dewsbury, Heckmondwike, and Holmfirth, and the villages and townships in the large and populous parishes of Batley, Birstall, Calverley, Guiseley, Kirkburton, Kirkheaton, Almondbury, Mirfield; and all others in and near the Yorkshire woollen district; etc. Sheffield: William White; 1858.

White W. Directory of Bradford, Halifax, Wakefield, Bingley, Keighley, Otley, Saddleworth, Todmorden, Skipton, Settle, Pontefract, Knottingley, Aberford, Sherburn, Castleford, Harrogate, Knaresborough, Tadcaster, Wetherby, Ripon, Haworth, Eccleshill, Shipley, Brighouse, Elland, and all the parishes and villages in and near those populous districts of the West Riding, forming the great seats of the worsted manufacture, being part II. of the clothing district directory (11th ed). Sheffield: William White, 1866.

White W. White's general and commercial Directory of Leeds, Bradford, Huddersfield, Halifax, Wakefield, Dewsbury, Batley, Keighley, Bingley, Ilkeley, Otley, Skipton, Todmorden, Holmfirth, Saddleworth, and all the villages and parishes in and near those populous districts of the West Riding, forming the great seats of the woollen and worsted manufactures (12th edn). Sheffield: William White, 1870.

Wilkins RH. Neurosurgical classics-XII. J Neurosurg. 1963;20(10):904–5.

Wilkins RH. The West Riding Lunatic Asylum, 1871–1876: extraordinarily productive research in an obscure institution. Neurosurgery. 1997;41(3):722–3.

[Willett A.]. Address of Alfred Willett President at the Annual Meeting, March 1st, 1904. Med Chir Trans. 1904a;87:cvii-cl.

[Willett A.]. Address of Alfred Willett President of the Royal Medical and Chirurgical Society of London at the Annual Meeting, March 1st, 1904. London/Dorking: Adlard and Son; 1904b.

Williams SWD. On the treatment of melancholia attonita, with refusal of food, by the continuous current. Lancet. 1873;1(2578):127–8. (25th January)

Williams M. History of Crichton Royal Hospital 1839–1989. Dumfries: Dumfries and Galloway Health Board; 1989.

Wilson G. The Brown Animal Sanatory Institution. J Hyg (Lond). 1979;83(1):171–97.

Wood J. A culture of improvement: knowledge, aesthetic consciousness, and the conversazione. Nineteenth Century Studies. 2006;20:79–97.

Woods OT. Tubercular meningitis in an adult idiot: no tubercle found in lungs. BMJ. 1874;2(706):32. (11th July)

Woods OT. Notes of a case of tubercular meningitis in an adult without tubercles in the lungs. J Ment Sci. 1874–1875;20(April 1874):92–4.

Worboys M. Allbutt, Thomas Clifford. In: Bynum WF, Bynum H, editors. Dictionary of medical biography. Westport: Greenwood Press; 2007. p. 108–9.

Wright TG. Cholera in the asylum. Reports on the origin and progress of pestilential cholera, in the West-Yorkshire Lunatic Asylum, during the autumn of 1849, and on the previous state of the Institution. A contribution to the statistics of insanity and of cholera. London: Longman, Brown, Green, and Longmans; 1850.

Wynter R. 'Horrible dens of deception': Thomas Bakewell, Thomas Mulock and anti-asylum sentiments, c.1815–60. In: Knowles T, Trowbridge S, editors. Insanity and the lunatic asylum in the nineteenth century. London: Pickering and Chatto; 2015. p. 11–27.

Yeats W. On haematoma auris. BMJ. 1873;1(651):702–3. (21st June).

York GK, Steinberg DA. An introduction to the life and work of John Hughlings Jackson with a Catalogue Raisonné of his writings. (Medical history, supplement no. 26). London: The Wellcome Trust for the History of Medicine at UCL; 2006. [Also published as: York GK, Steinberg DA. An introduction to the life and work of John Hughlings Jackson with a catalogue raisonné of his writings. Med Hist Suppl 2006; (26): 3-157.]

Young RM. The functions of the brain: Gall to Ferrier (1808–1886). Isis. 1968;59(3):251–68.

Young RM. Mind, brain and adaptation in the nineteenth century: cerebral localization and its biological context from Gall to Ferrier. Oxford: Clarendon Press; 1970. [Reprint: Oxford: Oxford University Press, 1990.]

Index